Maternal Influences and Early Behavior

Maternal Influences and Early Behavior

Edited by
Robert W. Bell
Department of Psychology
Texas Tech University
Lubbock, Texas
and
William P. Smotherman
Department of Psychology
Oregon State University
Corvallis, Oregon

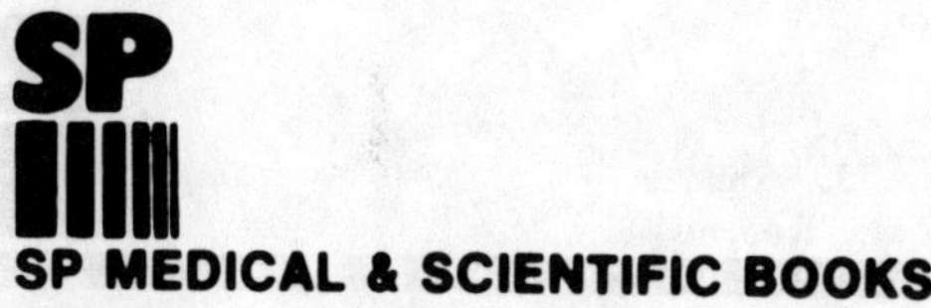

SP MEDICAL & SCIENTIFIC BOOKS
New York • London

SPECTRUM PUBLICATIONS, INC.
175-20 Wexford Terrace, Jamaica, N.Y. 11432

Library of Congress Cataloging in Publication Data
Main entry under title:

Maternal influences and early behavior.

Includes index.
1. Parental behavior in animals. 2. Animals, Infancy of. 3. Mother and child. 4. Rodents—Behavior. 5. Primates—Behavior. I. Bell, Robert Wayne, 1931– II. Smotherman, William P.
[DNLM; 1. Child behavior. 2. Mother-child relations.
WS105.5 F2M425]
QL762.M37 599'.05'6
ISBN 0-89335-059-1

Contributors

ROGER BAKEMAN, Ph.D.
Department of Psychology
Georgia State University
Atlanta, Georgia

ROBERT W. BELL, Ph.D.
Department of Psychology
Texas Tech University
Lubbock, Texas

JOSEPHINE V. BROWN, Ph.D.
Department of Psychology
Georgia State University
Atlanta, Georgia

CHRISTOPHER L. COE, Ph.D.
Department of Psychiatry
and Behavioral Sciences
Stanford School of Medicine
Stanford, California

DANIEL D. CUBICCIOTTI, III, Ph.D.
Department of Psychobiology
and Physiology
Stanford Research Institute
International
Menlo Park, California

VICTOR, J. DeGHETT, Ph.D.
Department of Psychology
SUNY-Potsdam
Potsdam, New York

VICTOR H. DENENBERG, Ph.D.
Department of Biobehavioral
Sciences
The University of Connecticut
Storrs, Connecticut

MARK J. DOLLINGER, Ph.D.
Department of Biobehavioral
Sciences
The University of Connecticut
Storrs, Connecticut

MARGARET P. FREESE, Ph.D.
Department of Psychology
University of Alabama
in Birmingham
Birmingham, Alabama

RONALD GANDELMAN, Ph.D.
Department of Psychology
Rutgers-The State University
New Brunswick, New Jersey

JOHN C. GURSKI, Ph.D.
Department of Psychology
Ft. Hays State University
Ft. Hays, Kansas

MICHAEL B. HENNESSY, Ph.D.
Department of Psychiatry
and Behavioral Sciences
Stanford School of Medicine
Stanford, California

WILLIAM R. HOLLOWAY, Jr., Ph.D.
Department of Psychiatry
University of Rochester
Medical Center
Rochester, New York

RICHARD A. HOLM, Ph D.
Regional Primate Research
Center
University of Washington
Seattle, Washington

JANICE R. HORVAT, Ph.D.
Department of Psychiatry
and Behavioral Sciences
Stanford School of Medicine
Stanford, California

JOEL N. KAPLAN, Ph.D.
Department of Psychobiology
and Physiology
Stanford Research Institute
International
Menlo Park, California

SARAH, J. KILPATRICK, Ph.D.
Department of Psychology
University of Chicago
Chicago, Illinois

ANNALIESE F. KORNER, Ph.D.
Department of Psychiatry
and Behavioral Sciences
Stanford School of Medicine
Stanford, California

NELLIE K. LAUGHLIN, Ph.D.
Department of Anesthesiology
Palo Alto Veterans Hospital
Palo Alto, California

SEYMOUR LEVINE, Ph.D.
Department of Psychiatry
and Behavioral Sciences

Stanford School of Medicine
Stanford, California

LYNDA M. McGINNIS, Ph.D.
102 Putnam Street
Watertown, Massachusetts

SALLY P. MENDOZA, Ph.D.
Department of Psychiatry
and Behavioral Sciences
Stanford School of Medicine
Stanford, California

HOWARD MOLTZ, Ph.D.
Department of Psychology
University of Chicago
Chicago, Illinois

JAY S. ROSENBLATT, Ph.D.
Institute of Animal Behavior
Rutgers-The State University
Newark, New Jersey

GENE P. SACKETT, Ph.D.
Regional Primate Research
Center
University of Washington
Seattle, Washington

GILLIAN SALES, Ph.D.
Department of Zoology
King's College-University
of London
London, England, U.K.

JOHN PAUL SCOTT, Ph.D.
Department of Psychology
Bowling Green State University
Bowling Green, Ohio

HAROLD I. SIEGEL, Ph.D.
Institute of Animal Behavior
Rutgers-The State University
Newark, New Jersey

JANE C. SMITH, Ph.D.
Department of Zoology
King's College-University
of London
London, England, U.K.

WILLIAM P. SMOTHERMAN, Ph.D.
Department of Psychology
Oregon State University
Corvallis, Oregon

EVELYN B. THOMAN, Ph.D.
Department of Biobehavioral
Sciences
The University of Connecticut
Storrs, Connecticut

SANDRA G. WIENER, Ph.D.
Department of Psychiatry
and Behavioral Sciences
Stanford School of Medicine
Stanford, California

Preface

This book is intended to bring together the contributions of many years of investigations from a number of laboratories involved in the systematic investigation of mother-offspring interactions and the attendant consequences for development. A similar book (Rheingold, 1963) is now more than a decade old. The value of such a book is attested to by the burgeoning interest in the subject matter since the publication of that earlier volume.

The importance of the mother-infant dyad has been recognized by scientests and parents alike since time immemorial. Pioneering writers such as Sigmund Freud, with his emphasis upon the expression of biological "needs" by the developing infant, and John B. Watson, with his emphasis upon the mother's role as a conditioner-trainer of her offspring, have been followed (in time, not emphases) by such investigators as Konrad Lorenz, with his now-classic studies of imprinting, Jean Piaget's sequential analyses of the development of intellect, and Harry Harlow's ingenious studies of attachment.

The present volume reflects the influences of these earlier investigators. It is comparative, psychobiological, and represents a blend of the "experimental" approach characteristic of those trained in experimental psychology and the "natural history" approach more often represented in the work of ethologists. Sequential analyses of developmental changes in the mother-offspring relationship characterize virtually all of the work reported herein.

The first nine chapters examine various facets of the mother-infant dyad in rodent species. The first two chapters focus upon parturition and the initial 12 hours of post-parturient life in the rat (*Rattus norvegicus*), the first emphasizing the adaptive quality of maternal behavior during that developmental period and the second the rapid development of behavioral competence of the young during that same developmental span. Chapter 3 introduces the complexity and detailed analyses involved in understanding the changing relationships of mother and young in the gerbil (*Meriones unguiculatus*). Chapters 4, 5, and 6 examine specific features of the young as they influence maternal behaviors; suckling by young as an eliciting and maintenance factor for aggression by mouse dams (*Mus musculus*), ultrasounds by young of many species of rodents as a controlling agent for maternal attention, and the changing characteristics of young rats as they influence the excretion of a hepatic-derived pheromonal attractant by the mother. Chapter 7 presents a developmental model of maternal behavior in the rat based upon 20 years of systematic investigation and integrates many of the conclusions of the earlier chapters. Chapters 8 and 9 point out the potential role of differential mother-infant interactions as confounding, and possibly explanatory, factors in related areas of developmental investigations; effects of early experience involving extrinsic stimulation of infant rodents and the study of malnutrition occurring during early development, respectively. These last two chapters present designs for unconfounding what has appeared to be inherently confounded and should prove useful for investigators in the research areas discussed.

Chapters 10 through 14 examine selected aspects of the mother-infant dyad in several species of infrahuman primates. Chapter 10 integrates the earlier chapters with succeeding ones through a comparative analysis of mother-infant interactions in rats and squirrel monkeys (*Saimiri sciureus*) and concludes that despite the very obvious species differences, modulation of arousal appears to be a primary factor for understanding these interactions in both species. Chapter 11 details the developmental changes in cues utilized by infant squirrel monkeys in recognizing their mothers and the role of early experience in the formation of social preferences. Chapter 12 examines the effects of prenatal and postnatal events upon social development in the pigtail macaque (*M. nemestrina*) comparatively with earlier studies utilizing rhesus monkeys (*Macaca mulata*) to highlight the need for genetic x environment designs in developmental research. Chapter 13 presents detailed analyses of developmental trends in mother-offspring interactions for four pairs of chimpanzees (*Pan troglodytes*). Chapter 14 provides a bridge to the subsequent chapters with a comparative analysis of the effects of mother-infant separation on nonhuman and human primates.

Chapters 15 through 17 illustrates the adaptation of many of the observational procedures developed in comparative laboratories to the study of human newborns and their maternal environment. Chapter 15 describes an ingenious procedure for providing compensatory stimulation akin to that normally provided by the intrauterine environment for premature infants and points to the clinical application of these procedures. Chapter 16 examines patterns of mother-infant interactions utilizing samples of infants which are known to differ markedly in their characteristics, full-term and premature infants. Chapter 17 presents a systematic model for the study of dyadic interactions between mother-infant pairs of humans which can be adapted to a variety of research programs.

Chapter 18 concludes the book with a truly comparative survey of one aspect of mother-infant interactions; the consequences and adaptive significance of multiple-mothering. Examining species ranging from mice to lions (*Panthera leo*) to humans, the authors provide a comparative, evolutionary framework for understanding the multiplicity of patterns of maternal styles, the potential variability evident in most species, and the adaptive significance of this variability.

Despite the obvious differences in behaviors exhibited by the range of species discussed in the various chapters, and the attendant differences in procedures, specific behavioral outcomes, and interpretive vocabulary associated with the study of disparate species, the editors have been impressed by the similarities of the various investigators' work. In contrast to the typical study of mother-infant dyads of 1-2 decades ago, when the scrutiny of the investigator was almost invariably focused upon the mature (e.g. mother) member of the dyad, virtually all of the work reported in this volume emphasizes the dyad, with the immature (e.g. infant) member influencing the nature of the interaction fully as much as the mother (this is so evident that the book easily could have been retitled "Infantile Influences and Maternal Behavior"). A second similarity is the emphasis upon the sequential and ever-changing nature of the dyad and the attendant reliance upon direct observations, in lieu of the more familiar and traditional (at least in psychology) automated equipment systems and "Fisherian" statistical designs. The third similarity, in contrast to earlier decades, is the notable reduction in appeals to presumed "learning contingencies" as a central explanatory construct.

The editors would like to express appreciation to the contributors for their time and efforts and to the publishers for their patience and support. There are some contributors whithout whose efforts this volume probably would never have been conceived, even though their names do not appear among the listing of contributors. The early epigeneticists such as Zing-Yank Kuo, T. C. Schneirla and Frank Beach made lasting impressions both upon their students and colleagues and those who, in turn, have been influenced by those collaborators. Donald Hebb virtually invented the sub-discipline of

Developmental Psychobiology and was greatly influential in the focus on developmentally-early events as necessary for an understanding of developmentally-later events. Finally, Harriet Rheingold's book, to which we alluded earlier, provided the proximate stimulus for the present volume.

Robert W. Bell
William P. Smotherman

REFERENCES

Rheingold, H. (ed.). *Maternal Behavior in Mammals*. J. Wiley & Sons, Inc., New York (1963).

Contents

Maternal Influences and Early Behavior

1 Parturition in the Rat: Description and Assessment

William R. Holloway, Jr.
Mark J. Dollinger
Victor H. Denenberg

The period of parturition occupies only a small portion of the rat's life; rarely is the actual delivery longer than 150 minutes. Yet this very narrow time span is a major focal point for both the pregnant female and her newborn young. In the mother, one finds major physiological changes occurring. For example, serum levels of progesterone and estrogen undergo marked fluctuations (Grota and Eik-Nes, 1967; Labhsetwar and Watson, 1974; Yoshinaga et al., 1969); the neurohumoral content of the neurohypophysis decreases significantly (Fuchs and Saito, 1971); the secretory activity of the anterior pituitary is elevated (Labhsetwar and Watson, 1974; Linkie and Niswender, 1972; Nagasawa and Yanai, 1972); and catecholaminergic systems in the hypothalamus show major alterations in their functional capacities (Moltz et al., 1975).

Morphological alterations of the female also occur. Loss of tissue and fluid volume accompany the expulsion of the conceptus mass and, at the same time, there is a tremendous increase in the functioning of the mammary tissue. By the birth of the first pup, the mammary glands are engorged with colostrum, and the DNA and RNA contents of the tissue are increasing at a rapid rate (Munford, 1963a,b,c).

The changes experienced by the fetus during this period are no less dramatic. Within a very few minutes after birth, the newborn shifts from a relatively stable, buffered intrauterine existence, to a situation where it must breathe air and ingest nutrients. Many internal processes increase in activity at the time of birth (Adolph, 1970), and several organ systems, including the brain, grow rapidly during the early postnatal hours (Holloway et al., 1978). Similarly, the behavioral competence and capabilities of the newborn change rapidly soon after birth (see Chapter 2).

In contrast to the remainder of the lactational period, the mother's behavioral changes during the parturitional and perinatal period have received little attention. Descriptions of the parturitional behavior patterns of females have been limited to qualitative observations (e.g., Wiesner and Sheard, 1933; Rosenblatt and Lehrman, 1963; Slotnick, 1975). Even though the behavioral interactions between the mother and her young during the perinatal period are critical for the establishment of long-term maternal responsiveness (Bridges, 1975, 1977), only a few studies have adequately assessed the importance of this period for the newborn with the objective of relating the behavioral environment afforded by the mother to the biological needs of the newborn rat (Denenberg et al., 1963; Denenberg et al., 1976).

The following presentation will provide a detailed look at the behavioral events characterizing the initial maternal environment experienced by a newborn rat. We will begin with a quantitative analysis of the mother's behavioral changes during and soon after parturition and will later show the importance of these highly ordered behavior patterns for the normal development of the young.

METHODOLOGICAL PROCEDURE

All animals described below were Purdue-Wistar rats, born and reared in our own closed breeding colony. See Denenberg (1977) for a description of the breeding and housing conditions. Pregnant rats were placed into clear plexiglas cages several days prior to delivery. Then on the expected day of parturition (typically 23 days after a positive sperm smear), each female was watched periodically for the presence of intense uterine contractions. When these were frequent, indicating the impending birth of a pup, behavior observations were initiated.

The observer sat approximately three feet from the rat's cage and wore an earplug attached to a tone generator which produced a beep every ten seconds. During each 10-second epoch, the behaviors exhibited by the parturient female were recorded (Denenberg et al., 1976). The observation period encompassed the entire parturition (from the birth of the first through the birth of the last pup), plus the 60 minutes immediately following the last birth in the litter.

Behaviors Recorded

We recorded a total of 23 behaviors which essentially included all of the behaviors exhibited by female rats during parturition. These are listed in Table 1. In addition, the delivery of each pup and the expulsion of each placenta were noted.

Several of the most characteristic behaviors are represented in Figures 1–7. In all of the illustrations, note the clustering of the pups under the mother,

TABLE 1
The Maternal Behaviors Observed and Their Definitions

Behavior	*Definition*
Nurse	Mother nurses one or more pups
Lick Pup	Mother licks one or more pups
Sniff Pup	Mother sniffs one or more pups
Pup Retrieval	Mother moves a pup into the nest or if the pups are in the nest, picks them up either in the forepaws or mouth
Zero Pup Contact	Mother out of contact with all pups at the beginning of a 10-second epoch
Lordosis Contraction	Contractions characterized by arching of back and stretching-out of body
Vertical Contraction	Contractions characterized by an upward bulging of the flanks
Intermediate Contraction	Any contraction which fits neither of the above descriptions
Pull	Mother pulls with her teeth at the anogenital region
Placentaphagia	Mother eats placenta or umbilical cord
Groom Anogenital Groom Head Groom Dorsal Groom Ventral	Mother self grooms specified region
Sniff	Any sniffing not directed at pups
Mouthe	Any mouthing not involving eating
Nest Build	Mother moves nesting material
Eat-Drink	Mother eats the food pellets or drinks the water
Twitch	Mother exhibits a spontaneous jerk originating at her ventral surface
General Activity	Mother locomotes about cage
Quiet	Absence of all the above behaviors during the entire 10-second epoch, except for Nurse and Zero Pup Contact

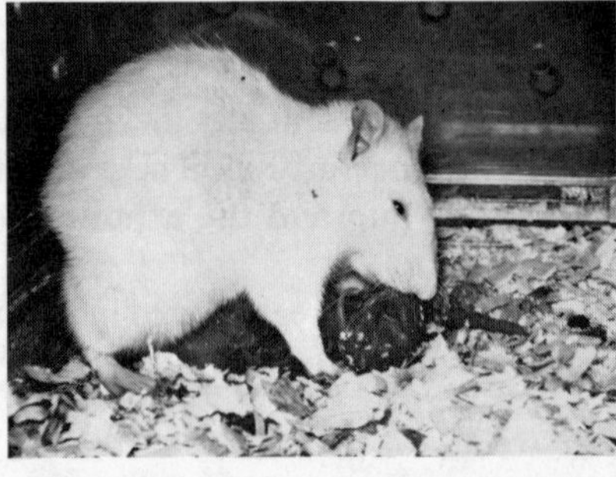

FIG. 1. This picture depicts the mother licking a pup. This is the prevalent behavior early in parturition.

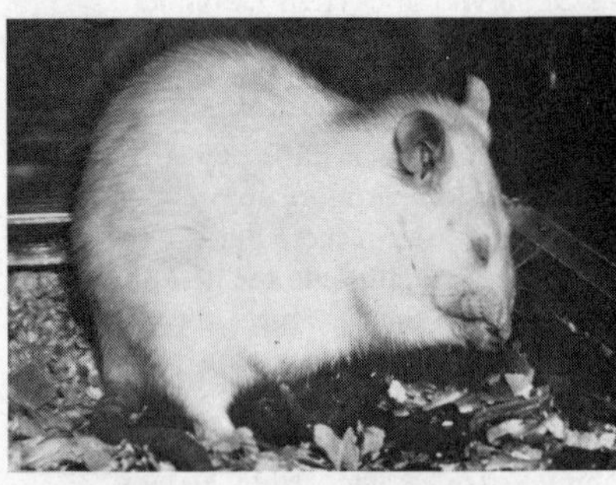

FIG. 2. Here the mother is shown grooming her head. Groom Head is often seen in conjunction with the cleaning of the birth fluids from the forepaws.

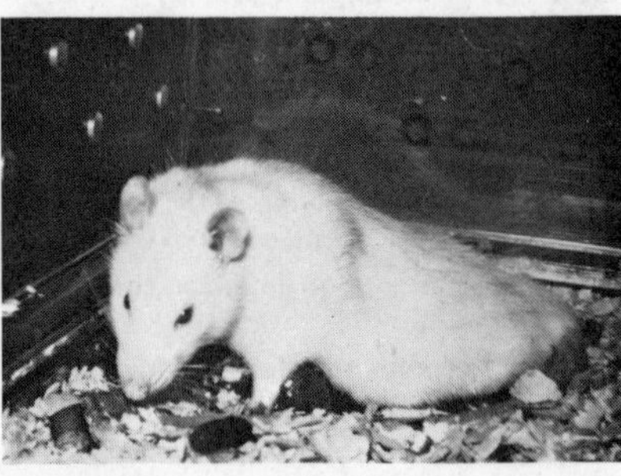

FIG. 3. This illustration shows the mother in a Lordosis Contraction. Note the characteristic arching of the back.

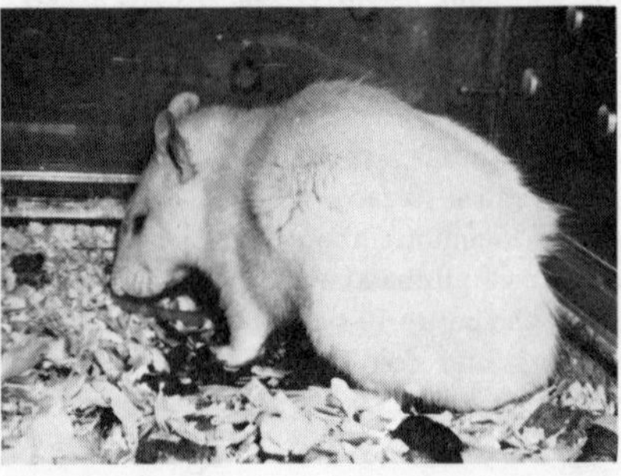

FIG. 4. In this picture the mother is in a Vertical Contraction. Note the characteristic bulging of the flanks. Pup births are closely associated with this type of contraction.

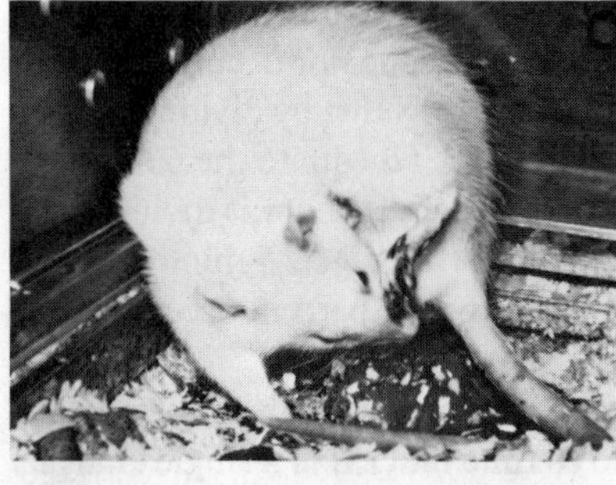

FIG. 5. Here we see the mother grooming in the anogenital region. The raising of the rear leg to facilitate access to the anogenital area is the most common posture associated with Groom Anogenital and Pull.

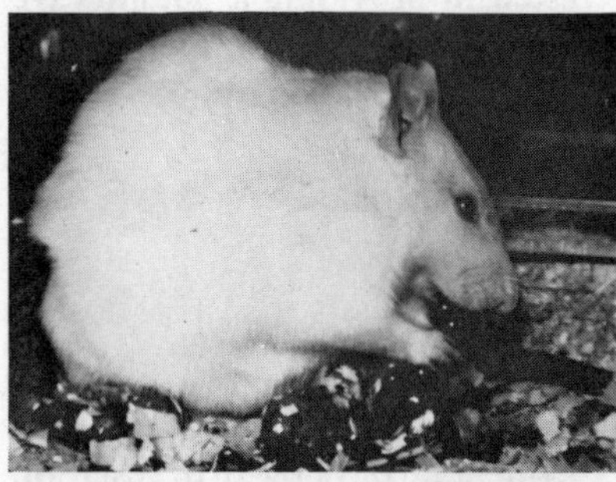

FIG. 6. This picture depicts the mother engaging in Placentaphagia. The placenta is typically held between the forepaws, similar to a food pellet.

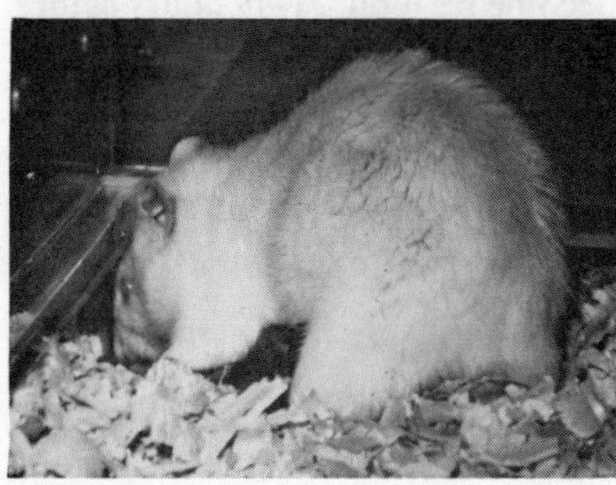

FIG. 7. In the final illustration the mother is settled over the pups, Nursing. After the birth of the last pup in the litter this is the prevalent behavioral pattern of the newly parturient mother.

even in the absence of a large nest, a feature common to nearly every normal parturition we observed.

Data Analysis

While the average delivery lasted 95 minutes, the range of parturition lengths was 35–180 minutes. Thus, it was necessary to find a way to adjust for these varying lengths so that the results could be pooled for statisical analysis. We equated for differences in parturitional length by dividing each delivery into equivalent, 10% time blocks (these ranged from 3.5 to 18.0 minutes). We then counted the number of epochs in which each behavior occurred during each 10% period and converted this to a percentage value by dividing by the total number of epochs per 10-percent time block. To equate the 60-minute period following the last birth with the period of delivery, it was divided into six, 10-minute periods (virtually identical with the average 9.5 minute length of each equivalent time unit during parturition) and the percent occurrence of each behavior in each time block was tabulated.

Coding the data in this way enabled us to analyze the delivery period (10 time blocks) anad the post-delivery period (6 time blocks) in a single analysis with 16 time points. Since we were interested in providing a quantitative description of the behavioral events occurring during parturition, the best fitting regression lines were generated from polynomial equations.

DESCRIPTION OF NORMAL PARTURITIONAL BEHAVIORS

The impending occurrence of parturition is first noted by the occurrence of weak, low amplitude uterine contractions, evident on days 18–20 of gestation (Fuchs, 1969). The contraction patterns become periodic 24–48 hours before delivery, and the contraction intervals are of a fairly long duration. True labor, which is charcterized by frequent, intense uterine contractions, begins 1–5 hours before the first birth (Boer et al., 1975; Fuchs, Nagasawa and Yanai, 1972). With the birth of the first pup, a series of highly integrated, organized behavior patterns is initiated.

Pup and Placenta Births

Figure 8 presents the percentage of an idealized litter of eleven pups born during each of the 10 equivalent time units of parturition. The number of births drops off sharply early in delivery, showing a nadir during the second equivalent time unit. Subsequently, there is a progressive increase in the percentage of the litter born throughout the remainder of the parturition. This increase in birth rate during the latter half of parturition also has been reported by Nagasawa and Yanai (1972).

The pattern of placenta deliveries is similar to that of pups born, although the curve is shifted somewhat to the right, reflecting the delay we frequently observed between the birth of a pup and the expulsion of its placenta (often as much as 15-20 minutes).

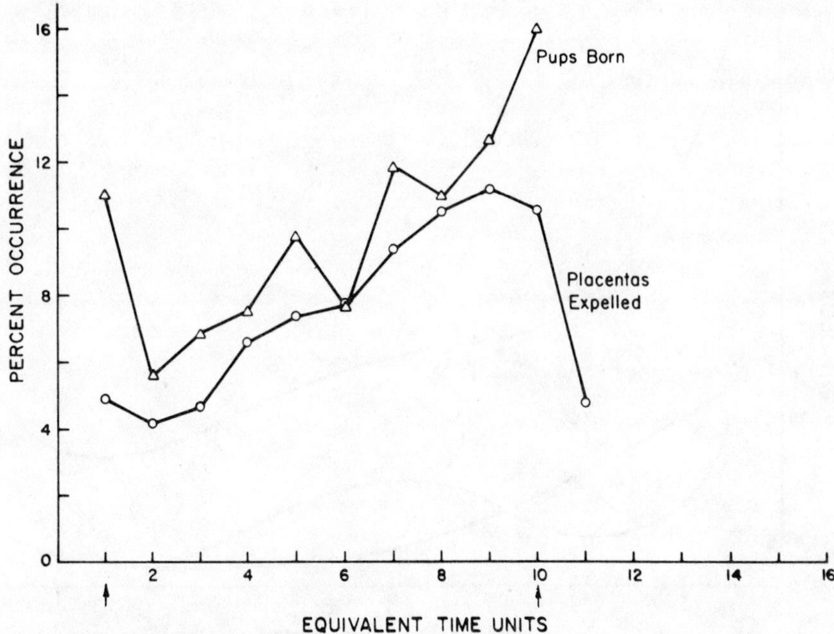

FIG. 8. The percent occurrence of Pups Born and Placentas Expelled. The two arrows designate the birth of the first and last pup in the litter, respectively.

Phases of Parturition

We were able to discern six clusters of behaviors based on their regression properties. Five of these characterized behavior patterns had significant time trends during parturition. The sixth cluster included behaviors with low percentages of occurrence, and all failed to show any significant time trend. These five groupings reflect sequential phases of parturition which are described by the temporal patterns exhibited by the various behaviors, beginning with those that peak within minutes after the first birth and ending with those having their maxima during the 60 minutes following the last birth.

Initiation Phase

Three behaviors were found to have their maximal occurrence soon after the first birth: Lick Pup, Sniff and Groom Head. Figure 9 presents the theoretical curves generated from the regression coefficients for these three behaviors. At the top of that figure are 11 circles to represent the time of

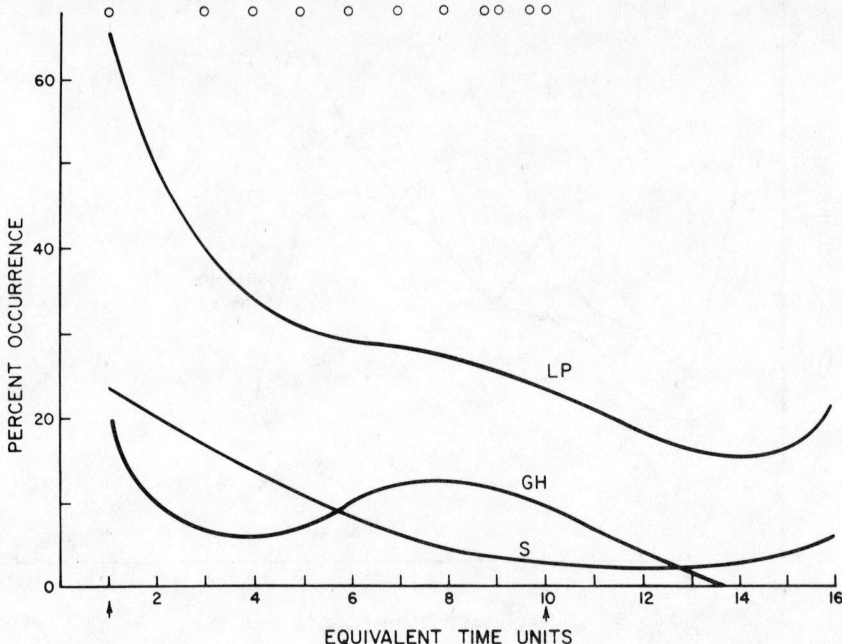

FIG. 9. The percent occurrence for Lick Pup (LP), Groom Head (GH), and Sniff (S). The circles at the top designate the time of occurrences of the births of an average litter of 11 pups.

occurrence of the births of an average litter (mean number of pups per litter in our colony = 10.9). Lick Pup was a very predominate behavior of the mother early in parturition, occurring in 65% of the epochs during the first time block, then dropping off during the remainder of the delivery period and reaching a minimum 40 minutes after the last pup was born. Sniff, while occurring at much lower frequencies than Lick Pup, showed virtually the same temporal pattern. Groom Head had the characteristic high incidence soon after the first birth followed by a decline; however, a second maximum is observed during the eighth time interval, close to the end of parturition. The occurrence of these behaviors in high amounts early in parturition reflects, in all probability, a response to the combined novelty of the first pups, placentas and the associated birth fluids.

Contraction Phase

A second cluster of behaviors have their peaks during the third to fifth time intervals, coincident with the third to fifth births (Figure 10). These behaviors serve as a transition from the pup-oriented nature of the Initiation phase to

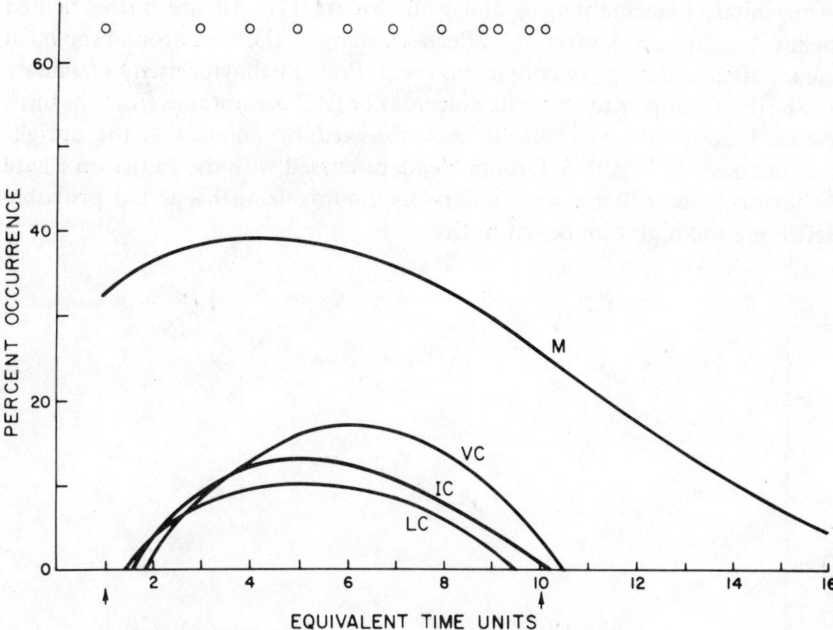

FIG. 10. The percent occurrence for Mouthe (M), Vertical Contraction (VC), Intermediate Contraction (IC), and Lordosis Contraction (LC).

the birth-oriented behaviors of the third phase, discussed below, and reach their maxima when the frequency of pup birth is relatively low. Three of the behaviors are contractions—Vertical, Intermediate, and Lordosis Contraction—while the fourth, Mouthe, is a very generalized behavior. As can be seen in the figure, the contraction behaviors reach their peaks sequentially. Lordosis Contraction, the predominant contraction observed prior to the first birth, is first, perhaps facilitating the movement of pups down the uterine horns and into the birth canal. Intermediate Contraction is next, providing a transition to the third type, the Vertical Contraction. This one is nearly always associated with the birth of a pup or a placenta. The high incidence of Mouthe during this period may reflect some unknown association with contraction events or may indicate the presence of fetal membranes or placental remnants in the mother's mouth. The occurrence of these behaviors during this period sets the stage for the following Birth-Oriented phase.

Birth-Oriented Phase

This phase encompasses the last half of parturition and is the period when the majority of the litter is born. Three behaviors peak at this time: Groom

Anogenital, Placentaphagia, and Pull (Figure 11). All are birth-oriented behaviors. Groom Anogenital reflects cleaning of the area around the birth canal, often occurring in conjunction with Pull, a behavior used to facilitate the birth of a pup or to extricate placentas or fetal membranes from the birth canal. Placentaphagia typically was observed by animals in the upright posture, seen in Figure 6. Groom Head, discussed with the Initiation Phase behaviors (Figure 9), has a secondary maximum during this period, probably reflecting the high number of births.

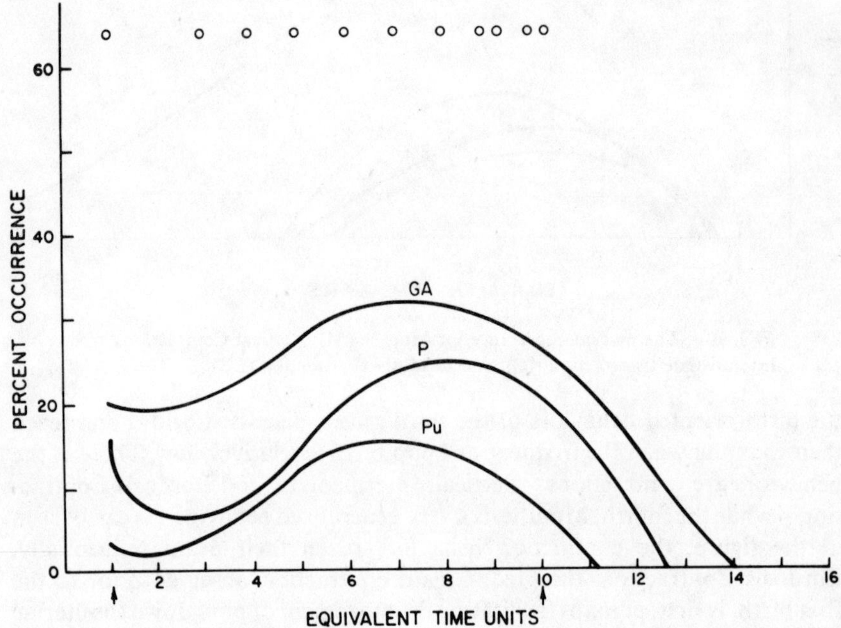

FIG. 11. The percent occurrence for Groom Anogenital (GA), Placentaphagia (P), and Pull (Pu).

Termination Phase

The birth of the last pup is characterized by an increase in the occurrence of Sniff Pup (Figure 12). This behavior, often associated with Pup Retrieve and Nest Build, is directed toward organizing the nest. It serves as a transition between the Birth-Oriented Phase and the final, Nursing Phase.

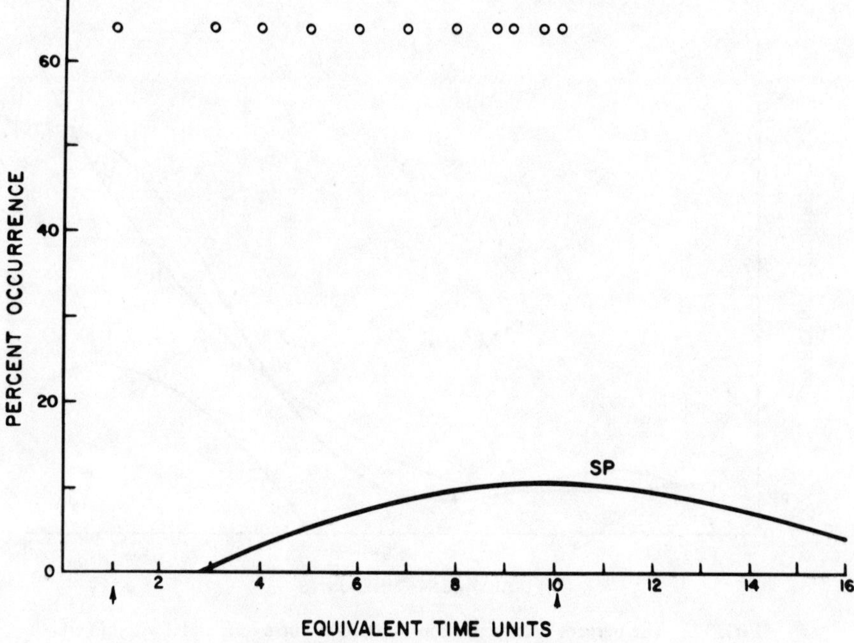

FIG. 12. The percent occurrence for Sniff Pup (SP).

Nursing Phase

This phase is marked by maternal inactivity and quiescence. Quiet, Nurse, and Twitch, the three behaviors characteristic of this phase, are rarely observed during the period of delivery (Figure 13). However, soon after the last birth, they begin to increase rapidly, reaching 50–60% occurrence for Quiet and Nurse within 60 minutes. Twitch, thought to reflect nipple attachment by the pups, reaches its maximum approximately 40 minutes after the last pup is born. The high correlation between the incidence of Nurse and Quiet suggests that the rapid initiation of suckling by the newborn pup is dependent on the mother's quiescence.

Aphasic Behaviors

Seven of the behaviors we observed did not have significant time trends and, in addition, occurred at very low levels: Groom Dorsal, Groom Ventral, Zero Pup Contact, Pup Retrieve, Nest Build, General Activity, and Eat-

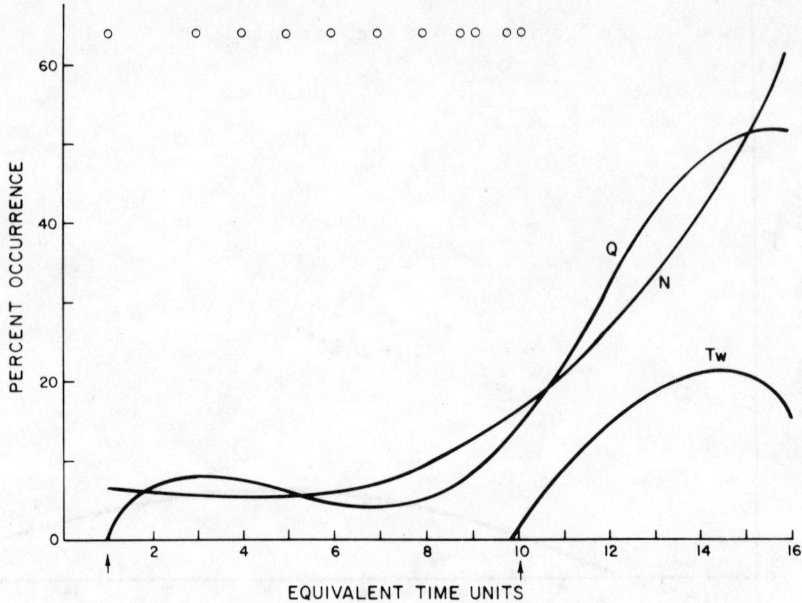

FIG. 13. The percent occurrence for Quiet (Q), Nurse (N), and Twitch (Tw).

Drink. Since these behaviors are all an integral part of the rat's behavioral repertoire, their low incidence may indicate that they are not needed for the successful completion of a normal delivery.

Summary

It is evident from these results that the parturient female exhibits well structured, precise behavioral patterning during her parturition. Most behaviors occur to some extent throughout the delivery period. However, it is their precise temporal patterning which reflects the highly ordered state characteristic of the parturitional process, an order closely tied to the pup births. Figure 14 provides a composite representation of the phases described above. An initial high incidence of pup-oriented behavior (Lick Pup) immediately follows the first birth. Transitional—internally oriented—behaviors (Contractions, Mouthe) characterize the lull in births during the early half of parturition. The rise in birth-oriented behaviors (Groom, Pull, Placentaphagia) accompanies the increasing rate of pup and placental deliveries during the last half of the delivery. The transition from the final birth to the beginning of the Nursing Phase, during which time the mother Sniffs Pup, is brief. Within 20–30 minutes following the last birth, the female

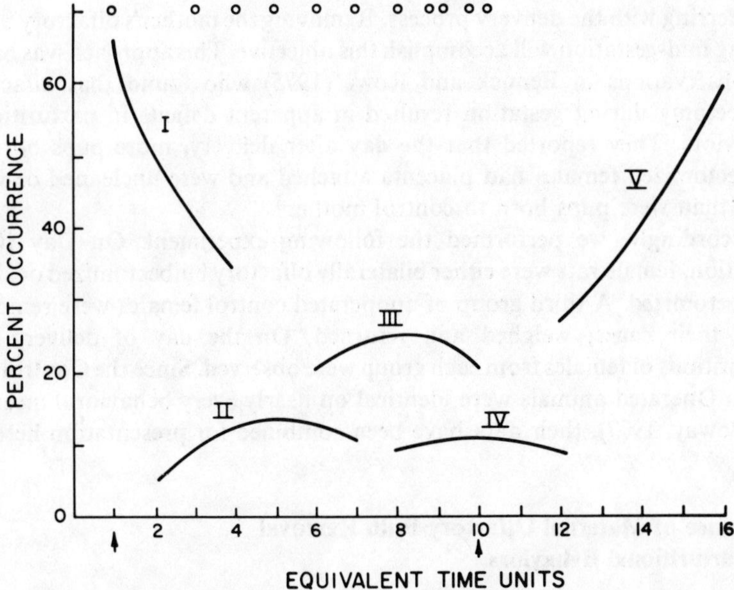

FIG. 14. Composite of the major behavioral phases identified during parturition in the rat, beginning with the Initiation Phase and extending to the final, Nursing Phase. Theoretical curves for the behaviors Lick Pup (I), Intermediate Contraction (II), Placentaphagia (III), Sniff Pup, (IV), and Nurse (V) are used as representative behaviors of the 5 phases. Only that portion of each curve falling within its phase is presented.

has again returned to pup-oriented behaviors, settling over the litter and becoming quiet and nursing.

IMPLICATIONS OF THE PARTURITIONAL BEHAVIOR PATTERNS FOR PUP DEVELOPMENT

It is a reasonable hypothesis that one major function of the highly ordered behaviors observed at the time of parturition is to insure the successful birth of live young. Thus, it is important that birth membranes be cleaned from the pup's head; that contraction patterns be regular and consistent; and that the mother become quiescent following delivery so that the motorically limited young can reach, attach to, and—more importantly—remain attached to a nipple.

A question which arises from these findings is: Does this orderly progression of behaviors exhibited by the parturient female also influence the pups subsequent development? One way to answer that question is to disrupt the temporal sequencing of the parturitional behaviors without directly interferring with the delivery process. Removing the mother's olfactory bulbs during mid-gestation will accomplish this objective. This approach was based on observations of Benuck and Rowe (1975) who found that olfactory bulbectomy during gestation resulted in apparent deficits in parturitional behaviors. They reported that the day after delivery, more pups born to bulbectomized females had placenta attached and were uncleaned or were dead than were pups born to control mothers.

Accordingly, we performed the following experiment. On Day 10 of gestation, female rats were either bilaterally olfactory bulbectomized or sham bulbectomized. A third group of unoperated control females were removed from their cages, weighed and returned. On the day of delivery, the parturitions of females from each group were observed. Since the Control and Sham Operated animals were identical on nearly every behavioral measure (Holloway, 1977), their data have been combined for presentation here.

Influence of Maternal Olfactory Bulb Removal on Parturitional Behaviors

There were no effects of the surgical treatment on either the rate of pup births or placentas expelled, indirectly suggesting the absence of differential prenatal effects. However, the Bulbetomized females were found to differ from the Controls on nearly every behavior measured. These findings are summarized below using the same headings as used to describe the normal parturitional sequence.

Initiation Phase

Two behaviors associated with the Initiation phase—Lick Pup and Groom Head—occurred significantly more in Control females while Sniff, a more generalized behavior, had a higher incidence in Bulbectomized females (Figure 15). The pattern of all three behaviors is consistent with the hypothesis that the Bulbectomized female is very insensitive to the focal parturitional event.

Contraction Phase

The Bulbectomized females differed from normal animals on only two of the Contraction Phase behaviors. They had higher percentages of Lordosis and Intermediate Contractions while not differing from Controls in the incidence of Mouthe and Vertical Contraction (Figure 16).

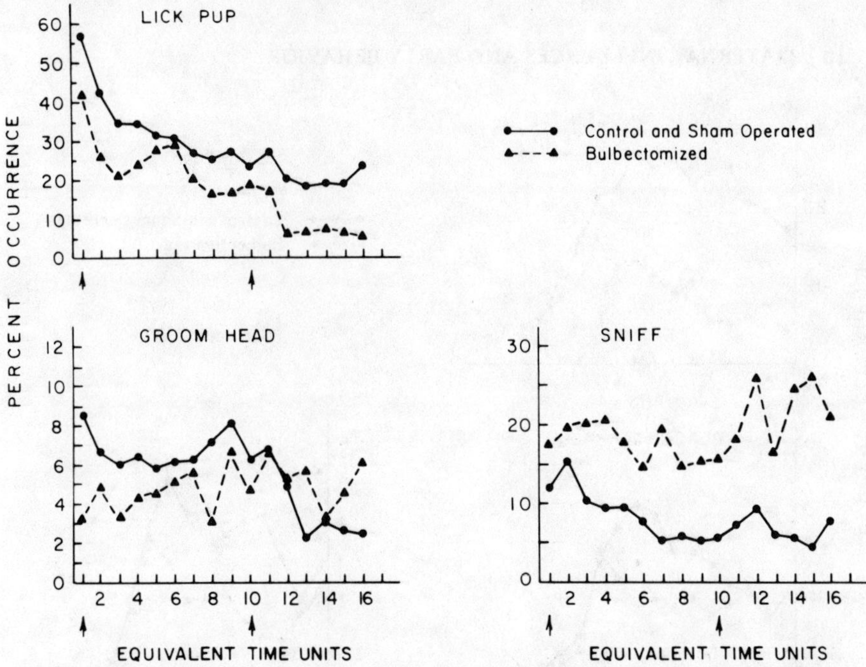

FIG. 15. The percent occurrence of Lick Pup, Groom Head and Sniff in Control and Bulbectomized mothers during parturition.

FIG. 16. The percent occurrence of Mouthe, Vertical Contraction, Lordosis Contraction and Intermediate Contraction in Control and Bulbectomized mothers during parturition.

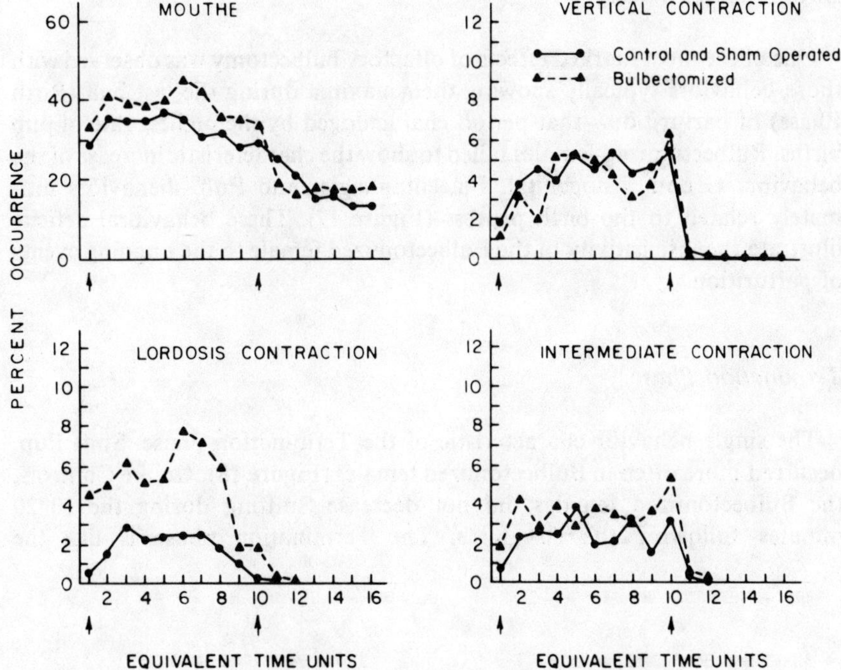

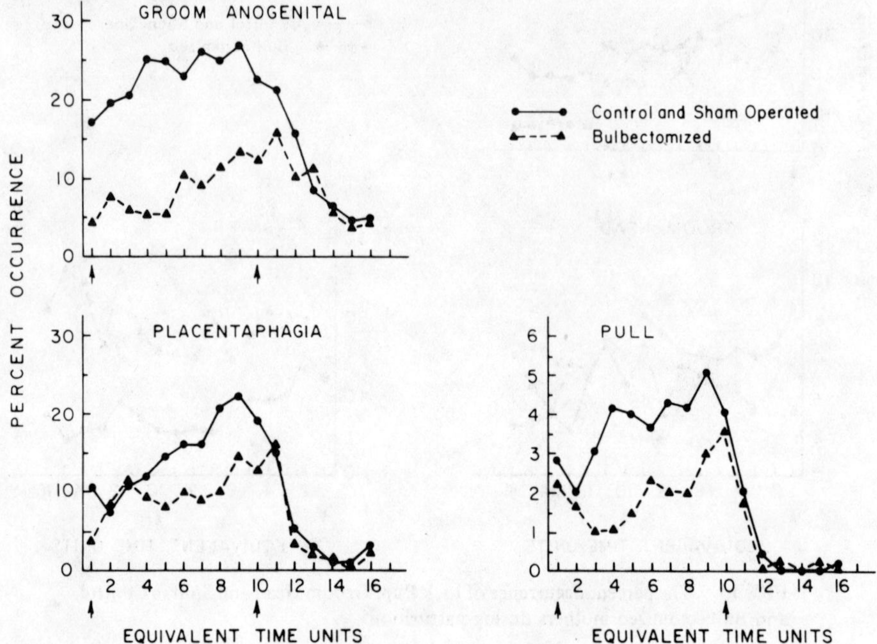

FIG. 17. The percent occurrence of Groom Anogenital, Placentaphagia, and Pull in Control and Bulbectomized mothers during parturition.

Birth-Oriented Phase

One of the most marked effects of olfactory bulbectomy was observed with those behaviors typically showing their maxima during the last half (Birth Phase) of parturition—that period characterized by the highest rate of pup births. Bulbectomized females failed to show the characteristic increase of the behaviors Groom Anogenital, Placentaphagia, and Pull—behaviors intimately related to the birth process (Figure 17). These behavioral deficits illustrate the insensitivity of the Bulbectomized female to the ongoing events of parturition.

Termination Phase

The single behavior characteristic of the Termination phase, Sniff Pup, occurred more often in Bulbectomized females (Figure 18). Unlike Controls, the Bulbectomized females did not decrease Sniffing during the 10–20 minutes following the last birth. The Termination phase is like the

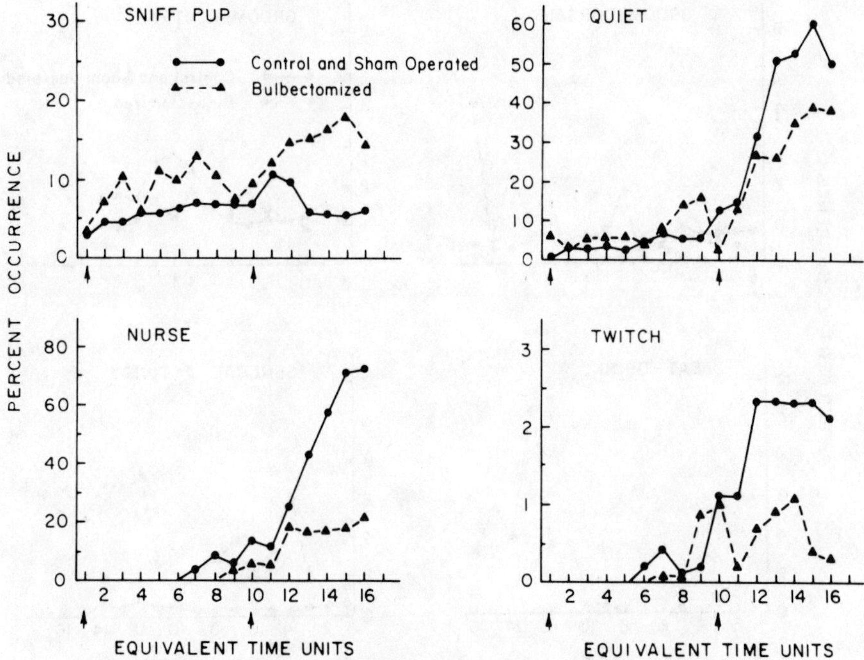

FIG. 18. The percent occurrence of Sniff Pup, Quiet, Nurse and Twitch in Control and Bulbectomized mothers during parturition.

Contraction phase in that both are transitional periods, and the Bulbectomized females appear unable to make a smooth shift from one phase to another.

Nursing Phase

The Nursing phase was quite attenuated in Bulbectomized females. While Controls sharply increased their frequencies of Quiet, Nurse, and Twitch following the last birth, Bulbectomized animals showed much smaller increases in these behaviors (Figure 18).

Aphasic Behaviors

A final indication that the Bulbectomized female is unresponsive to the parturitional process involves the relatively high incidence of those behaviors which were aphasic among Controls (Groom Dorsal, Groom Ventral, Eat-

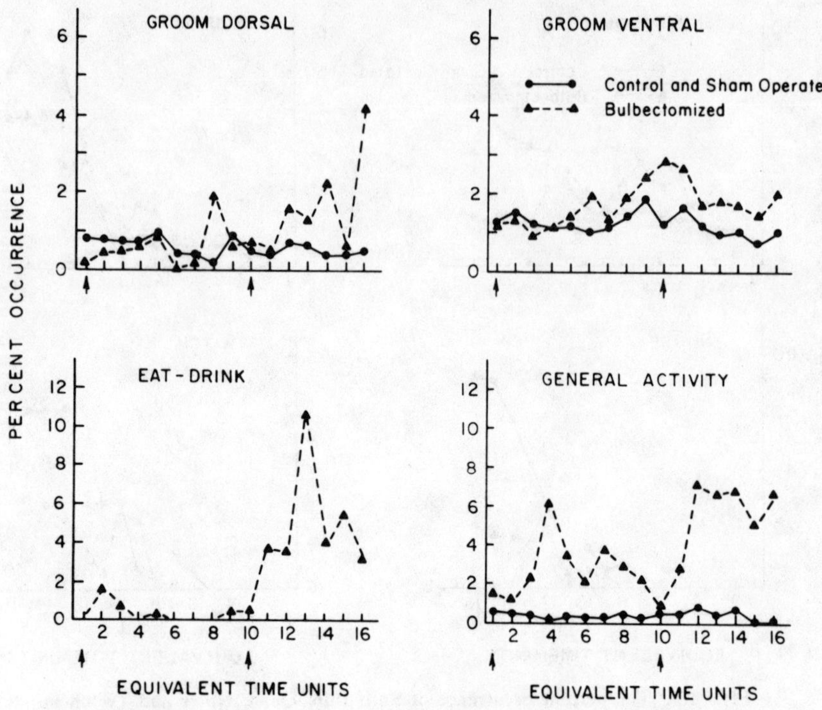

FIG. 19. The percent occurrence of Groom Dorsal, Groom Ventral, Eat-Drink and General Activity in Control and Bulbectomized mothers during parturition.

Drink, General Activity, Pup Retrieve, Nest Build, and Zero Pup Contact). In most instances, these differences occurred only in certain periods during parturition. Groom Dorsal, Groom Ventral and Eat-Drink had their highest incidence primarily during the 60 minutes following the last birth (Figure 19). In contrast, the behaviors General Activity (Figure 19), Pup Retrieve, Nest Build, and Zero Pup Contact (Figure 20) occurred with higher frequencies soon after the first birth and again following the last birth in the litter.

Summary

It is apparent that the parturitional behaviors expressed by Bulbectomized mothers differ from the normal females. The most characteristic feature of their delivery pattern is the much higher incidence of non-pup-oriented behaviors, and correspondingly, the significantly lower levels of pup- and birth-oriented behaviors. The Bulbectomized females simply behave inappropriately in the nest situation. Although they engage in the same behaviors as the Controls, the temporal patterning are markedly different. The pup and

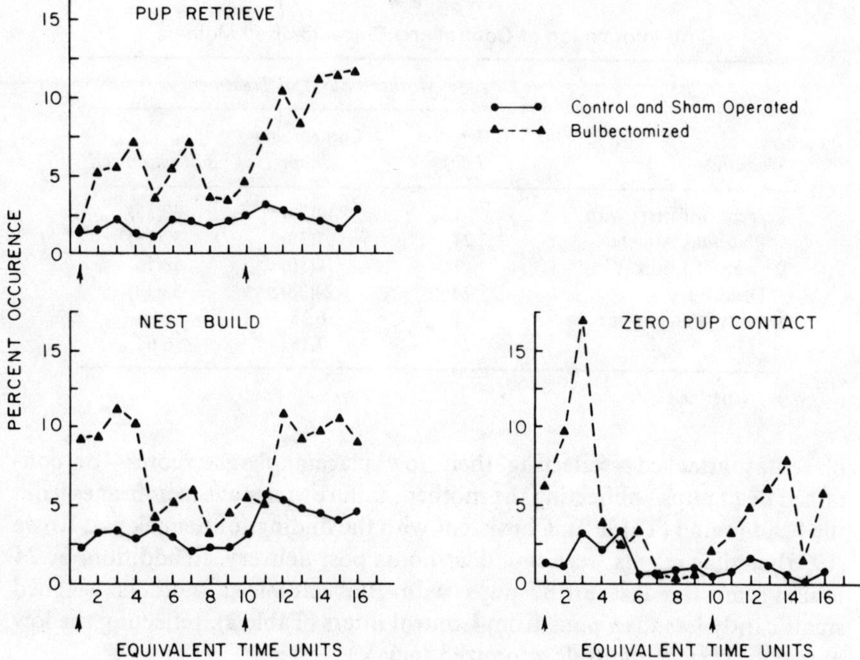

FIG. 20. The percent occurrence of Pup Retrieve, Nest Build and Zero Pup Contact in Control and Bulbectomized mothers during parturition.

placental births are not the focal points of the female's behaviors. Whether these effects are due to an olfactory deficit or to central effects resulting from the olfactory bulb removal cannot be determined from these data. It is worth noting that despite the aberrant parturitional environment experienced by pups born to Bulbectomized females, in no instance was a pup observed to be born dead. Further, one hour following the last birth in the litter, the body weights of pups born to Bulbectomized females did not differ from Control pups.

CONSEQUENCES OF AN ABNORMAL PARTURITIONAL ENVIRONMENT

Immediate Effects

The immediate effects of experiencing the aberrant parturitional behavior patterns were evident in several ways. One hour after the last birth, more litters born to Bulbectomized mothers contained pups which still had

TABLE 2
Birth Information of Control and Bulbectomized Mothers

		Mother's Surgical Treatment	
Measure	*Litter Age (Hr)*	*Control and Sham*	*Bulbectomized*
Percent of Litters with	1	14(30)*	80(15)
Placentas Attached	24	5(38)	32(19)
Percent of Litters with	1	17(30)	53(15)
Dead Pups	24	24(38)	53(19)
$\bar{X}$ Body Weight (gm)	1	6.38	6.61
	24	7.18	6.67

*N per cell

placentas attached—reflecting their low placentaphagia scores—or contained dead pups—reflecting the mother's failure to remove membranes from the head region (Table 2). Consistent with the findings of Benuck and Rowe (1975) similar results were found 24 hours post-delivery. In addition, by 24 hours after the last birth, pups with Bulbectomized mothers weighed significantly less than pups from Control litters (Table 2), reflecting the low nursing scores of the Bulbectomized females.

Long-Term Effects

In addition to the immediate effects noted above, are there long-term effects on the pups which can be attributed to the aberrant parturition? We addressed this issue in a very simple way. Either 1 or 24 hours following the last birth, four healthy pups from each litter were fostered to a control mother who had been nursing her own litter from 24 to 48 hours. Thus, any subsequent development difference observed among pups born to Bulbectomized or Control females could be attributed to the parturitional and early postnatal environments experienced by the pups. At weaning (Day 21) the pups were removed from their foster mother, weighed, and the number of live pups recorded. One female was placed into a standard laboratory cage and tested for activity in the open field on Days 25–28 of life (Denenberg, 1969).

The results showed that there were long-term effects. First, fewer pups born to Bulbectomized females survived to weaning than pups born to the two groups of Control mothers (Table 3). Interestingly, the weaning weights of the survivors did not differ. Secondly, pups from Bulbectomized females had a different pattern of activity in the open field. Whereas the Controls decreased their activity over the four test days, the pups from Bulbectomized mothers

TABLE 3
Survival Probability at Weaning of Pups Born to Control and Bulbectomized Mothers

	Natural Mother's Surgical Treatment	
Litter Age When Fostered	*Control and Sham*	*Bulbectomized*
Hour 1	89%(92*)	64%(44)
Hour 24	99%(143)	77%(62)

*N per cell

maintained the same level on all days (Figure 21). These results imply that the parturitional and perinatal environment experienced by a rat pup greatly influences its subsequent survival probability and behavioral expression. However, before this can be taken as a serious hypothesis, it is necessary to establish that the results could not be due to events occurring prior to the onset of the parturitional phase. We now turn to that issue.

Control for the Specific Effects of Olfactory Bulb Removal

Although the Sham Operated group controlled for the effects of surgical trauma during gestation, the possibility remained that the removal of the olfactory bulbs and the resultant neuronal degeneration and damage may have affected the pups in utero. Hence, the behavioral and survival differences observed in pups from Bulbectomized mothers may have been due to prenatal effects.

We tested this as follows: Pregnant female rats were subjected to bilateral olfactory bulbectomy, sham bulbectomy, or were not disturbed, on Day 10 of gestation, just as in the earlier experiment. On Day 23 of pregnancy, the expected day of delivery, the pups were delivered by cesarean section and subsequently fostered to control lactators (four pups from each litter). Prior research has shown that cesarean-delivered pups do not differ from normally delivered animals in their survival probability, body weight or open-field behavior (Grota et al., 1966). Therefore, if the Bulbectomized group does not differ from Controls, we may conclude that the prenatal events up to the time of the cesarean section did not have a measurable effect, and from this draw a second conclusion, namely, that the significant effects shown in Table 3 and Figure 21 must be a function of the parturitional and perinatal environment.

At weaning, 84% of Control and Sham Operated pups were alive, and 89% of the Bulbectomized pups survived. These data compare favorably to the

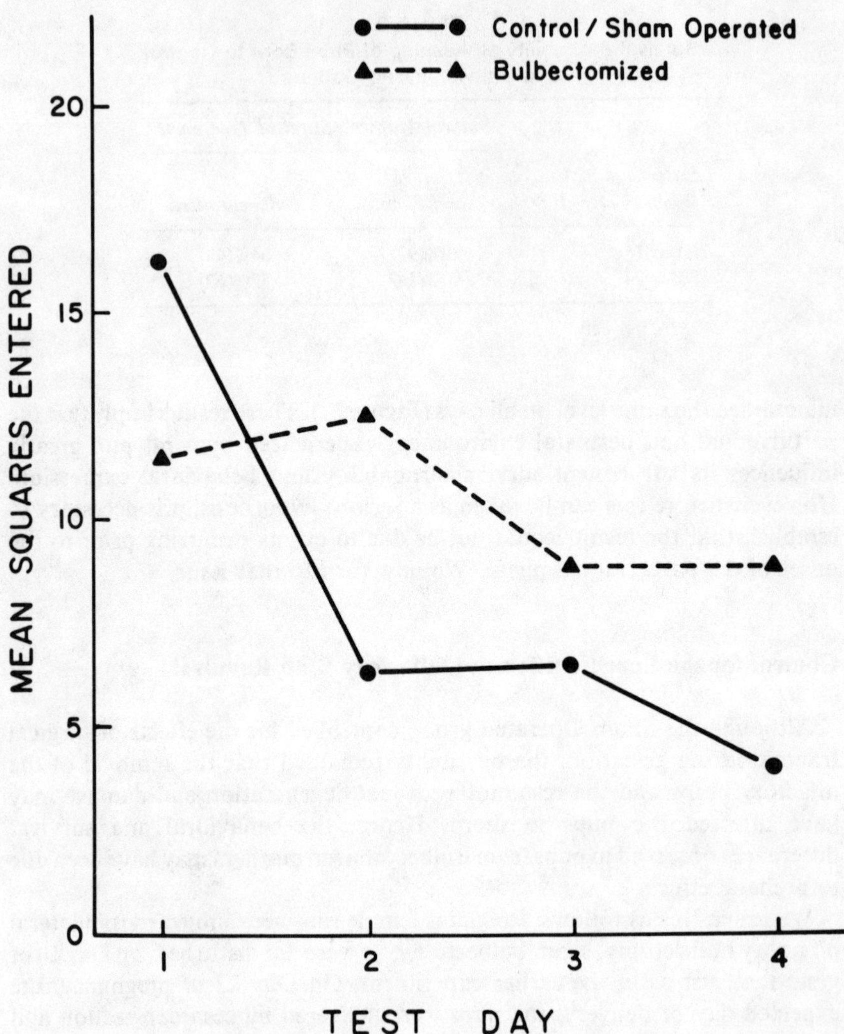

FIG. 21. Open-field activity of pups born to Bulbectomized or Control mothers.

Control data in Table 3 for the 1-Hour delivery group. Furthermore, the open-field activity pattern of all three groups—including the pups from Bulbectomized mothers—was virtually identical to those of the Control group from the previous experiment (see Figure 21).

Since we have been able to eliminate the differences in survival probability and open-field activity found previously through use of a cesarean delivery technique, we may conclude that the differences previously found are a function of the parturitional and perinatal environment of a bulbectomized mother.

ROLE OF THE EARLY POSTNATAL HOURS IN PUP DEVELOPMENT

In addition to the work focusing on the parturitional environment, we have performed a series of experiments focusing on the 12 hours after birth (Denenberg et al., 1963; Denenberg et al., 1976; Dollinger, 1977). In 1963, Denenberg et al. provided evidence that the maternal environment experienced by rat pups during their first 12 hours of life significantly influenced their subsequent growth and survival probability. One hour following the last birth, pups either remained with their own mother or were given to a 10-day lactating female. Eleven hours later, all pups were fostered to 10-day lactators. At weaning, pups who had been with their own mother during the first 12 hours of life weighed more and had higher survival probabilities than their littermates who had been with a 10-day lactator during the same period. Since all pups were reared by 10-day lactators from Hour 12 onward, these results showed that some aspects of the maternal environment of the 10-day lactator during the early postnatal hours was deleterious to the newborn rat.

Recently, we repeated this experiment, recording the maternal behaviors of the newly parturient females and 10-day lactators when given pups 1 hour old (Denenberg et al., 1976). One hour following the last birth in a litter, four pups were placed with their own mother and four littermates were placed with a 10-day lactator. During the 1-hour period following the fostering, the behaviors of each female rat during successive 10-second epochs were recorded. Ten-day lactators were found to be much more active with the newborn than were newly parturient females. They licked pups more, groomed themselves more and were out of pup contact more than the 1-hour lactators. This high activity was reflected in much lower levels of Quiet and consequently fewer episodes of Nursing by the 10-day lactators. These behaviors resulted in decreased body weights at Hour 12 for pups who had been with the 10-day lactators (7.5 vs. 6.7). At Hour 12 of life each litter of pups was given to a 10-day lactator. At weaning, pups who had been with a 10-day lactator during Hours 1–12 of life still showed the lowered body weight evident at Hour 12 (45.7 vs. 39.5). These results nicely replicated the early work and further showed the importance of the maternal behavior patterns experienced by newborn pups on their subsequent development.

DISCUSSION

These two series of experiments, one focusing on the parturitional period and one on the early postnatal hours, clearly implicate the maternal environment during the perinatal period as a determinant, not only of immediate survival, but also of long-term developmental trends.

In both instances, behavior patterns which were incompatible with the needs of the pup resulted in deleterious effects on the young, even after fostering to control females soon after birth. These findings mesh nicely with what is known about the perinatal physiology of the rat. The endogenous energy stores of the pup are limited primarily to its liver glycogen deposits (Hahn and Koldovsky, 1966). Within 12 hours following birth, these stores are depleted and the pup enters a hypoglycemic state (Dawkins, 1963). Thus, the newborn rat is very dependent on external sources of energy, especially during the early postnatal hours. The milk of the newly parturient female contains very high levels of readily metabolizable fat (24%), more than double that found during mid-lactation (Luckey et al., 1954). Since the pups are relatively immobile under normal nest conditions, the female must behave in a manner to facilitate the rapid attachment of pups to her nipples, and their subsequent ingestion of milk. This behavior pattern is characterized, as noted above for normal females, by a rapid settling over the pups, with associated quiescence. The pups attach and begin nursing shortly thereafter.

The behavior patterns of both the Bulbectomized females and the 10-day lactators are totally inappropriate for the rapid initiation of nursing by newborn. Bulbectomized females engage primarily in non-pup-oriented behaviors and are very active. One consequence of this behavior pattern is that the pups are unable to attach successfully to a nipple. The 10-day lactator engages in pup-oriented behaviors, but at much higher frequency than normally experienced by the newborn. Also her behavior is characterized by higher levels of activity than the newly parturient female, levels characteristic of her interactions with her own 10-day-old pups. Thus, the behaviors exhibited by the newly parturient females during parturition and the early postnatal period are ultimately related to the biological needs of the newborn; they show the high degree of synchrony which can, and must, exist during the earliest postnatal moments.

These data support a very important hypothesis, namely, that the early postnatal hours are important for the normal growth and development of the young of an altricial species. The perinatal period is already known to be important for the formation of social bonds and a viable mother-infant relationship in many precocial animals including the goat (Klopfer, 1971), the sheep (Collias, 1956) and the cow (Neindre and Garel, 1976). Removal of the young from the mother for periods ranging from 5 minutes in one case, up to several hours in others, typically results in complete or near total rejection of the young animal by its mother. Our results suggest that the important emphasis placed on this period should be extended to altricial species as well. Work presented elsewhere in this volume (Chapter 2) also indicate that the newborn is capable of complex behavioral interactions with its environment soon after birth. Consequently, any manipulation which alters the stimulus properties of the newborn is readily observed in the resulting mother-infant interaction patterns. Thus, a highly synchronous relationship is present at birth in the rat, a relationship which is ultimately tied to the successful growth and development of the young.

REFERENCES

Adolph, E. F. Physiological stages in the development of mammals. *Growth 34,* 113–124 (1970).

Benuck, I. and Rowe, F. A. Central and peripherally induced anosmia: Influences on maternal behavior in lactating female rats. *Physiol. Behav. 14,* 439–447 (1975).

Boer, K., Lincoln, D. W., and Swaab, D. F. Effects of electrical stimulation of the neurohypophysis on labor in the rat. *J. Endocrin. 65,* 163–176 (1975).

Bridges, R. S. Long-term effects of pregnancy and parturition upon maternal responsiveness in the rat. *Physiol. Behav. 14,* 245–250 (1975).

Bridges, R. S. Parturition: Its role in the long term retention of maternal behavior in the rat. *Physiol. Behav. 18,* 487–490 (1977).

Collias, N. E. The analysis of socialization in sheep and dogs. *Ecology 37,* 228–239 (1956).

Dawkins, M. J. R. Glycogen synthesis and breakdown in fetal and newborn rat liver. *Ann. N. Y. Acad. Sci. 111,* 203–211 (1963).

Denenberg, V. H. Open-field behaviour in the rat: What does it mean? *Ann. N. Y. Acad. Sci. 159,* 852–859 (1969).

Denenberg, V. H. Assessing the effects of early experience. In *Methods of Psychobiology, Vol. 3,* R. D. Myers, ed., Academic Press, New York: (1977), pp. 127–147.

Denenberg, V. H., Grota, L. J., and Zarrow, M. X. Maternal behavior in the rat: Analysis of cross-fostering. *J. Reprod. Fert. 5*, 131–141 (1963).

Denenberg, V. H., Holloway, W. R., and Dollinger, M. J. Weight gain as a consequence of maternal behavior in the rat. *Behav. Biol. 17*, 51–60 (1976).

Dollinger, M. J. The importance of the early postnatal period in the rat (*Rattus norvegicus*). Unpublished doctoral dissertation, University of Connecticut, 1977.

Fuchs, A. R. Uterine activity in late pregnancy and during parturition in the rat. *Biol. Reprod. 1*, 344–353 (1969).

Fuchs, A. R. and Saito, S. Pituitary oxytocin and vasopressin content of pregnant rats before, during, and after parturition. *Endocrin. 88*, 574–578 (1971).

Grota, L. J., Denenberg, V. H., and Zarrow, M. X. Normal versus cesarean delivery: effects upon survival probability, weaning weight, and open-field activity. *J. Comp. Physiol. Psychol. 61*, 159–160 (1966).

Grota, L. J. and Eik-Nes, K. B. Plasma progesterone concentration during pregnancy and lactation in the rat. *J. Reprod. Fert. 13*, 83–91 (1967).

Hahn, P. and Koldovsky, O. *Utilization of Nutrients During Postnatal Development*. Pergamon Press, London: (1966).

Holloway, W. R. Developmental changes in the behavior of the mother rat and her pups during the early postnatal period. Unpublished doctoral dissertation, University of Connecticut, 1977.

Holloway, W. R., Dollinger, M. J., and Denenberg, V. H. Body and organ growth in the newborn rat. *Biol. Neonate, 33,* 113–118 (1978).

Klopfer, P. Mother love: What turns it on? *Amer. Sci. 59*, 404–406 (1971).

Labhsetwar, A. P. and Watson, D. J. Temporal relationship between secretory patterns of gonadotropins, estrogens, progestins, and prostaglandin-F in peri-parturient rats. *Biol. Reprod. 10*, 103–110 (1974).

Linkie, D. M. and Niswender, G. D. Serum levels of prolactin, leutinizing hormone, and follicle stimulating hormone during pregnancy in the rat. *Endocrin. 90*, 632–637 (1972).

Luckey, T. D., Mende, T. J., and Pleasants, J. The physical and chemical characterization of rats' milk. *J. Nutr. 54*, 345–359 (1954).

Moltz, H., Rowland, D., Steele, M., and Halaris, A. Hypothalamic norepinephrine concentration and metabolism during pregnancy and lactation in the rat. *Neuroendo. 19*, 252–258 (1975).

Munford, R. E. Changes in the mammary glands of rats and mice during pregnancy, lactation and involution. 1. Histological structure. *J. Endocrin. 28*, 1–15 (1963 a).

Munford, R. E. Changes in the mammary glands of rats and mice during pregnancy, lactation, and involution. 2. Levels of deoxyribonucleic acid and alkaline and acid phosphatases. *J. Endocrin. 28*, 17–33 (1963 b).

Munford, R. E. Changes in the mammary glands of rats and mice during pregnancy, lactation and involution. 3. Relation of structural and biochemical changes. *J. Endocrin. 28*, 35–44 (1963 c).

Nagasawa, H. and Yanai, R. Changes in serum prolactin levels shortly before and after parturition in rats. *Endo. Jap. 19*, 139–143 (1972).

Neindre, P. L. and Garel, J. P. Existence of sensitive period for the development of maternal behavior after parturition in domestic cattle. *Biol. Behav. 1,* 217–221 (1976).

Rosenblatt, J. S., and Lehrman, D. Maternal behavior in the laboratory rat. In *Maternal Behavior in Mammals*, H. L. Rheingold, ed. John Wiley & Sons, Inc., New York: (1963), pp. 8–57.

Slotnick, B. M. Neural and hormonal basis of maternal behavior in the rat. In *Hormonal Correlates of Behavior, Vol. 2. An Organismic View*, B. Eleftheriou and R. L. Sprott, eds. Plenum Press, New York: (1975), pp. 585–656.

Wiesner, B. and Sheard, N. *Maternal Behavior in the Rat*. Oliver and Boyd, London: (1933).

Yoshinaga, K., Hawkins, R. A., and Stoker, J. F. Estrogen secretion by the rat ovary in vivo during the estrous cycle and pregnancy. *Endocrin. 85*, 103–112 (1969).

2

The Development of Behavioral Competence in the Rat

Mark J. Dollinger
William R. Holloway
Victor H. Denenberg

An understanding of the development of the mother-infant unit necessitates the study of both the behavior of the newly parturient female and of the newborn young. Parturition heralds not only the onset of maternal behavior (see Chapter 1) is also provides the newborn with its first postnatal experiences. In precocial mammals, such as the sheep and lamb, these first postnatal experiences are crucial for the acceptance of the newborn by the mother. Indeed, separation for as short a time as the first five minutes after birth is sufficient to result in the newborn's rejection (Klopfer, 1964). In precocial birds, such as the duck and chick, the early postnatal experiences are responsible for the neonate's recognition of its mother—a process commonly referred to as "imprinting" (Lorenz, 1934).

While the importance of the early postnatal environment has been well documented for numerous precocial species, it has received little attention in the study of altricial species. The information which is available on the early postnatal period in altricial animals provides a description of the newborn's inadequacies on the morphological and physiological levels, and the limitations of both its motor and sensory capabilities. The newborn rat's brain has achieved only about 10% of its adult weight (Himwich, 1975). While neurogenesis is completed prenatally except for the cerebellum, hippocampus and olfactory bulbs (Altman and Das, 1966), the nerve axons are poorly myelinated (Jacobson, 1963) and synaptogenesis in much of the brain is incomplete (Armstrong-James and Johnson, 1970). Many of the enzyme systems necessary for the degradation of food stuffs are not mature at birth (Hahn and Koldovsky, 1966), and the intestinal wall has not achieved closure

(Daniels et al., 1972). The motor skills of the newborn rat are limited primarily to head raising, with little ability to move from one location to another (Altman and Sudarshan, 1976; Bolles and Woods, 1964).

The newborn rat is also limited in its ability to perceive its environment by the immaturity of its sensory systems. The pup is born hairless, thereby compromising its ability to thermoregulate. In addition it is born both preaudial and previsual (Salas and Schapiro, 1970; Schapiro and Norman, 1967). The sensory systems which appear to be functional at birth are the somatosensory and the olfactory. The functioning of the somatosensory system is evident by the presence of a thermotactic response (Fowler and Kellogg, 1975) and its response to noxious stimuli. The functional ability of the olfactory system is seen in the quieting and the home-orientation responses to maternal odors at Day 2, which is the youngest age tested to date (Schapiro and Salas, 1970; Scherzenie and Hsiao, 1977), and by the importance of appropriate odors on the ventral surface of the lactator for the elicitation of nipple attachment (Teicher and Blass, 1977).

Thus, the picture of the newborn rat which emerges is one of marked immaturity as most levels of biological organization. This view of the newborn rat as a decidedly incompetent organism has also been accepted as an appropriate description of its behavioral repertoire, suggesting that the pup plays an inconsequential role in the establishment of the mother-infant unit. However, very little work has been directed toward the assessment of the newborn rat's behavior. Recent research investigating aspects of the rat's behavior during the first 10 days of life has found that the perinatal and neonatal pup behaves in a surprisingly competent fashion, which is necessary for and facilitates its survival. The purpose of this chapter is to describe a series of experiments from our laboratory on this topic as well as review other recent literature.

SECTION I: METHODOLOGICAL ISSUES

In order to assess the question of behavioral competence in the young rat, an appropriate behavioral measure must be utilized. This behavioral measure must be one that can be perceived and elicited. These requirements exclude visual and auditory stimuli and those tasks requiring motor skills. In addition, it is preferable for the measure to be within the naturally occurring behavioral repertoire of the species. This permits a broader interpretation of the results.

The behavior of the newborn pup in attaching to the mother's nipple meets all these criteria. Nipple attachment is a component of suckling, which is a naturally occurring behavior within all mammalian species. Also, the behavior is found to occur shortly after birth, (Rosenblatt and Lehrman, 1973; Chapter 1). Another important feature of suckling behavior is that it can be measured independent of maternal influences in an experimental setting, thus allowing us to bypass the mother's behavior which is known to strongly influence the behavior of the young (See Section VII).

The technique which we employ to assess nipple attachment is a modification of the procedure developed by Drewett et al. (1974). A lactating dam is anesthetized with a pentabarbitol based anesthetic, thereby excluding the possibility of milk letdown during the test (Lincoln et al., 1973). The anesthetized dam is laid on her back in a plastic tub, exposing the nipple lines. Pups are then held individually at a nipple (see Figure 1). Each pup receives three test trials. During the intertrial interval (2–6 minutes) the pup is placed into a moist warming oven maintained at 35°C. Each trial lasts either two minutes or until the nipple is secured. Attachment is readily discernable by the presence of a seal around the nipple (see Figure 2).

This procedure of measuring the pup's nipple attachment to an anesthetized lactator is relatively simple, yet is a precise measure of one of the

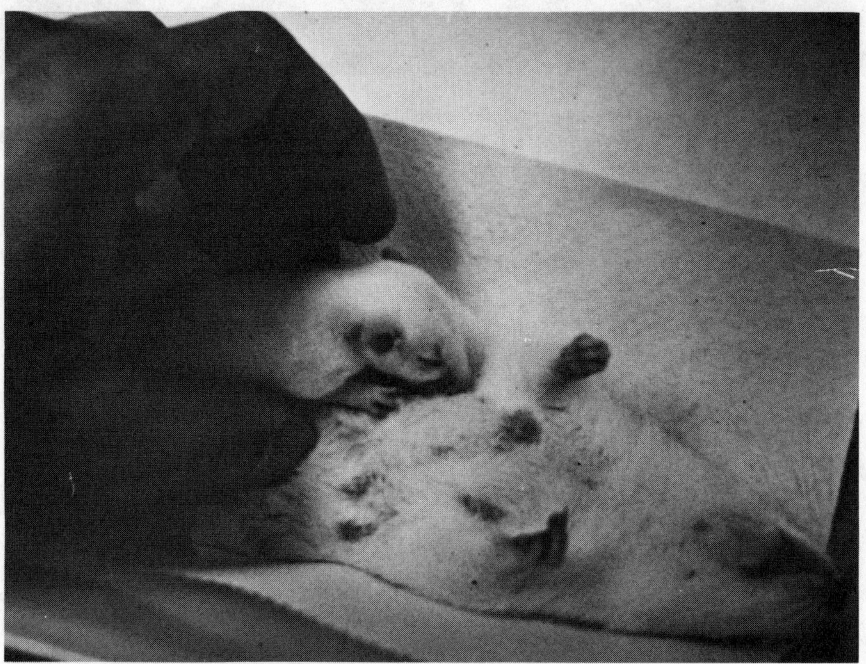

FIG. 1. This picture depicts the hand held suckling test. The pup is gently held at an axillary nipple of an anesthetized lactating dam.

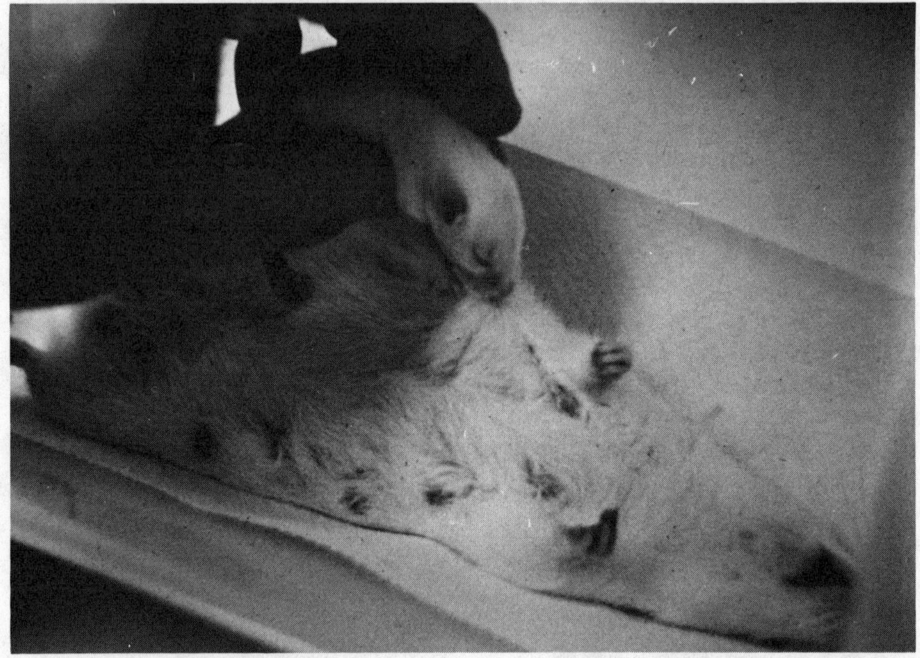

FIG. 2. This picture depicts the seal which the pup forms around the nipple. The presence of a seal when the pup is removed from the nipple provides an easily discernable criterion for attachment.

most important behavioral activities of the young animal. This measure was used to study various features of the pup's behavioral competence in adapting to postnatal life.

SECTION II: NIPPLE ATTACHMENT DURING THE FIRST 24 HOURS OF LIFE

The Developmental Course During the First Day

The first issue we addressed was whether systematic changes in the pup's behavior occur during the perinatal period. We investigated this by assessing the pup's nipple attachment at 1, 12, and 24 hours of life. We found that 1-hour old pups are inefficient in attaching to the nipple—only 21% attach even once out of the three test trials. However, by 12 hours the incidence of nipple attachment improves markedly to 82%, and remains high at 24 hours (70%) (see Figure 3).

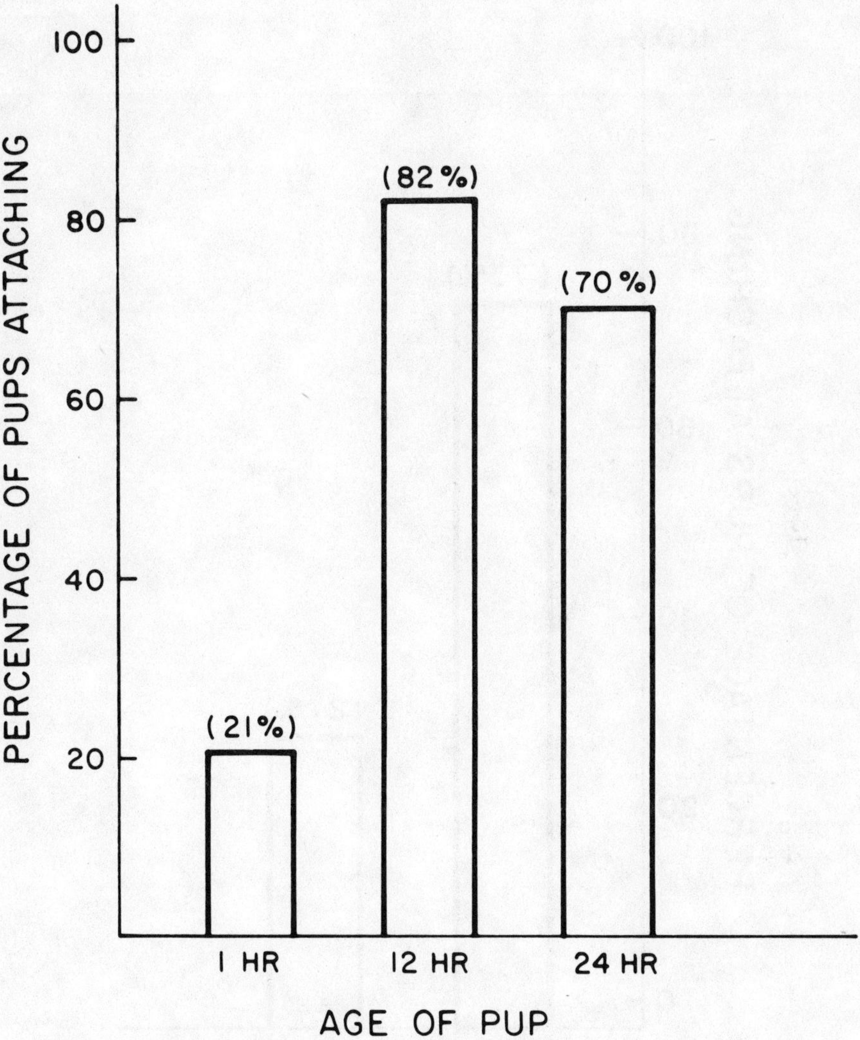

FIG. 3. Percentage of pups attaching to the nipples of an anesthetized lactator at Hour 1, Hour 12, or Hour 24 of life.

Testing a Maturational Hypothesis

The sharp increase in the nipple attachment during the first 12 hours raises the question of what is the mechanism mediating this transition. The first hypothesis we investigated was whether the increase from Hour 1 to Hour 12 is a function of maturational changes.

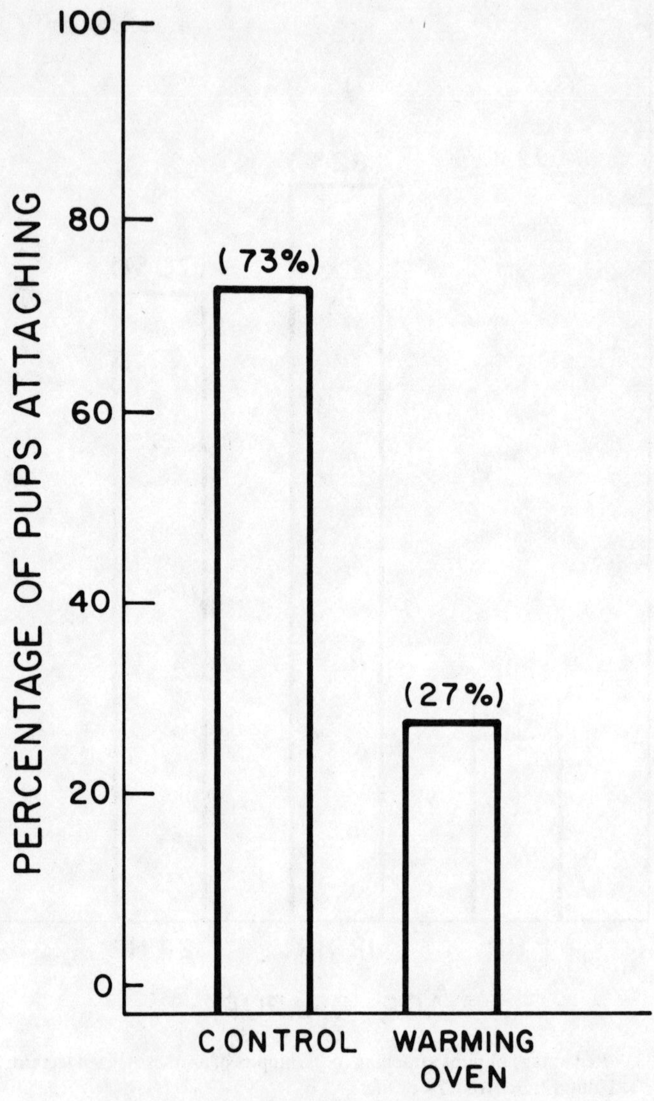

FIG. 4. Percentage of pups attaching which were either reared with their mother from Hour 1–12 (Control), or were deprived from Hour 1–12 (Warming Oven).

We tested this by rearing littermates from Hours 1–12 either with their own mother (Control group), or in a moist warming oven maintained at 35°C. Thus, when the two groups of pups were tested at Hour 12, they differed in their experiental history but not in their chronological age. So, if the increase in nipple attachment was mediated by maturational changes, the Warming Oven pups and their Control littermates should not differ. However, we found that Control pups had a much higher incidence of attachment than did Warming Oven pups—73% vs. 27%, respectively (see Figure 4).

The Role of Nipple Experience

The level of attachment exhibited by the Warming Oven pups was strikingly similar to the Hour-1 pups (21% and 27% respectively). One dimension along which these two groups are similar is the extent of their maternal exposure and the concomitant nipple experience, suggesting that nipple experience may be the mechanism responsible for the increase in nipple attachment we see during the first 12 hours of life.

We tested this hypothesis by generating three groups of 1-Hour old pups. We again had a Control and a Warming Oven group; in addition we had a group of pups which were exposed to a lactator whose nipples had been surgically ligated the preceding day (Ligation group). Since the maternal behavior of the ligated females is indistinguishable from the Control lactator (Dollinger et al., 1978), the Control and Ligation groups differ only in their acquisition of milk, and the Warming Oven and Ligation groups only in their experiential histories. Thus, if nipple experience is the mechanism mediating the increase in attachment from Hour 1 to Hour 12, the Ligated group should exhibit the same high levels of attachment as the Control group.

The results were consistent with this hypothesis. Pups in the Ligation group had a high incidence of attachment (67%) similar to that of the control group (83%) and much higher than the Warming Oven group (8%) (see Figure 5).

In addition to providing strong support for the experiential hypothesis, the high attachment percentage seen in the Ligation group eliminates the possibility that the low incidence of attachment of the Warming Oven rats was a function of debilitation, since both groups lost the same amount of weight from Hour 1 to Hour 12.

The Role of Non-Nipple Maternal Experience

The Warming Oven pups in the previous experiment had less suckling experience than either of the other two groups. However, they also differed

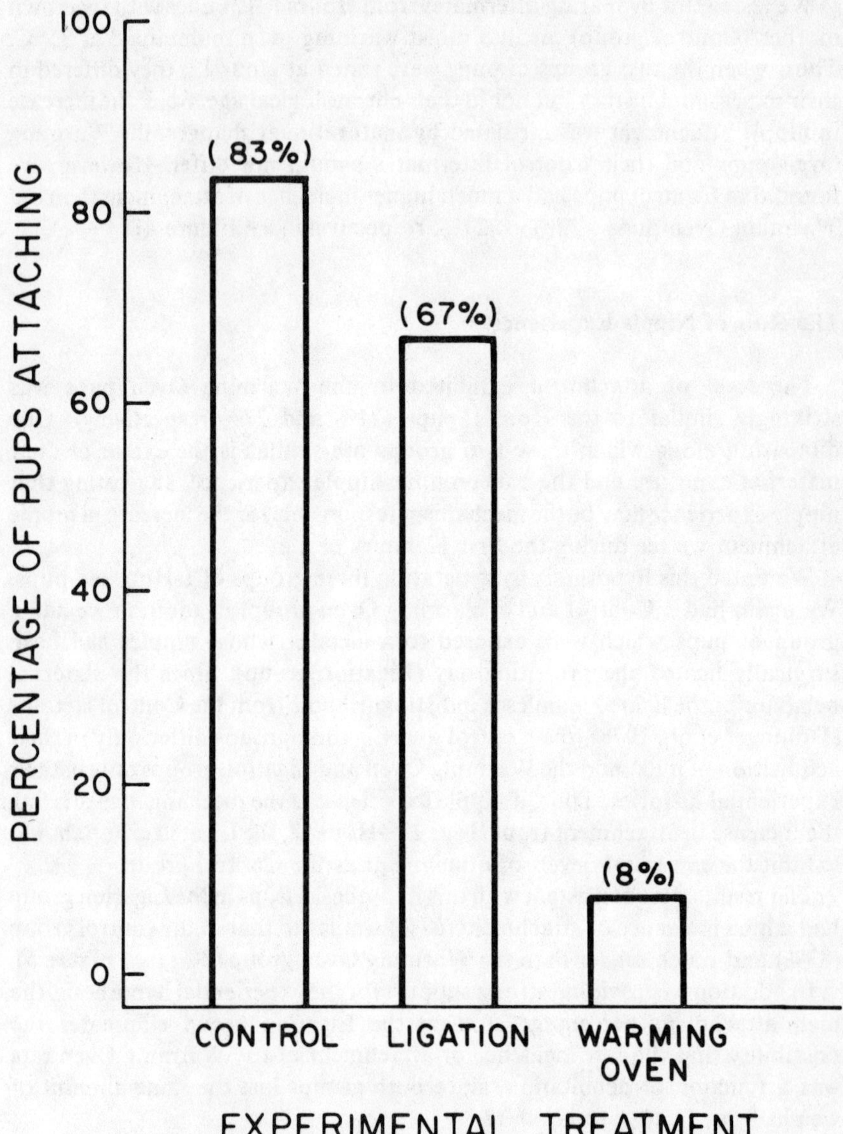

FIG. 5. Percentage of Pups attaching which were either reared with a 24–48 Hour lactator from Hour 1–12 (Control), or were reared from Hour 1–12 with a 24–48 Hour lactator whose nipples had been ligated (Ligation), or were deprived from Hour 1–12 (Warming Oven).

from the other groups in another important respect: they did not receive *any* maternal attention while the other pups were exposed to other aspects of the maternal environment not associated with suckling, such as maternal licking and exposure to maternal odors. Thus, there is a second interpretation of the results of the prior experiment: perhaps exposure to these more general properties of the maternal environment is responsible for the increase in nipple attachment.

We tested this hypothesis by placing pups between Hour 1 and 12 with a lactator who had been Thelectomized the day prior (nipples removed through cauterization). Since the maternal behavior of the Thelectomized female is the same as Control mothers (Moltz et al., 1967; Rosenberg et al., 1970), the maternal environment of Thelectomized and Control pups differed only in the nipple exposure, while the Thelectomized and Warming Oven groups differed in exposure to the general properties of the maternal environment. Thus, if exposure to the general properties is sufficient to mediate this increase, the Thelectomized group should have a similar attachment incidence as the Control group.

The results, however, are inconsistent with this hypothesis. The attachment incidence of the Thelectomized group is much lower than that of the Control group and is similar to the Warming Oven group. Thus, exposure to the general properties of the maternal environment from Hour 1 to Hour 12 of life does not constitute a sufficient set of experiences to result in high levels of attachment at Hour 12 (see Figure 6).

Conclusions

These results demonstrate an improvement in nipple attachment from Hour 1 to Hour 12 of life. The higher levels of attachment is dependent upon suckling experience but independent of milk acquisition which is normally associated with suckling. The improvement in attachment from Hour 1 to Hour 12 demonstrates that the rat's behavior is modifiable from the earliest postnatal hours and suggests that learning may be employed as a behavioral strategy during the perinatal period.

SECTION III: THE DEVELOPMENT OF RESPONSIVENESS TO DEPRIVATION

The normal response to food and water deprivation in adults is to seek out and consume the needed nutrients. The analogous response in the neonate is to seek out the nipple and attach to it. However, the results from Section II

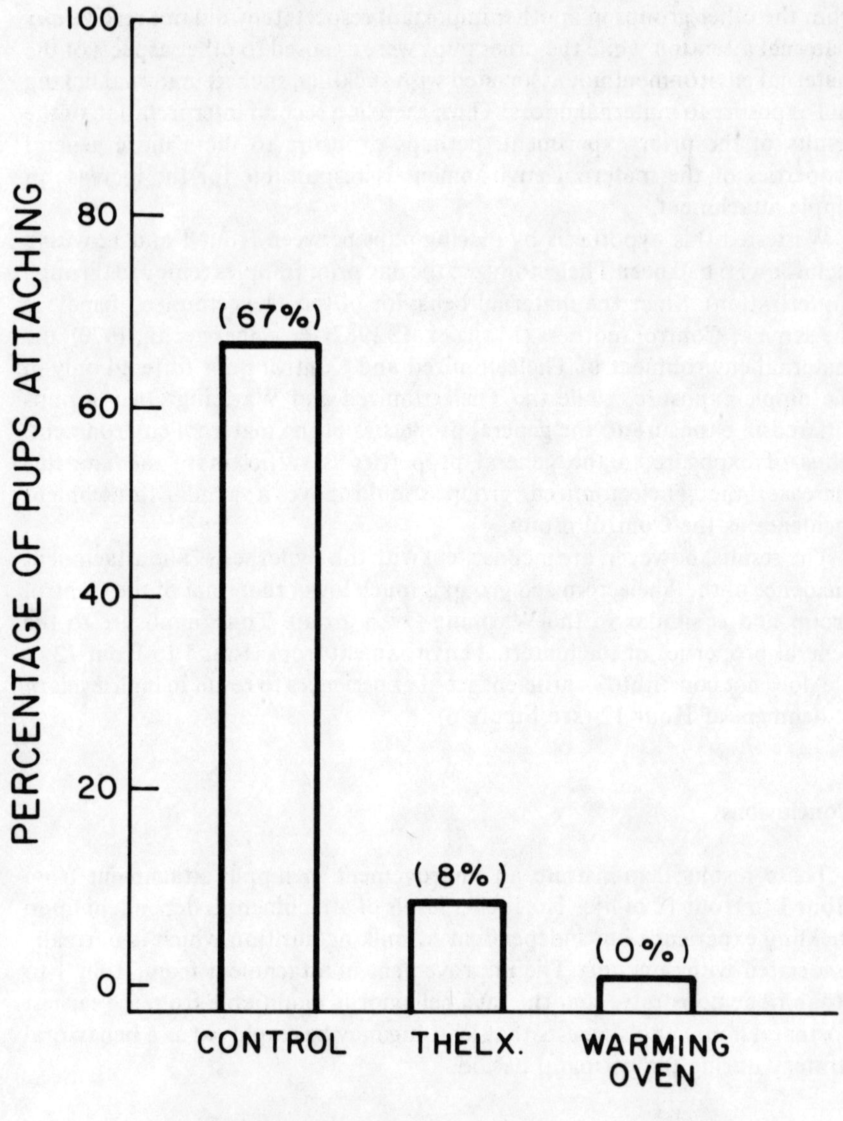

FIG. 6. Percentage of pups attaching which were either reared with a 24–48 Hour lacator from Hour 1–12 (Control), or were reared from Hour 1–12 with a 24–48 hour lactator whose nipples had been surgically removed (Thelx.), or were deprived from Hour 1–12 (Warming Oven).

indicate that the 12-hour-old pup does not respond to 11 hours of deprivation by attaching more quickly. Indeed, prior to acquiring the necessary nipple experience, deprivation results in an increased latency to attach. These results raise the question as to when does this adult form of responsiveness to deprivation first appear.

22 Hours of Deprivation

We first deprived 24-hour-old and 9-day-old pups for 22 hours. Following the deprivation period the deprived animals and their littermate controls were tested for nipple attachment. We found that both 24-hour and 9-day-old pups respond to 22 hours of deprivation with a decrease in the latency to attach. Thus, by 24 hours of age suckling behavior appears to be under nutritional control (see Figure 7).

11 Hours of Deprivation

While the 24-hour-old pup and the 9-day-old pup respond similarly to 22 hours of deprivation, this does not preclude the possibility that there are age-related differences in the sensitivity to deprivation. Indeed, in two other strains of rats responsiveness to deprivation does not appear to be established until the end of the second week of life (Hall et al., 1975, 1977). We tested this hypothesis by exposing 24-hour-, 36-hour-, and 9-day-old pups to 11 hours of deprivation.

Neither 24- nor 36-hour-old pups responded to 11 hours of deprivation with a decrease in attachment latency. However, as with 22 hours of deprivation, 9-day-old pups did decrease their attachment latencies significantly (see Figure 8).

These experiments indicate that while sensitivity to deprivation is present by 24 hours of life, the sensitivity to deprivational cues is still maturing. Indeed the mechanisms responsible for the sensitivity to deprivation may be different in young and old pups (see Section VI). The immaturity of the young pup's nutritional control over intake is also evident from its behavior once it has attached to the nipple. While at about 15 days of age the deprived pup will shift from one nipple to another (presumably in search of milk), the young pup will remain attached to the same nipple for long periods of time (Hall et al., 1975). In addition, pups 10 days of age or older will leave the nipple following several milk ejections while the young pup remains steadfastly attached until it practically chokes from the milk-loaded stomach (Hall and Rosenblatt, 1977).

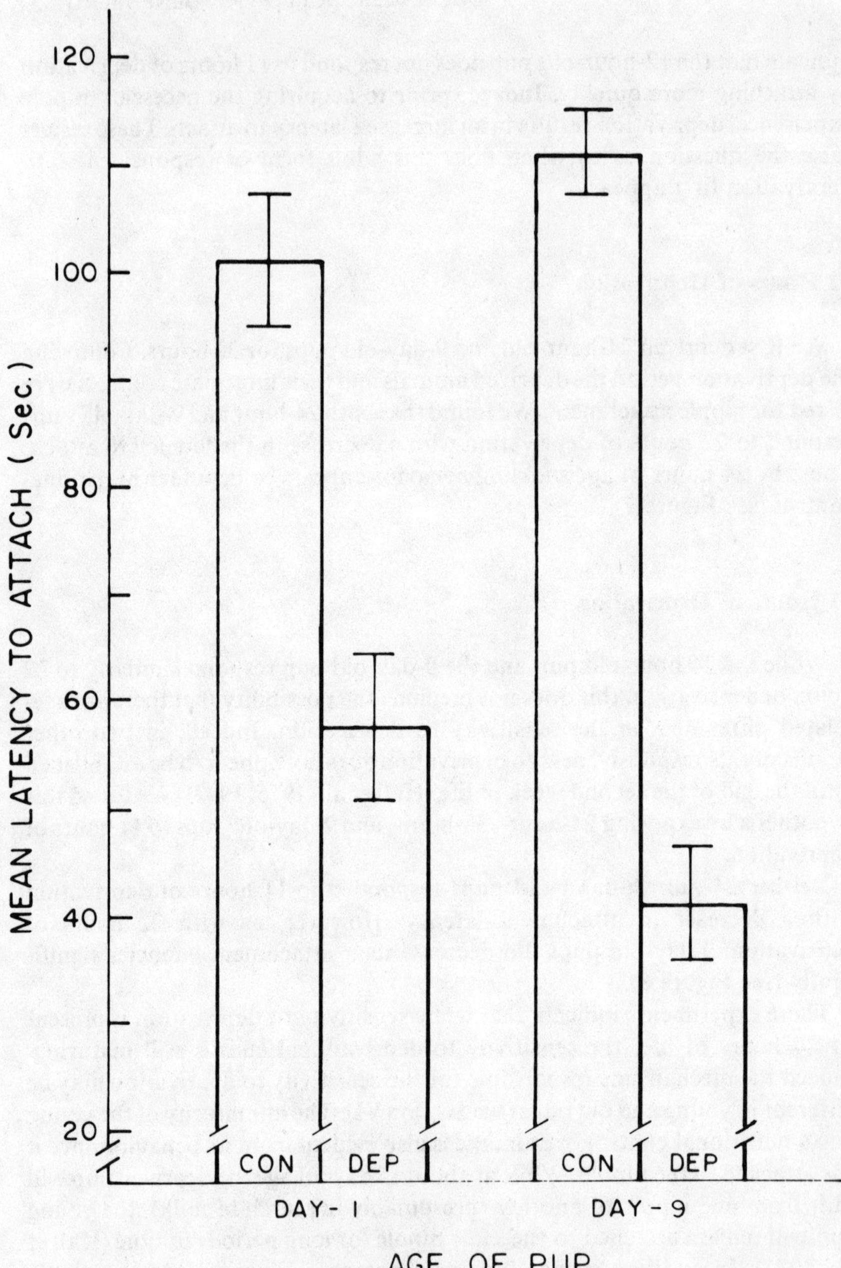

FIG. 7. Mean latency to attach of 1-day old and 9-day old pups which were either with their mothers the proceeding 24 hours (Control), or were placed into a moist warming oven at 35°C (Deprived). Standard errors are depicted.

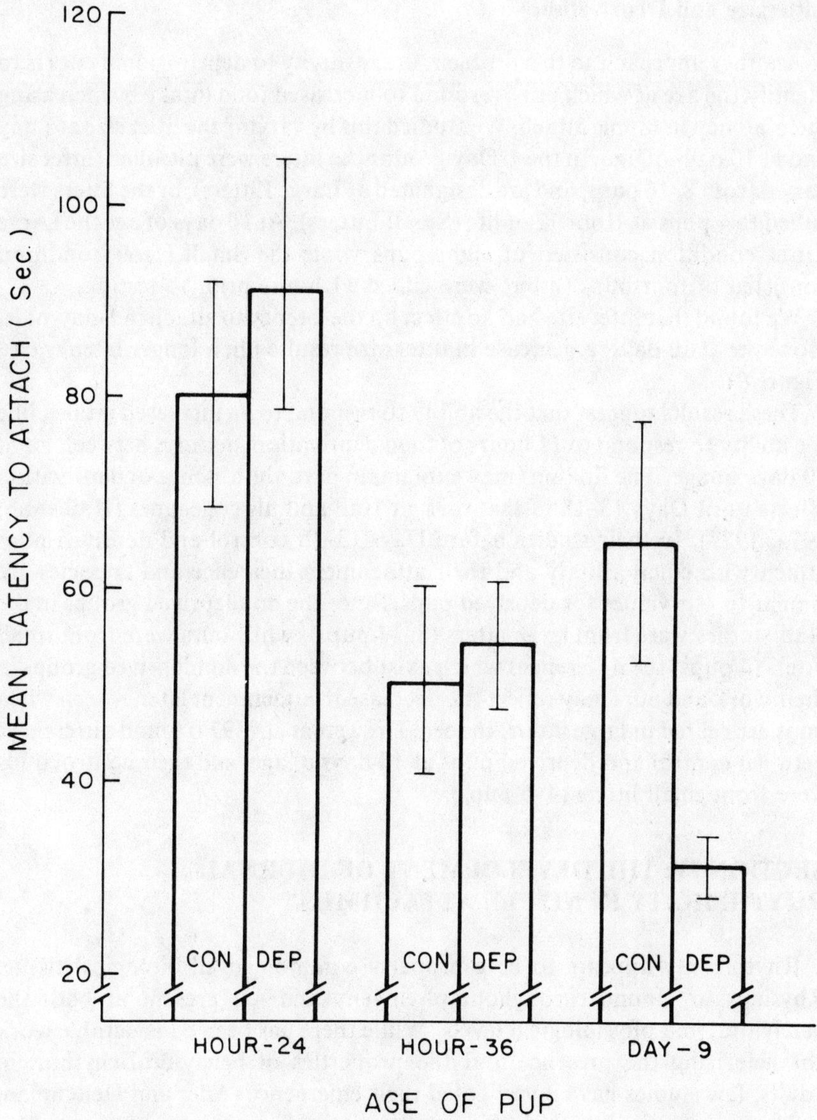

FIG. 8. Mean latency to attach of 24-hour, 36-hour, and 9-day old pups which were either with their mother the preceeding 11 hours (Control) or were placed into the warming oven (Deprived). Standard errors are depicted.

Littersize and Deprivation

Another approach to this problem of sensitivity to deprivational cues is to identify the age at which pups respond to increased food intake by increasing their latency to nipple attach. We studied this by varying the litter size at 1 day and at 10 days of age. In the 1-Day groups the litters were unculled (litter size varied from 8–16 pups, and are designated as Large Litters), or the litters were culled to 4 pups at Hour 12 of life (Small Litters). At 10 days of age the Large Litter condition consisted of eight pups while the Small Litter condition consisted of four pups (litters were culled 11 hours prior to testing).

We found that litter size had no effect on the latency to attach in 1-day-olds. However at 10 days, a decrease in litter size resulted in a longer latency (see Figure 9).

These results suggest that the ability to respond to an increased intake, like the ability to respond to 11 hours of food deprivation, matures between 1 and 10 days of age. The findings may explain, in part, the absence of deprivation effects until Days 13–15 in the work in Hall and his colleagues (Hall et al., 1975, 1977). In their studies before Days 13–15 control and deprived pups attach with equal affinity and their attachment incidence and latencies are similar to our values for deprived pups. Since the nondeprived groups in the Hall studies were from large litters (8–14 pups), while ours were from small litters (4 pups) the differences which exist between the nondeprived groups in their work and ours may reflect the decrease in attachment latency seen when pups are reared in large litters. Indeed, Drewett at al. (1974) found differences between control and deprived pups at 10 days of age, and their control pups were from small litters (4–5 pups).

SECTION IV: THE DEVELOPMENT OF DIURNAL RHYTHMICITY IN NIPPLE ATTACHMENT

Rhythmicity appears to be a property common to all biological tissue. Rhythms are found throughout phylogeny and are present at both the behavioral and physiological levels. While there has been considerable work characterizing the presence and the properties of behavioral rhythms in adults, few studies have investigated their emergence (Ader and Deitchman, 1970). Since nipple attachment occurs soon after birth, this provides us with a means to investigate behavioral rhythmicity from the earliest postnatal hours.

The Development of Rhythmicity

We tested pups which were 1, 3, 5, and 10 days of age during either the light portion or the dark portion of their day/night cycle. The pups were tested against like-aged lactators which were in the same part of the light/dark cycle

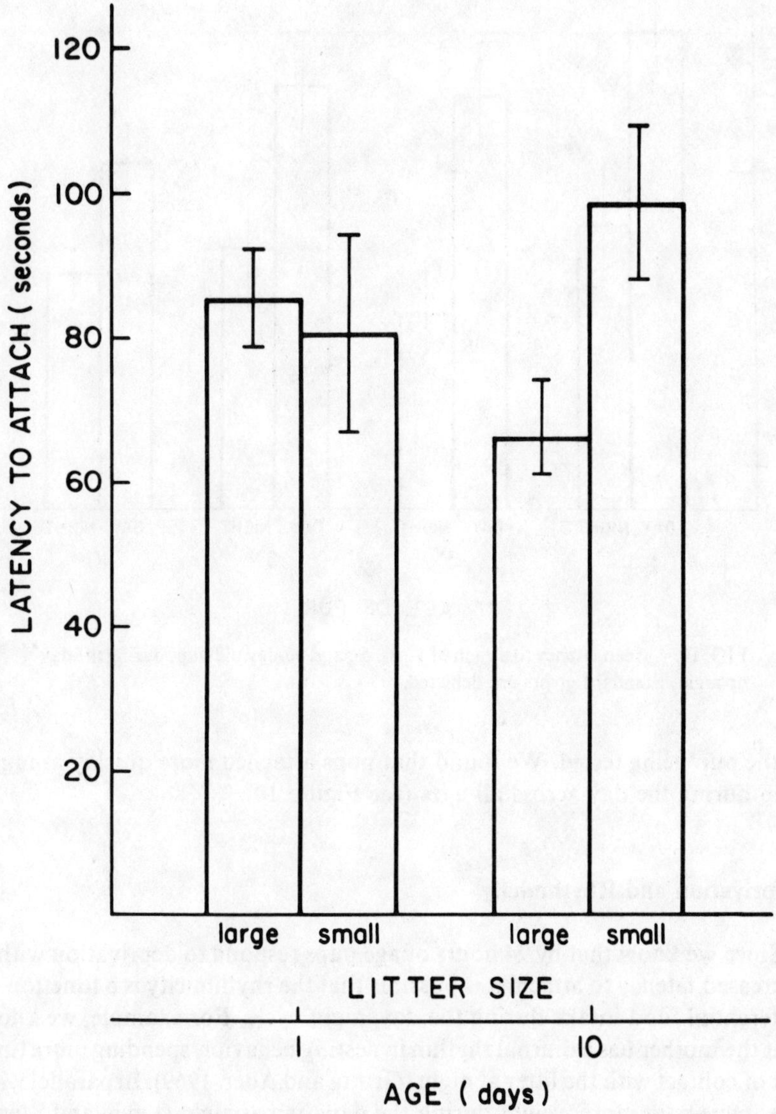

FIG. 9. Mean latency to attach of 1-day and 10-day old pups from either large or small litters. Standard errors are depicted.

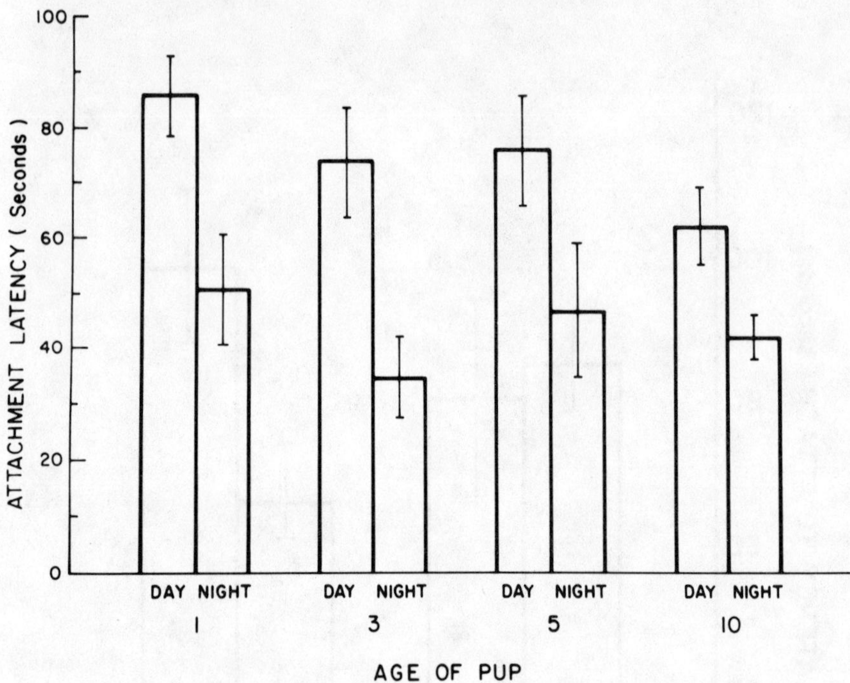

FIG. 10. Mean latency to attach of 1-, 3-, 5-, and 10-day old pups during the day or night. Standard errors are depicted.

as the pup being tested. We found that pups attached more quickly at night than during the day across all ages (see Figure 10).

Deprivation and Rhythmicity

Since we know that by 24 hours of age pups respond to deprivation with a decreased latency to attach, it is possible that the rhythmicity is a function of differential food intake during the day/night cycle. For example, we know that the mother has a diurnal rhythm in nesting behavior, spending more time out of contact with the litter at night (Grotta and Ader, 1969). In parallel with this, pups gain more weight during the day than at night (Levin and Stern, 1975).

To investigate the deprivational hypothesis we weighed the stomach and intestines (with contents) of 10-day-old pups four hours into either their day or night cycle. Contrary to the hypothesis, the organ weights were at least as heavy in the night group as in the day group (see Table 1).

TABLE 1
Mean Stomach and Intestine Weights of 10-Day Old Pups From Either the Day or Night Cycle

	Day	*Night*
Stomach Weight with contents (mg)	819.1	1043.9
Intestine Weight with contents (mg)	1018.1	1144.5

Rhythmicity Differences in Lactators

Another possible mechanism for the day/night differences is changes in the lactator during the different portions of the cycles. Several studies have established the importance of the properties of the lactator's ventral surface for nipple attachment (Hofer et al., 1976; Teicher and Blass, 1976, 1977). In addition, the integrity of the pup's olfactory system appears to be an important determinant of attachment in both the rat (Singh and Tobach, 1975; Singh et al., 1976), and the mouse (Cooper and Cowley, 1976). Thus, cyclic changes in the properties of the lactator's ventral surface, rather than changes in the pup's behavior, could be the cause of the rhythmic nipple attachment.

We addressed this hypothesis by testing 3-day-old pups, which were in either their day or night cycle, against a lactator which was either in her day or night cycle. If changes in the mother were responsible for the rhythmic nipple attachment, then pups should attach more quickly to test mother's in their night cycle, regardless of their own cycle.

However, we found that pups attach more quickly at night than during the day regardless of the test lactator's cycle (see Figure 11).

Conclusions and Implications

These experiments show that the rhythmic changes are a direct function of the pup's behavior.

The presence of a behavioral rhythm by 24 hours of age raises some interesting issues. First of all, is the rhythm exogenously or endogenously controlled, that is, is the rhythm a function of some entraining stimulus in the environment, such as the mother's behavior, or is it modulated by internal cues. Secondly, if the control is endogenous it raises the issue of the neural structures serving as the biological clock. While the suprachiasmatic nucleus has been implicated as the mediating structure for many diurnal rhythms in

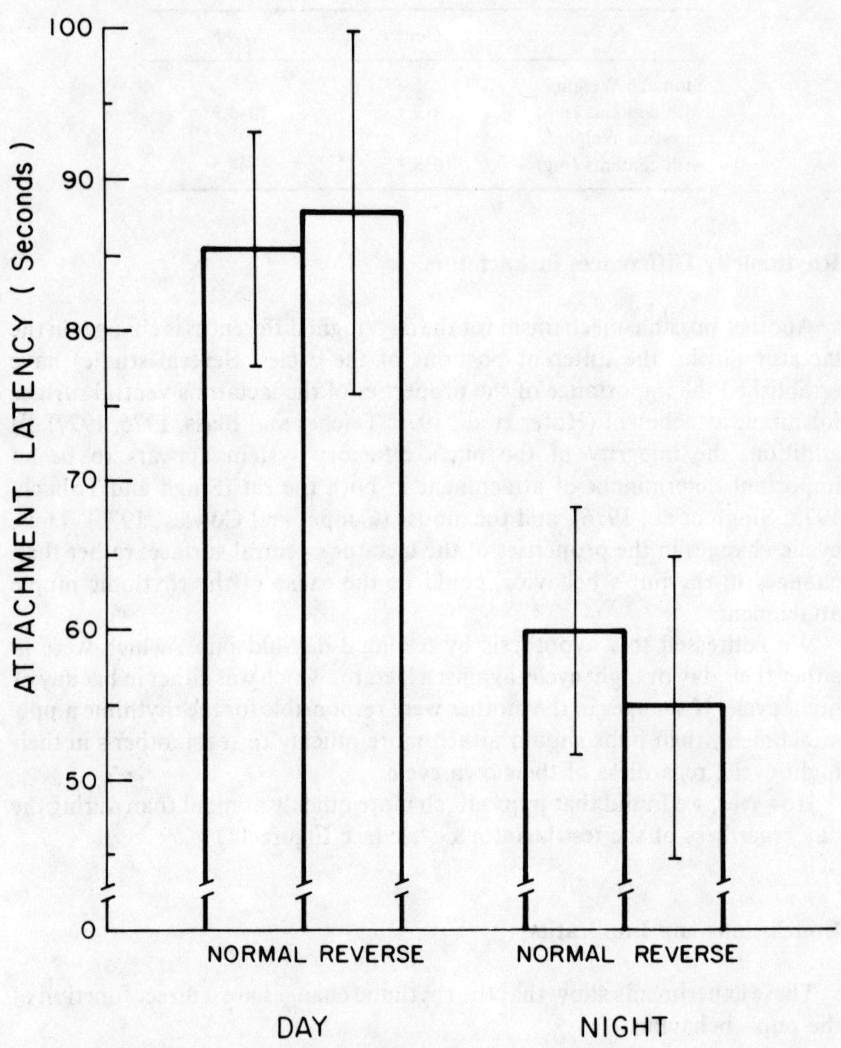

FIG. 11. Mean latency to attach of 10-day old pups tested during the day or night portion of their light/dark cycle. The test lactators were either in Normal or Reverse segments of their light/dark cycle. Standard errors are depicted.

the adult (Moore and Eichler, 1976), this structure does not appear to mature until about day 5 (Lenn et al., 1977; Stanfield and Cowan, 1976).

SECTION V: THE DEVELOPMENT OF NIPPLE DISCRIMINATION

The sychrony between the needs of the pup and the behavior of the mother is a compelling feature of mother-infant interactions (cf. Chapter 1; Denenberg et al., 1976; Rosenblatt, 1974). While synchrony has been commonly addressed in terms of the mother's changing behavior during the lactational period, systematic changes in the pup's behavior may also be involved.

Mother-Pup Match and Mismatch

One way to test this hypothesis is to observe the pup's nipple attachment with lactators which are either matched with the pup's age or are mismatched. If the pup's behavior is a component of the mother-pup synchrony, then pups should attach more readily to the nipples of matched lactators than mismatched lactators. This is what we found. Pups did attach with a higher incidence to matched lactators than to mismatched lactators (differing in lactational status by at least seven days from the pup's age) except at Hour 1 and Day 10 (see Figure 12).

Effects of Increasing Deprivational Status

The Hour-1 and Day-10 differences may have been obscured by the low incidence of attachment which was found. Accordingly, we tested additional groups of 10-day pups under conditions which would result in higher baselines of attachment. This was done by subjecting them to 22 hours of food deprivation and by testing the pups during the dark portion of the day/night cycle.

When these groups were tested against matched and mismatched lactators, we found a lower latency to attach to the matched than the mismatched lactator (see Figure 13).

Conclusions

Our data show that the neonatal pup can discriminate between a nipple of an appropriate lactational status from one of a differing lactational status. The work of Teicher and Blass (1977) suggests there is also a matching in the

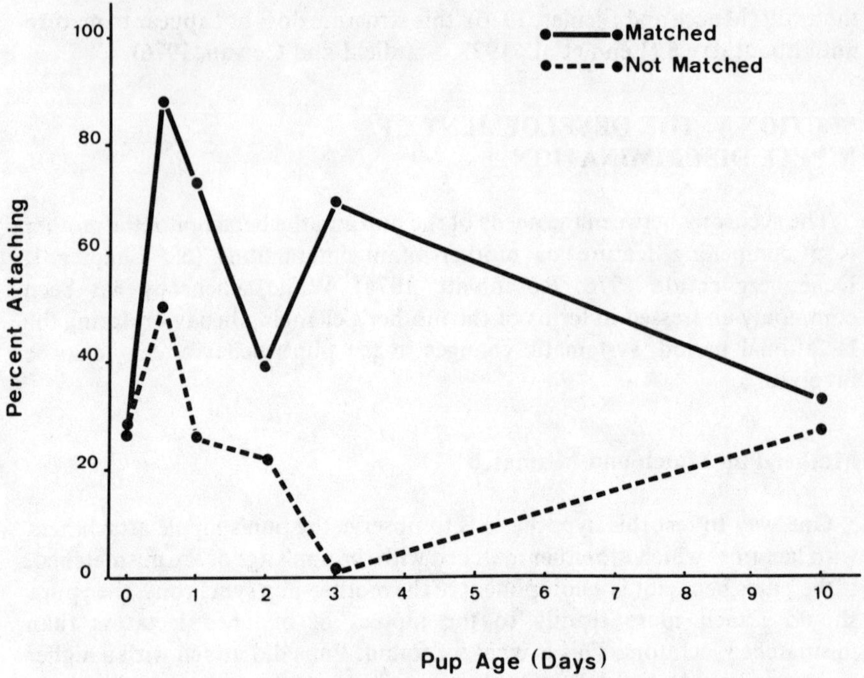

FIG. 12. Percentage of pups attaching at Hour 1, and Hour 12, and 1-, 2-, 3-, and 10-days of age. Pups were tested against lactators which were either of a lactation status similar to the pups age (Matched), or dissimilar by at least 7 days (Not Matched).

newborn pup; newborn pups attach more quickly to the test lactator when the amnionic fluid is present on the ventral surface than when it is removed. Thus, from birth onward the behavior of the pup is one basis for the synchrony between mother and pup.

SECTION VI: AGE-RELATED CHANGES IN BEHAVIORS AT THE NIPPLE

In the preceding sections we have identified several factors which influence nipple attachment. However, we have not as yet considered the nature of the behaviors which the pups exhibit at the nipple. The purpose of this section will be to describe the specific behaviors and to show age-related changes in the pups responses to the nipple.

As before, we again used our hand-held nipple attachment test. However,

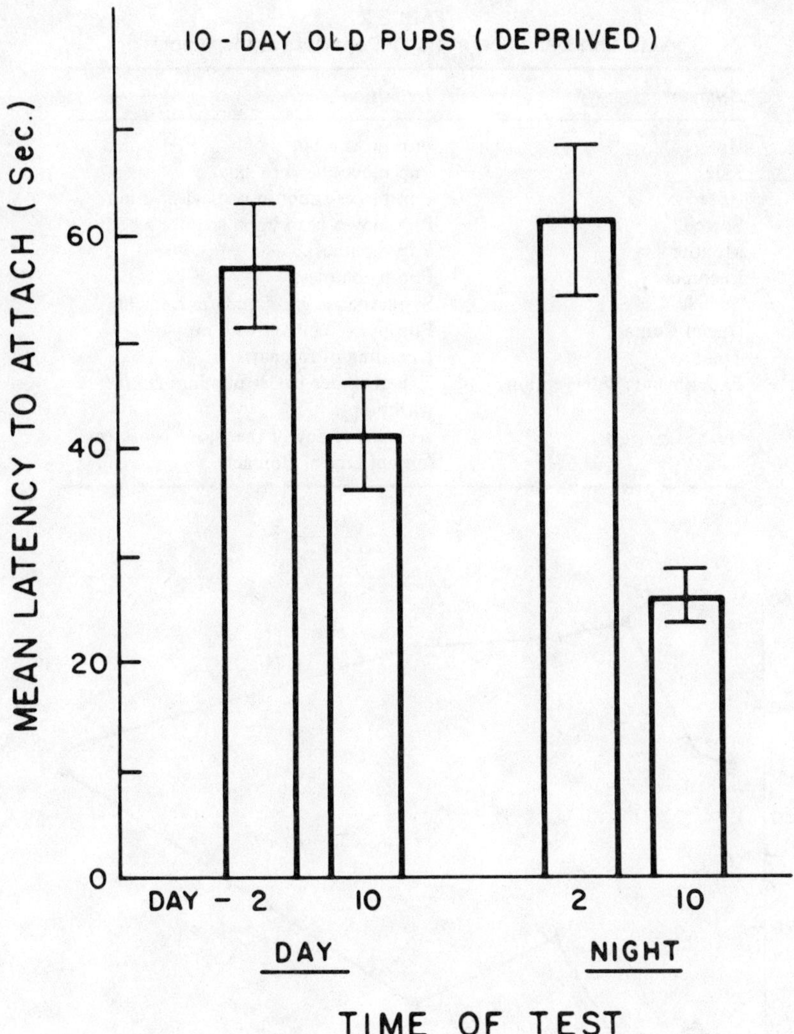

FIG. 13. Mean latency to attach of 10-day old deprived pups tested either during the day or night against either a 2- or a 10-day lactator.

in this experiment a second observer recorded the behaviors of the pup on a 20-channel Esterline-Angus recorder (Table 2 lists the behaviors).

Not surprisingly, the behaviors of pups which attach are quite different from those which do not attach. Behaviors associated with attachment include Search, Mouthe, Nose, Locomote, and Tread. In addition, the

TABLE 2
List and Definition of Pup's Behaviors at the Nipple

Behavior	*Definition*
Up	Pup raises head
Side	Pup moves head to side
Nose	Pup places snout in vertical position
Search	Pup moves head upon lactator's body
Mouthe	Pup mouthes
Locomote	Pup locomotes
Twitch	Spontaneous gross body movement
Out of Contact	Pup out of contact with nipple
Tread	Kneading of forepaws
Experimenter Intervention	Experimenter palces pup into contact with nipple
Quiet	Absence of any of the above behaviors (except Out of Contact)

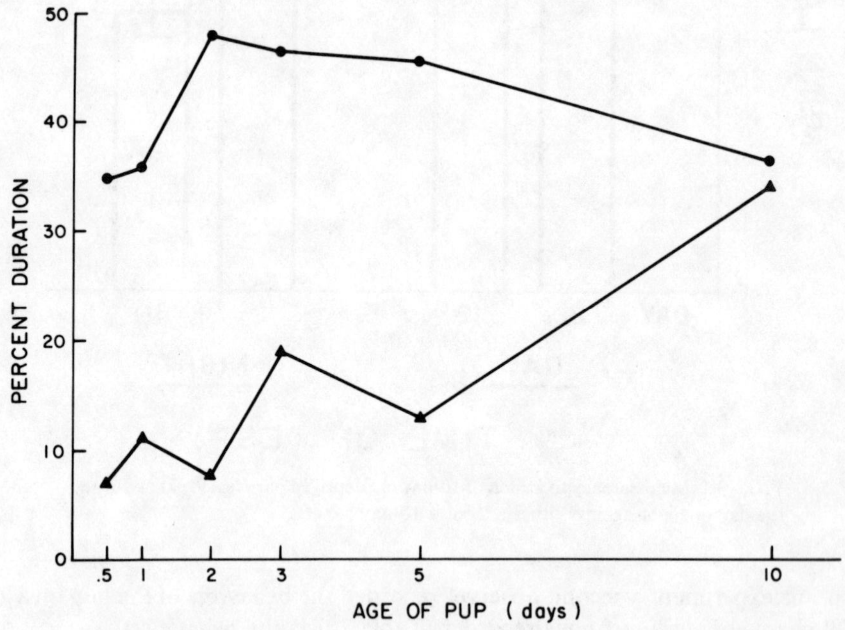

FIG. 14. Percent duration Search of pups which either attach or do not attach at Hour 12, and 1, 2, 3, 5, and 10 days of age. Attachers are depicted with circles and nonattachers with triangles.

expression of these behaviors are modulated by the age of the pup. For example, the behaviors Search and Locomote have a higher duration in attachers across all ages (see Figure 14), while the behavior of Tread does not reach a high duration until Day 10.

Pups which fail to attach have much higher duration of the variables Out of Contact, Side, Experimenter Intervention, Quiet, Twitch, and Up than do attachers. The nonattachment behaviors cluster into two groups. Out of Contact, Side, and Experimenter Intervention are "pure" nonattachment behaviors—they are present in higher amounts in nonattachers across all ages (see Figure 15), while the three other behaviors—Quiet, Twitch, and Up—have age-related trends. Quiet and Twitch are high during the early postnatal days, decreasing in frequency by Day 10 (see Figure 16), Search shows the opposite pattern, occurring in low amounts soon after birth and increasing on Day 10.

These findings provide a picture of the changing behavioral strategies of the

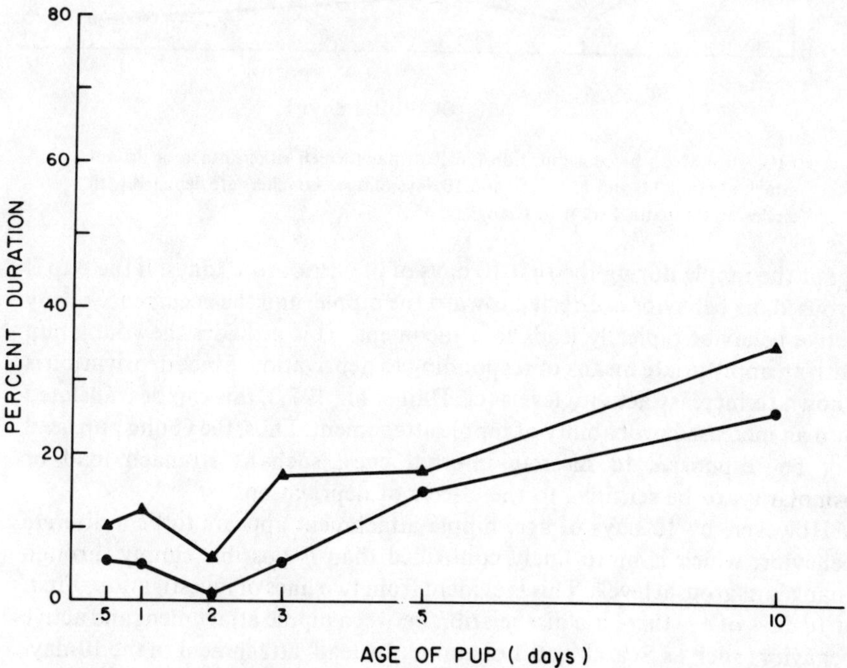

FIG. 15. Mean percent duration Out of Contact of pups which either attach or do not attach at Hour 12, and 1, 2, 3, 5, and 10 days of age. Attachers are depicted with circles and nonattachers with triangles.

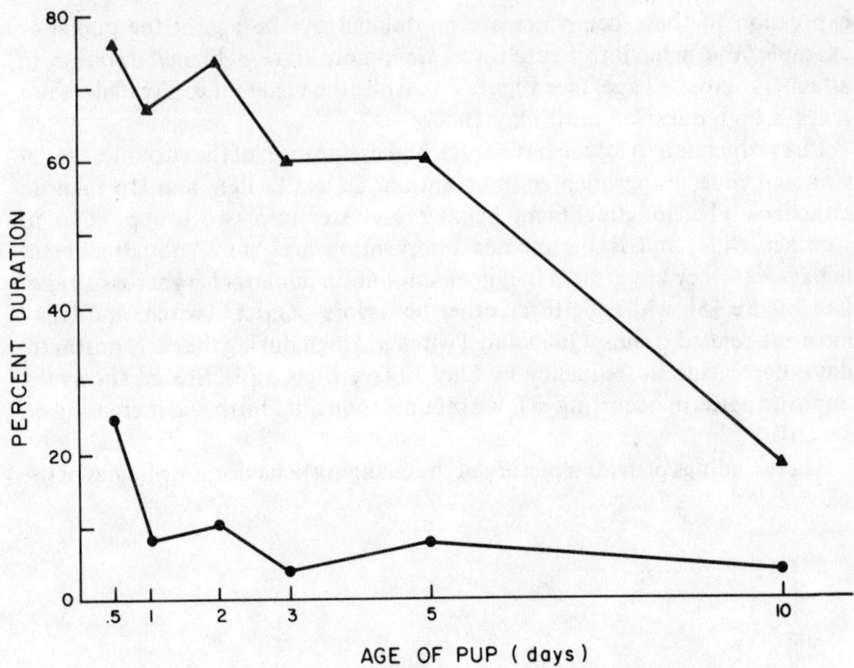

FIG. 16. Mean percent duration Quiet of pups which either attach or do not attach at Hour 12, and 1, 2, 3, 5, and 10 days of age. Attachers are depicted with circles and nonattachers with triangles.

rat at the nipple during the first 10 days of life. Prior to 10 days, if the pup is aroused, its behavior is directed toward the nipple, and the occurrence of any active behavior typically leads to attachment. This provides the young pup with an appropriate means of responding to deprivation. Since deprivation is known to increase activity levels (cf. Hall et al., 1977), this can be translated into an increased probability of nipple attachment. Thus, the young pup need not be responsive to discrete internal cues, such as stomach load or osmolarity, to be sensitive to the effects of deprivation.

However, by 10 days of age, nipple attachment appears to be a discrete behavior, which is more finely controlled than is possible simply through changes in arousal levels. This is evident from two lines of investigation. First, at 10 days of age there is a dissociation between nipple attachment and active behaviors such as Search and Locomote. Instead, attachment in the 10-day-old is of a different form than in the younger pup: when attaching, the 10-day-old quickly locates the nipple, then rapidly Noses, Mouthes, and Treads. The second line of evidence is that during the third week of life nutritional control of attachment emerges. The pup suppresses intake in response to stomach loading (Hall and Rosenblatt, 1976), and cellular dehydration (Bruno, 1977).

SECTION VII: TRANSITION FROM MATERNAL TO PUP CONTROL OF SUCKLING

There are a number of parameters which directly influence the young pup's nipple attachment including experiential history, deprivational status, nipple quality, day-night cycle, and developmental status. Since nipple attachment is one component of the more complex act of suckling, these results suggest that the pup's behavior may influence nursing in the interactive setting with the mother.

To study interaction we began by generating groups of 10-day-old and newborn pups. Littermates at each age either remained with their mother (Control groups) or were placed into a warming oven maintained at 35°C (Deprived groups). The pups were then tested in one of two settings. In one setting the latency to attach to an anesthetized dam was assessed using our standard preparation. In the second setting we measured the latency to nurse when pups were presented to conscious mothers. Four pups were fostered to either a 1- or a 10-day lactator. The latency for the first pup to attach to a nipple was determined through direct observation. The observation period was one hour in length and was divided into 360, 10-second epochs.

As found before deprived 10-day-old pups attach more quickly than control pups to the anesthetized dam (see right panel of Figure 17). Similarly, in the interactive setting, deprived pups also have a shorter latency to attach and this pattern is not influenced by the mother's lactational status (see left panel of Figure 17).

A different pattern is seen in the newborn. When 1-day-old pups are tested against a 1-day lactator, Control pups initiate nursing more quickly than Deprived—the same pattern is seen when tested against the anesthetized lactator (see middle and right sections of Figure 18). However, when tested with a 10-day lactator control pups attach somewhat slower than deprived pups. Furthermore, both groups attach more slowly to the 10-day lactator than to the 1-day lactator (see leftmost section of Figure 18).

These results suggest that in the newborn pup, the behavior of the mother is the primary determiner of nursing (for a more complete discussion of this issue see Denenberg et al., 1976), while in the 10-day-old mother-pup preparation it is the pup who is the principal determiner. When the behavior of the pup, independent of its mother, is compared to its behavior when interacting with its mother, a transition in the behavioral regulation of

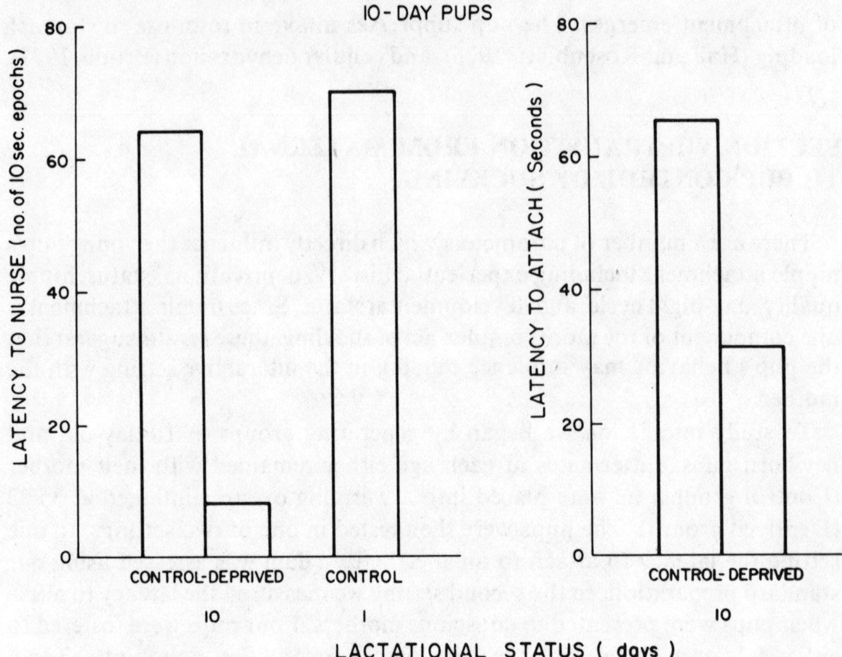

FIG. 17. The left panel depicts the mean latency to nurse of 10-day old control and 22-Hour deprived pups fostered to either a 1- or 10-day lactator. The right panel depicts the mean latency to attach of control and 22-Hour deprived 10-Day old pups.

nursing can be discerned between birth and 10 days of age. The locus of control shifts from the mother to the pup during this period.

SECTION VIII: SUMMARY AND CONCLUSIONS

The following picture emerges from our observations of factors influencing nipple attachment during the first 10 days of life. At 1 hour of life pups are inefficient at attaching to the nipple, with only 21% attaching even once out of three trials. However, by Hour 12 the attachment incidence has increased markedly. This increase is dependent upon nipple experience but is independent of the milk letdown normally associated with attachment.

As soon as the experiential requirements are fulfilled, other factors modulating attachment become evident. By 12 hours, pups are capable of attaching with a higher incidence to matched lactators than to mismatched lactators. Thus, one basis for the synchrony between mother and pup is the preference for the nipple of the like-aged lactator.

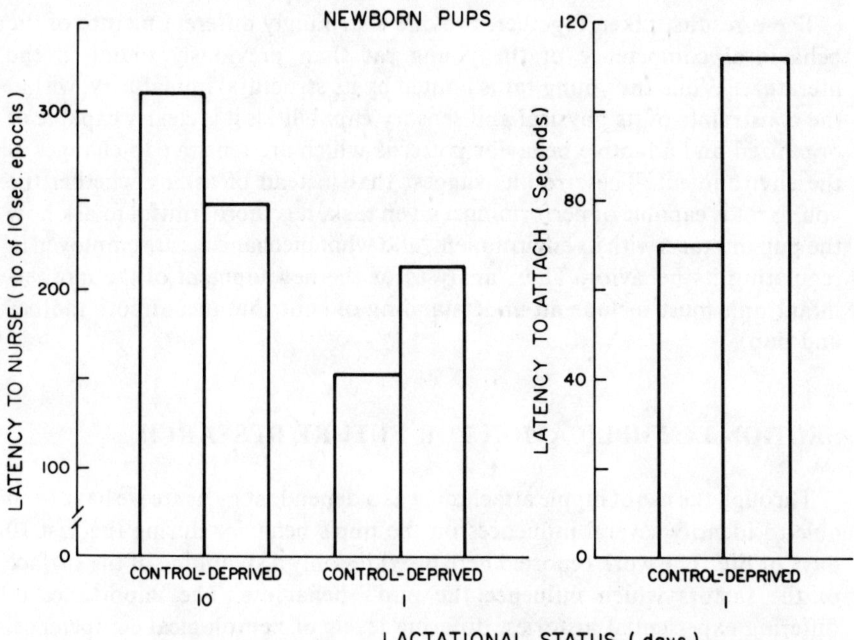

FIG. 18. The left panel depicts the mean latency to nurse of newborn pups fostered to either 1- or 10-day lactators, the right panel depicts the mean latency to attach of control and 11-Hour deprived newborn pups.

By 24 hours of life, pups show rhythmicity in nipple attachment, attaching more quickly at night than during the day. While the basis of this rhythmicity remains to be resolved, it is a direct property of the pup's behavior, and not related to periodic changes in the stimulus properties of the mother.

The development of the response to deprivation is more complex. By Hour 24, pups respond to 22 hours of deprivation with a decrease in the latency to attach. Thus, one aspect of the adult responsiveness to deprivation is present soon after birth. However, responsiveness to 11 hours of deprivation and to litter size does not develop until a somewhat later age suggesting that the control mechanisms are not fully mature.

In addition to the increasing number of factors which influence attachment during the first 10 days of life, there are also changes in the behaviors exhibited at the nipple. Attachment is closely associated with arousal in pups which are younger than 10 days of age—activity in the presence of a nipple invariably leads to nipple attachment. In the 10-day-old pup, attachment is a more discrete behavior associated with Mouthing, Treading, and Nosing at the nipple, behaviors which are associated with the act of swallowing the nipple.

These results, taken together, provide a strikingly different picture of the behavioral competence of the young rat than previously found in the literature. While the young rat is limited by its structural immaturity, within the constraints of its physical and sensory capabilities it is clearly capable of organized and adaptive behavior patterns which are sensitive to changes in the environment. These results suggest that instead of asking whether the young rat is capable of performing a given task, it is more fruitful to ask how the pup interacts with its environment, and what mechanisms are employed in regulating its behavior. Thus, analyses of the development of the mother-infant unit must include an understanding of contributions of both mother and pup.

SECTION IX: IMPLICATION FOR FUTURE RESEARCH

Through the use of nipple attachment as a dependent measure we have been able to identify several influences on the pup's behavior during the first 10 days of life. The work reported here provides only a skimming of the surface of the factors which influence the pup's behaviors. The importance of differing experiential histories, differing levels of neurological competence, and age-related changes should all prove to be fruitful areas for further investigation.

Thus, a thorough analysis of this important component of the young rat's behavioral repertoire will provide a broader understanding of behavioral development in the rat.

The use of dependent measures which are sensitive to the behavioral capabilities of the young rat provide new tools with which to investigate the neural correlates of behavioral development. Such questions as the identification of the neural mechanisms involved in the expression of nipple attachment becomes an interesting problem to pursue. Work of this nature could prove extremely valuable in unravelling the relationships between structure and function if the emergence of behavioral competence could be associated with the emergence of biochemical, anatomical, and electrophysiological competence in specific central nervous system structures.

REFERENCES

Ader, R. and Deitchman, R. Effects of prenatal maternal handling on the maturation of rhythmic processes. *J. Comp. Physiol. Psych. 71*, 492–496 (1970).

Altman, J. and Das, G. D. Autoradiographic and histological studies of postnatal neurogenesis. I. *J. Comp. Neurol. 126*, 337–390 (1966).

Altman, J., and Sudarshan, K. Postnatal development of locomotion in the laboratory rat. *Anim. Behav. 23*, 896–920 (1975).

Armstrong-James M. and Johnson, R. Quantitative studies of postnatal changes in synapses in rat superficial cerebral cortex. *Z. Zellfursch. Mikrosk. Anat. 110*, 559–568 (1970).

Bolles, R. C. and Woods, P. S. The ontogeny of behavior in the albino rat. *Anim. Behav. 12*, 427–441 (1964).

Bruno, J. P. Body fluid challenges inhibit nipple attachment in preweanling rats. Paper presented at the Eastern Psychological Association meeting, Boston, April (1977).

Cooper, A. J. and Cowley, J. J. Mother-infant interaction in mice bulbectomized early in life. *Physiol. Behav. 16*, 453–459 (1976).

Daniels, V. G., Hardy, R. N., Malinowski, K. W., and Nathanielsz, P. W. Adrenocortical hormones and absorption of macromolecules by the small intestine of the young rat. *J. Endocrinol. 52*, 405–406 (1972).

Denenberg, V. H., Holloway, W. R., and Dollinger, M. J. Weight gain as a consequence of maternal behavior in the rat. *Behav. Biol. 17*, 51–60 (1976).

Dollinger, M. J., Holloway, W. R. and Denenberg, V. H. Nipple attachment in rats during the first 24 hours of life. *J. Comp. Physiol. Psych. 92,* 619–626 (1978).

Drewett, R. F., Statham, C., and Wakerley, J. B. A. Quantitative analysis of the feeding behavior of suckling rats. *Anim. Behav. 22*, 907–913 (1974).

Fowler, S. J. and Kellogg, C. Ontogeny of thermoregulatory mechanisms in the rat. *J. Comp. Physiol. Psych. 89*, 738–746 (1975).

Grota, L. J. and Ader, R. Continuous recording of maternal behaviour in *Rattus norvegicus. Anim. Behav. 17*, 722–729 (1969).

Hahn, P. and Koldovsky, O. *Utilization of Nutrients During Postnatal Development*. Pergamon Press, Oxford (1966).

Hall, W. G., Cramer, C. P., and Blass, E. M. Developmental changes in suckling of rat pups. *Nature 258*, 318–320 (1975).

Hall, W. G., Cramer, C. P., and Blass, E. M. The ontogeny of suckling in rats: Transitions towards adult ingestion. *J. Comp. Psychol. Psych. 91*, 1141–1155 (1977).

Hall, W. G. and Rosenblatt, J. S. Developmental changes in the suckling behavior and intake control of rat pups. Paper presented at the annual meeting of the International Society for Developmental Psychobiology, Toronto, November (1976).

Himwich, W. A. Forging a link between basic and clinical research: Developing brain. *Biol. Psychiat. 10*, 125–139 (1975).

Hofer, M. A., Shair, H., and Singh, P. Evidence that maternal ventral skin substances promote suckling in infant rats. *Physiol. Behav. 17*, 131–136 (1976).

Jacobson, S. Sequence of myelinization in the brain of the albino rat. A. Cerebral cortex, thalamus and related structures. *J. Comp. Neurol. 121*, 5–29 (1963).

Klopfer, P. Mother love: What turns it on? *Am. Scient. 59*, 404–406 (1964).

Lenn, N. J., Beebe, B., and Moore, R. Y. Postnatal development of the suprachiasmatic hypothalamic nucleus of the rat. *Cell Tissue Res. 178*, 463–475 (1977).

Levin, R. and Stern, J. M. The ontogeny of nocturnal feeding in the rat. *J. Comp. Physiol. Psych. 89*, 711–721 (1975).

Lincoln, D. W., Hill, A., and Wakerley, J. B. The milk ejection reflex of the rat: An intermittent function not abolished by surgical levels of anesthesia. *J. Endocrinol. 57*, 459–476 (1973).

Lorenz, K. Der kumpan in der unwelt des vogels. *J. Ornithol., 83*, 137–213, 289–413 (1934), Translated in *Studies in Animal and Human Behaviour, Vol. I.*, R. B. Martin, Cambridge University Press, Harvard (1964).

Moltz, H. R., Geller, D., and Levin, R. Maternal behavior in the totally mammectomized rat. *J. Comp. Physiol. Psych. 64*, 225–229 (1967).

Moore, R. Y. and Eichler, V. B. Central neural mechanisms in diurnal rhythm regulation and neuroendocrine responses to light. *Psychoneuroendo. 1*, 265–279 (1976).

Rosenberg, K. M., Denenberg, V. H., and Zarrow, M. X. Mice (*Mus musculus*) reared with rat aunts: The role of rat-mouse contact in mediating behavioural and physiological changes in the mouse. *Anim. Behav. 18*, 138–143 (1970).

Rosenblatt, J. S. Views on the onset and maintenance of maternal behavior in the rat. In *Development and Evolution in Behavior*, L. R. Aronson, E. Tobach, J. S. Rosenblatt, and D. S. Lehrman, eds., Freeman, San Francisco (1970).

Rosenblatt, J. S. and Lehrman, D. S. Maternal behavior of the laboratory rat. In *Maternal Behavior in Mammals*, H. L. Rheingold, ed., John Wiley & Sons, Inc., New York (1963).

Salas, M. and Schapiro, S. Hormonal influences upon the maturation of the rat brain's responsiveness to sensory stimuli. *Physiol. Behav. 5*, 7–12 (1970).

Schapiro, S., and Norman, R. Thyroxine effects of neonatal administration on maturation, development, and behavior. *Science 155*, 1279–1281 (1967).

Schapiro, S. and Salas, M. Behavioral response of infant rats to maternal odor. *Physiol. Behav. 5*, 815–817 (1970).

Scherzenie, V. and Hsiao, S. Development of locomotion toward home nesting maternal in neonatal rats. *Develop. Psychobiol. 10*, 315–321 (1977).

Singh, P. J. and Tobach, E. Olfactory bulbectomy and nursing behavior in rat pups (Wister DAB). *Develop. Psychobiol. 8*, 151–164 (1975).

Singh, P. J., Tucker, A. M., and Hofer, M. A. Effects of nasal $ZnSO_4$ irrigation and olfactory bulbectomy on rat pups. *Physiol. Behav. 17*, 373–382 (1976).

Stanfield, B. and Cowan, W. M. Evidence for a change in the retinohypothalamic projection in the rat following early removal of one eye. *Brain Res. 104*, 129–136.

Teicher, M. H. and Blass, E. M. Suckling in newborn rats: Eliminated by nipple lavage, reinstated by pup saliva. *Science 193*, 422–425 (1976).

Teicher, M. H. and Blass, E. M. First suckling response of the newborn albino rat: The role of olfaction and amnionic fluid. *Science 198*, 635–637 (1977).

3
The Maternal Behavior of the Mongolian Gerbil

V. J. De Ghett

The Mongolian gerbil (*Meriones unguiculatus*) is a Cricetid rodent belonging to the subfamily Gerbillinae. It is one of the most abundant small mammals of China, Mongolia, and the adjacent parts of Russia (Allen, 1940). It inhabits the arid, sandy areas of Mongolia, North Korea, the Necca province of China, and the northern portions of the Sinkiang, Shensi, Ordos, and Shansa provinces of China (Bannikov, 1954; Gulotta, 1971; Rich, 1968; Tanimoto, 1943).

According to Allen (1940) and Tanimoto (1943), Mongolian gerbils are colonial rodents. They live in burrows dug in dry banks and ditches. The burrows have several entrances and may extend to a depth of 40–45 cm. in the summer and 110–150 cm. in the winter (Naumov and Lobachev, 1975). A nest chamber and several food storage areas are found in the burrow system (Gulotta, 1971; Tanimoto, 1943). Leont'ev (1963) reported that a single burrow might contain as many as 26 gerbils but that the typical number was about 5 or 6 gerbils. Additional information on the ecology of the species can be found in Gulotta (1971) and Naumov and Lobachev (1975).

The testes descend between 28 and 45 days of age and the vagina opens between 40 and 76 days of age (Nakai et al., 1960) but males are not considered to be sexually mature until 70 to 85 days of age and females are not considered to be sexually mature until 65 to 85 days of age (Marston and Chang, 1965). The estrus cycle of the mature female has been reported by some to be irregular (Marston and Chang, 1965; Theissen & Yahr, 1977) and by others to be a regular 4- to 6-day cycle (Barfield and Beeman, 1968; Vick & Banks, 1969; and my laboratory). Marston and Chang (1965) concluded that the vaginal smear had little value as an indicator of sexual activity. However, data from my laboratory indicate an obvious estrus phase of the cycle complete with cornified epithelial cells similar to those found during estrus in the laboratory rat and with a definitive lordosis response during the time when cornified epithelial cells are most numerous. The standard estrus, metestrus, diestrus, and proestrus phases of the cycle can be identified in the female Mongolian gerbil.

Male reproductive behavior has been examined by Kuehn and Zucker (1968). The reproductive pattern has been analyzed by Dewsbury (1972). According to Dewsbury's classification system, the male Mongolian gerbil fits into Pattern Number 13 with no lock, no thrusting, multiple intromissions, and multiple ejaculations. This is the same male reproductive pattern as the laboratory rat.

M. unguiculatus is polyestrus. A postpartum estrus is typical (Meckley and Gintner, 1972; Norris and Adams, 1971), and delayed implantation may occur if the female is lactating (Marston and Chang, 1965; Norris and Adams, 1971). Estimates of the duration of gestation may be inaccurate because of delayed implantation. Typical figures are about 24 days but a 20-day gestation period is occasionally observed. Litter sizes vary from 1 to 12 but litters of 4 to 6 young are most common.

The newborn Mongolian gerbil resembles other nonprecocial rodents at birth. At birth it weighs about 2.5 g, has closed eyelids, folded auditory pinnae, and it lacks body hair. The pinnae unfold between 3 and 6 days but evidence for hearing does not appear until 14 to 16 days. The eyes open between 15 and 20 days and the visual system appears functional at that time. Walking is first seen between 9 and 13 days. The young begin to eat solid food between 19 and 23 days and are usually weaned between 21 and 27 days. These data are from De Ghett (1972).

The purpose of the research described here was twofold. Although the Mongolian gerbil has been a popular research animal for sometime, we still lack information on many fundamental aspects of its behavior. The literature on parental care in this species is minimal. Elwood (1975, 1977) has examined certain aspects of paternal and maternal care in *M. unguiculatus* and has identified some reliable sex differences. Roper and Polioudakis (1977), in a study on the behavior of the Mongolian gerbil in a semi-natural environment, included some information about maternal care. In addition to providing some data on the maternal behavior of this species, another concern was to demonstrate the levels of quantitative interrelationships that exist among and between the behaviors. Maternal care is more than just a few behaviors such as latency to retrieve and retrieval time that change following the birth of a litter. It is a behavioral system or a set of behavioral systems whose design features have been molded by natural selection. From a sociobiological perspective, parental care provides a mechanism whereby the parents can individually insure the survival of their genes represented in the members of their litter. The survival of one's genes is of monumental importance. Complex interactions should exist among and between the behaviors we call parental care. Attention is focused in this paper on the maternal component of the parental system.

HOUSING AND MAINTENANCE

Eight litters of Mongolian gerbils were used in this study. The eight litters consisted of 45 young (22 males and 23 females) born to six multiparous females that had produced one normal litter before being included in the study. The litter size ranged from 3 to 8 (3, 5, 5, 6, 6, 6, 6, and 8) with an average litter size at birth of 5.625. All of the young survived the duration of the study.

The six breeding pairs had been formed by pairing individuals that were between 25 and 35 days old. These breeding pairs remained intact throughout the study. The only time the male was removed was during the daily testing period. The breeding pairs and their litters were maintained in clear plastic cages (48 × 27 × 16 cm) that had about 4 cm of San-I-Cel bedding and a generous supply of nest material ("Nestlets" Ancare Corp.). Food and water were available *ad lib.* The food (Teklad Hamster Diet Complete) was scattered on the cage floor and was supplemented weekly with wheat germ, rolled oats, barley, and carrots. The colony room was maintained on a normal day/night cycle with the lights coming on at 0500 hrs and going off at 1700 hrs (Eastern Standard Time). The room temperature was maintained at 23°C.

The daily testing, which is described below, was conducted between 1600 and 1700 hrs. This corresponded to the time of maximum activity in the colony and the time that all of the young in this study were born. The day of birth was recorded as Day 0 and testing began 24 hrs later on Day 1 and continued until Day 25.

MEASURES OF MATERNAL BEHAVIOR

1. *Percentage of Pups Suckling.* Careful observation of the undisturbed mother and pups revealed the number of pups actively suckling. The resulting data, expressed as percentages (Number/45 × 100), are presented in Figure 1.

2. *Percentage of Females Nursing.* These data were gathered at the same time as the percentage of pups suckling (measure #1). These data are also presented in Figure 1.

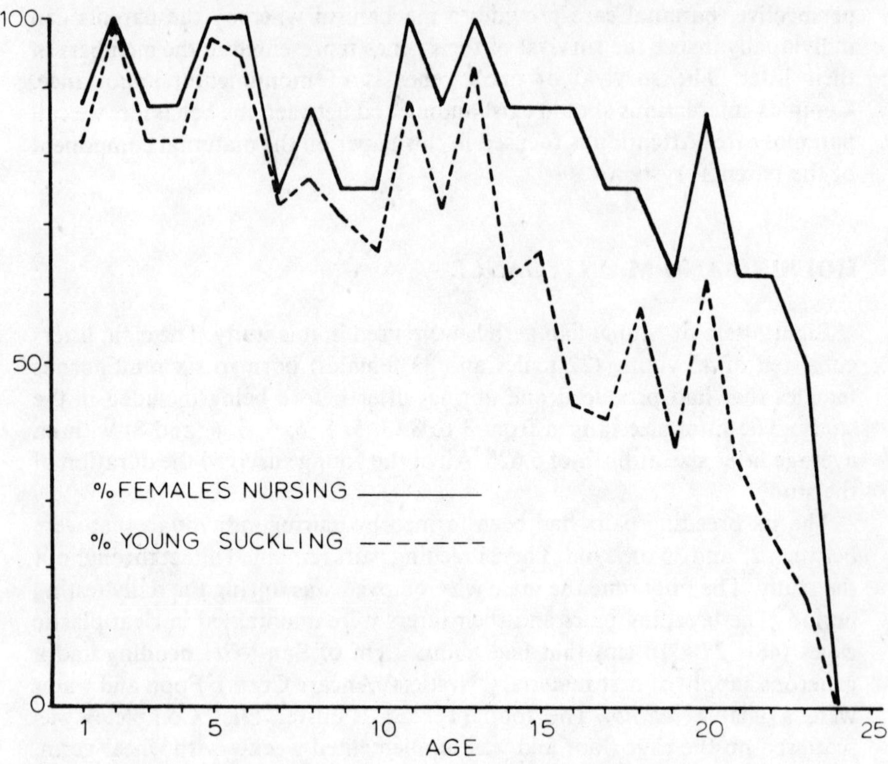

FIG. 1. The percentage of young suckling and mothers nursing before daily testing.

3. *Nest Condition*. The following values were assigned to various nest conditions: 0 = no nest or material scattered throughout the cage; 1 = trampled but localized nest material, 2 = a ring shaped nest with low sides; 3 = a ring shaped nest with medium sides; 4 = a ring shaped nest with high sides or a ball shaped nest. A daily mean score was calculated and these scores are shown in Figure 2.

4. *Reaction of Mother to Disturbance*. The cage top was removed following the recording of the above three measures. The female's reaction to this was scored as: 0 = no immediate reaction; 1 = a generalized alert response; 2 = an alert response together with a head turn and a whole body response; 3 = leaving the nest; and 4 = hiding the pups under the nest material. Daily averages were calculated and these are shown in Figure 3.

5. *Defense of the Young*. Approximately one minute after the cage top was removed the pups were removed by hand. The mother's reaction was scored

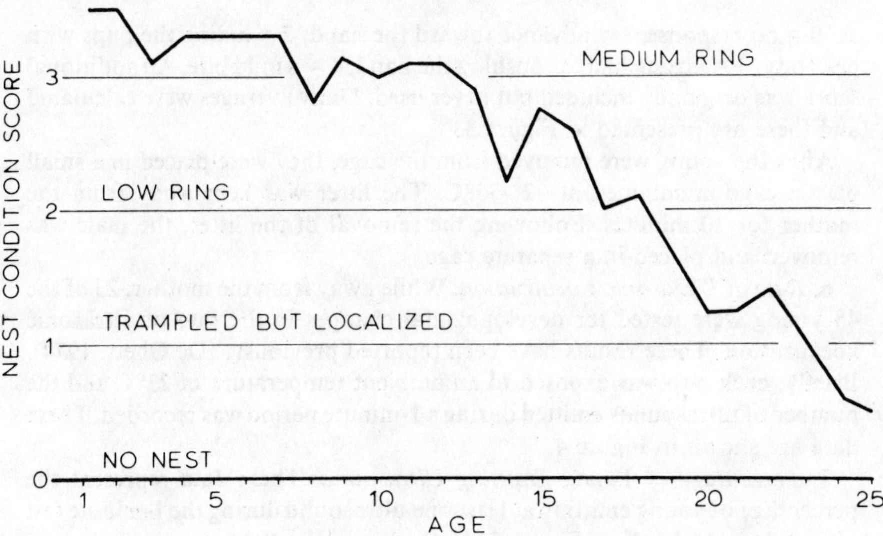

FIG. 2. The changes in the condition of the nest across the 25 days of observation and testing.

FIG. 3. The reaction of the mother to the disturbance caused by cage top removal and her defensive reaction to the removal of her litter.

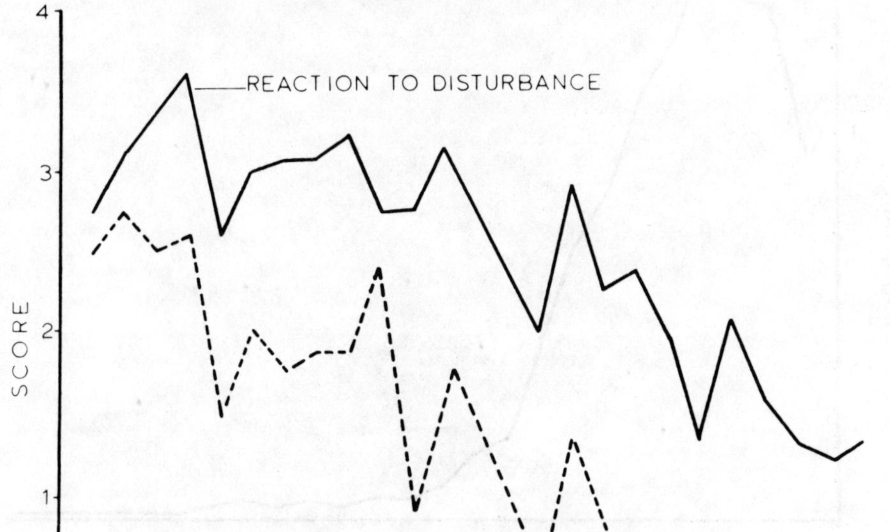

as: 0 = no response; 1 = advance toward the hand; 2 = hiding the pups with her body; 3 = nosing and/or pushing the hand; 4 = a mild bite. An additional score was originally included but never used. Daily averages were calculated and these are presented in Figure 3.

After the young were removed from the cage, they were placed in a small plastic cage maintained at 32°-35°C. The litter was kept away from the mother for 10 minutes. Following the removal of the litter, the male was removed and placed in a separate cage.

6. *Rate of Ultrasonic Vocalization.* While away from the mother, 23 of the 45 young were tested for developmental changes in the rate of ultrasonic vocalization. These results have been reported previously (De Ghett, 1974). Briefly, each pup was exposed to an ambient temperature of 23°C and the number of ultrasounds emitted during a 1-minute period was recorded. These data are shown in Figure 4.

7. *Percentage of Young Emitting Ultrasounds.* These data represent the percentage of young emitting at least one ultrasound during the 1-minute test period described below. Figure 5 shows these data.

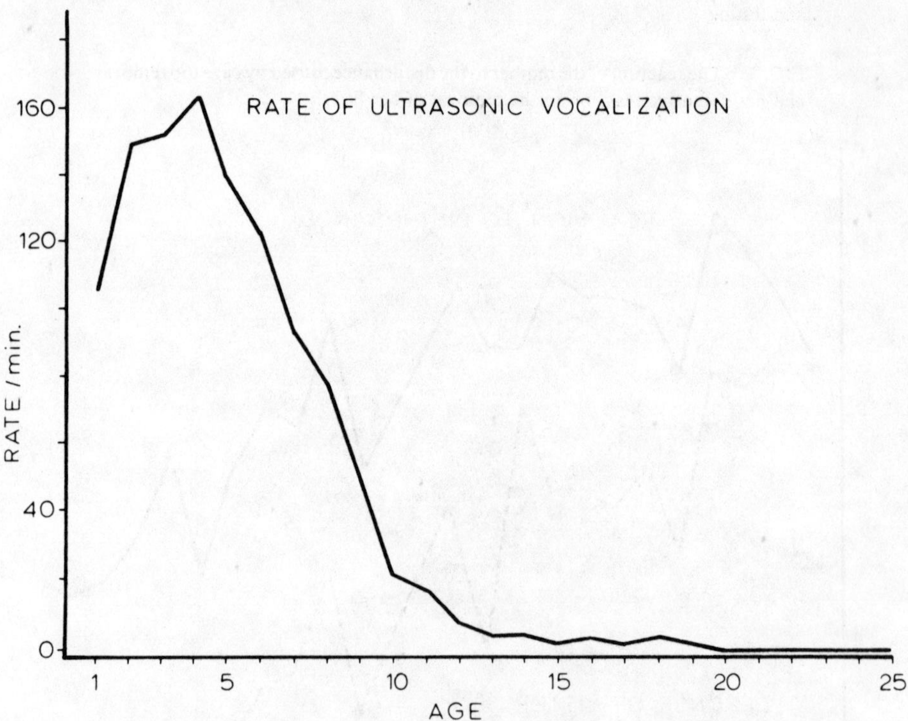

FIG. 4. The changes in the rate of ultrasonic vocalization. Redrawn from De Ghett (1974). Reprinted with permission of John Wiley & Sons, Inc.

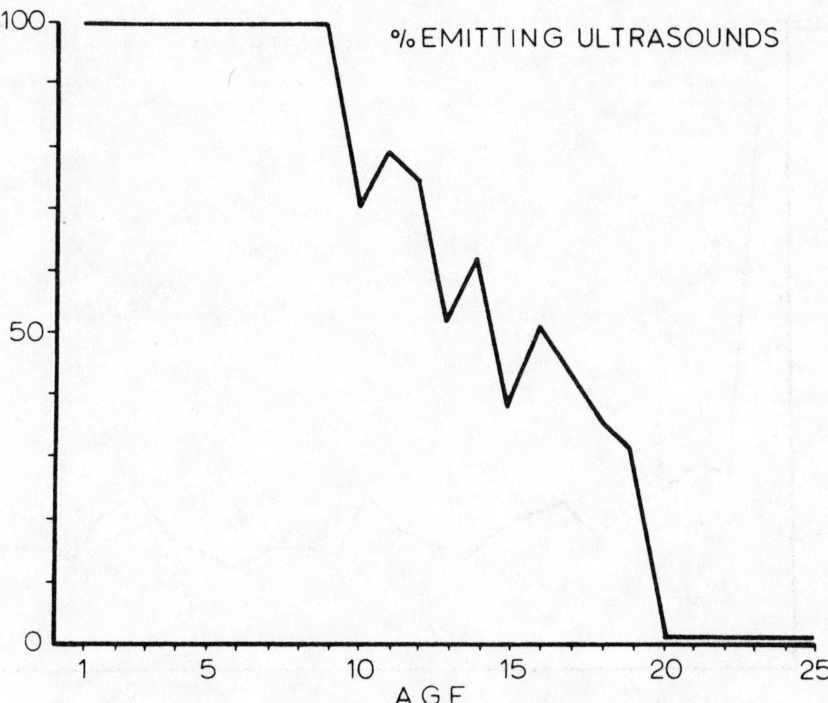

FIG. 5. The changes in the percentage of young emitting ultrasounds. Redrawn from De Ghett (1974). Reprinted with permission of John Wiley & Sons.

8. *Latency to Retrieve.* When 10 minutes had passed a single pup was returned to the home cage for the mother to retrieve. The pup was placed in the front center of the cage after the female was in the nest. The nest was always in a rear corner of the cage. The latency to retrieve the pup was measured in tenths of a second from the time the pup was placed in the cage to the time the female made physical contact with the pup. This latency measure was calculated on only one pup in each of the eight litters, the first member of the litter to be returned. The data in Figure 6 reflect the time it took females to leave an empty nest to retrieve a single pup each day. After this pup was retrieved, the remaining pups were returned one at a time but latency to retrieve was not measured for these pups.

The following five behaviors could be considered as behaviors associated with retrieval. They represent the actions of the maternal female following her initial contact with each pup. These behaviors were recorded for all of the pups in each litter including the single pup that was used to establish the latency measure (#8).

9. *Nosing During Retrieval.* This was a frequently observed behavior and consisted of nosing and sniffing the pup and probably represents olfactory

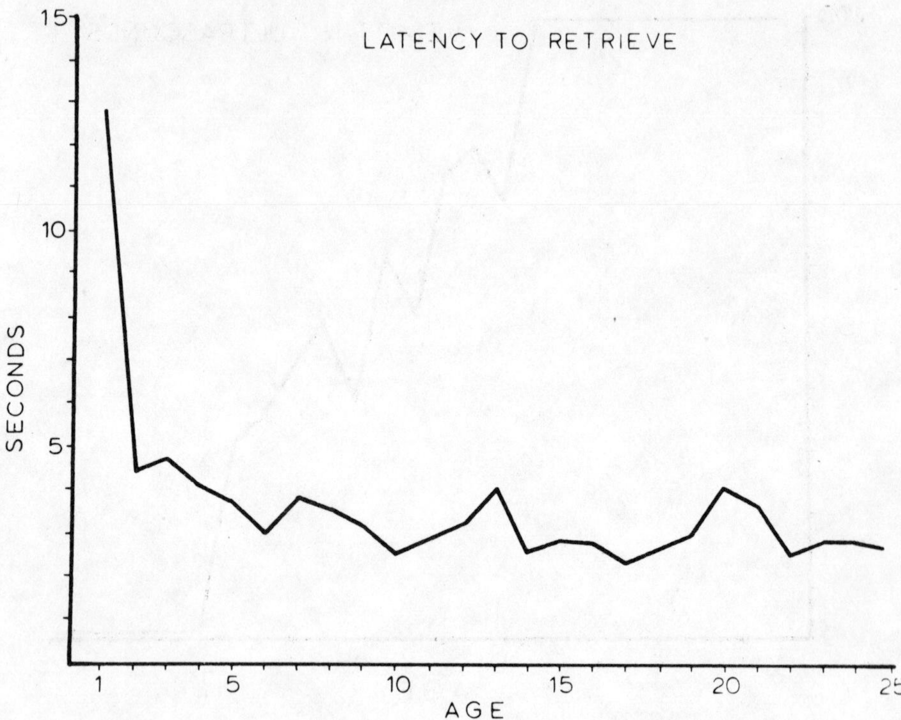

FIG. 6. The changes in the latency to retrieve the first pup returned to the cage on each day.

investigation. Figure 7 shows the percentage of young being nosed during retrieval.

10. *Licking During Retrieval.* The female often spent considerable time licking the pup before she attempted to retrieve it. Figure 7 shows the percentage of young being licked during retrieval.

11. *Hovering During Retrieval.* Hovering is the same behavior as is often referred to as assuming the nursing position. It often occurs independent of actual nursing. Figure 7 shows the percentage of young that were hovered over during retrieval.

12. *Nursing During Retrieval.* Occassionally the female would actually nurse the pup before she picked it up and returned it to the nest. Figure 7 shows the percentage of pups that were nursed under these circumstances.

13. *Nest Building During Retrieval.* As soon as a pup was returned to the nest some immediate nest building often occurred. This behavior of the female consisted of rather minor nest modifications. These data are shown in Figure 7.

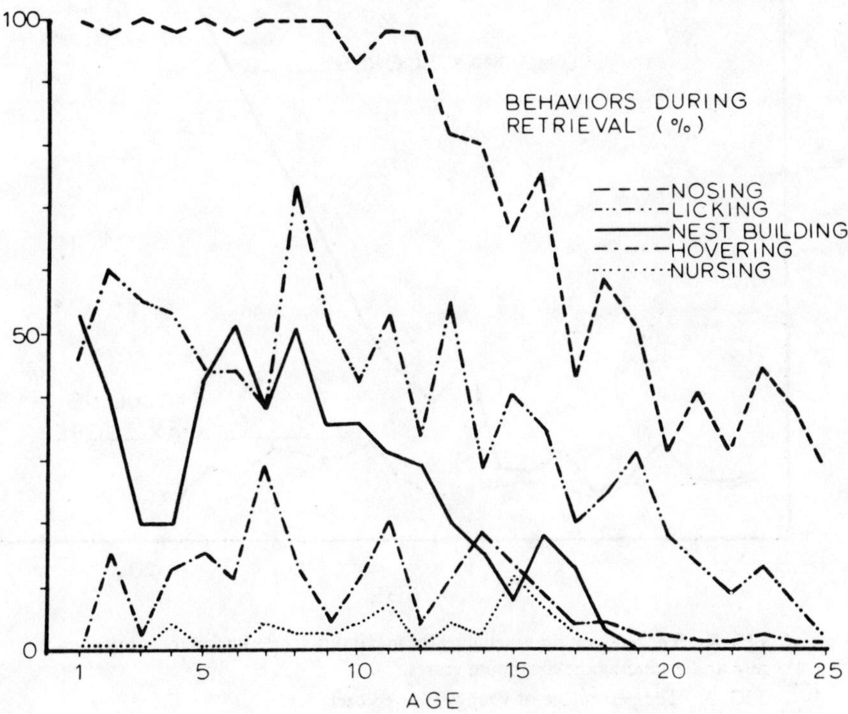

FIG. 7. The behavior of the mother during the retrieval of her pups.

14. *Retrieval Time (Maximum Scores Included).* This measure was the average time that it took the female to return each pup to the nest. It was mesured from when the pup was first picked up to when it was deposited in the nest. The female was given a maximum score of 60 seconds, if she returned to the nest without the pup. These data appear in Figure 8.

15. *Retrieval Time (Maximum Scores Excluded).* Figure 8 also shows the daily average retrieval time excluding the above mentioned maximum scores.

16. *Percentage of Young Retrieved.* The percentage of young retrieved per day is shown in Figure 9.

17. *Drops per Retrieval.* The average number of times each pup was dropped per successful retrieval is shown in Figure 10.

A 10-minute observation period followed the retrieval of all of the young back to the nest. During this time period, the behavior of the maternal female toward the young was observed and data on eight behaviors were recorded.

18. *Active Assembly Following Retrieval.* This behavior consisted of the gathering and positioning of pups under the female or near the female. These data are shown in Figure 11.

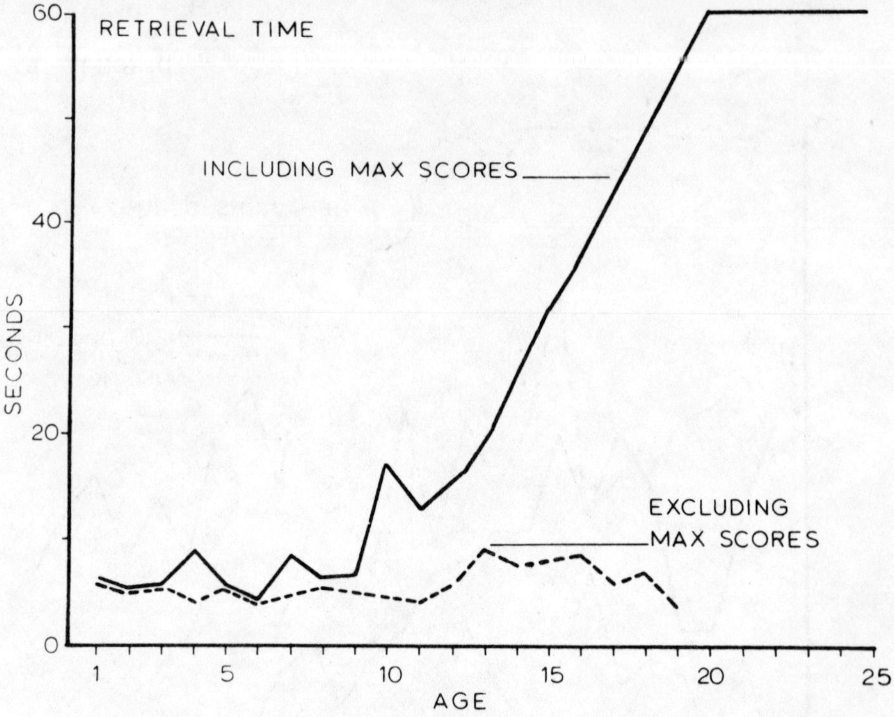

FIG. 8. The retrieval time including the maximum scores for failure to retrieve a pup and excluding the maximum scores.

FIG. 9. The percentage of young retrieved each day.

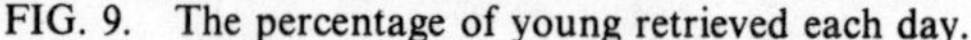

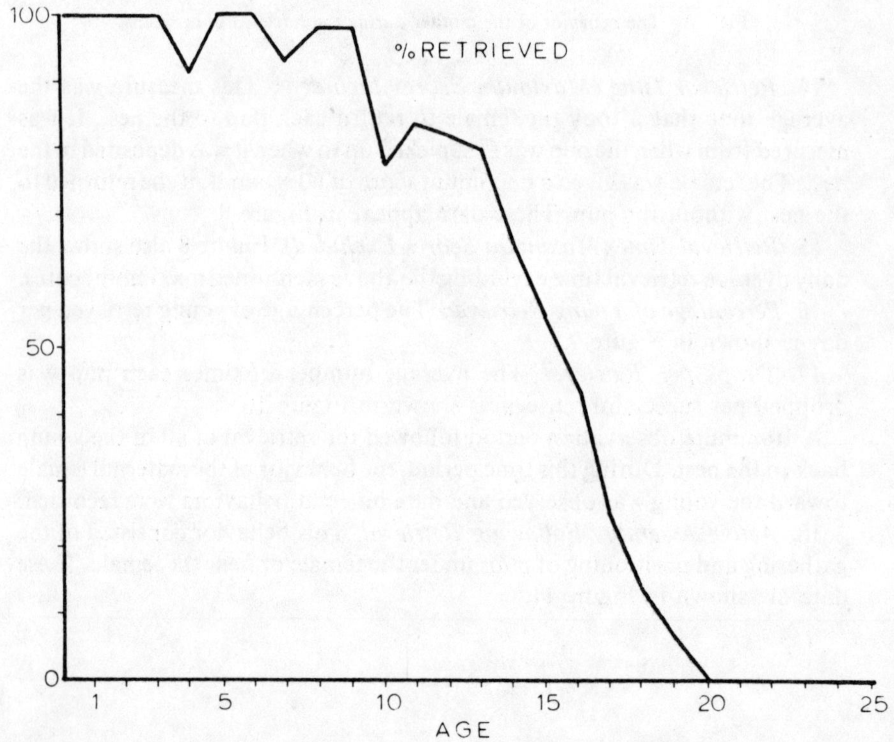

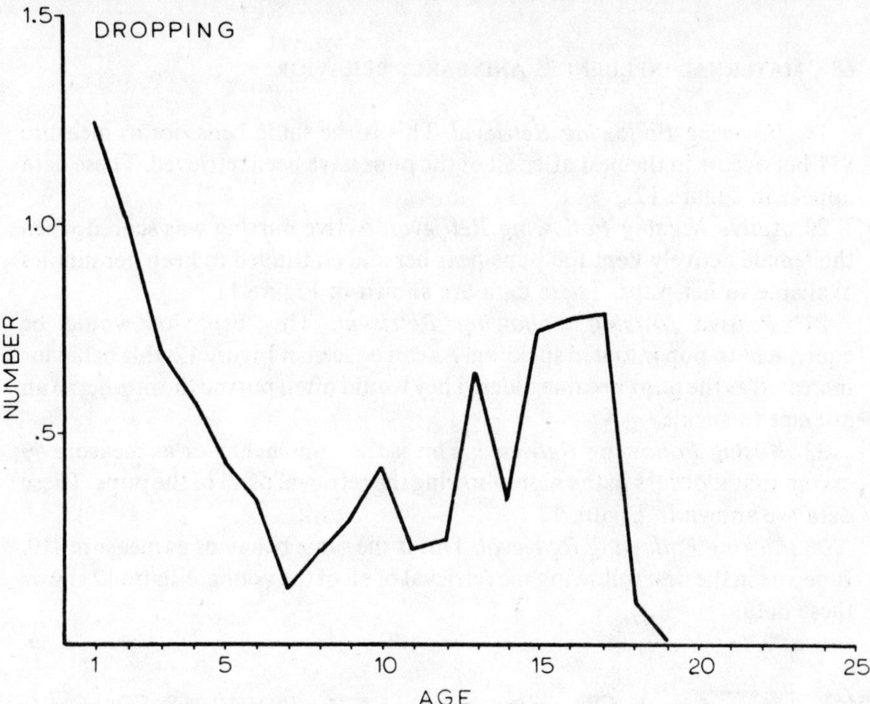

FIG. 10. The average number of drops per day of pups by the retrieving mother.

FIG. 11. The behavior of the mother following the retrieval of all of her pups. See also Figure 12.

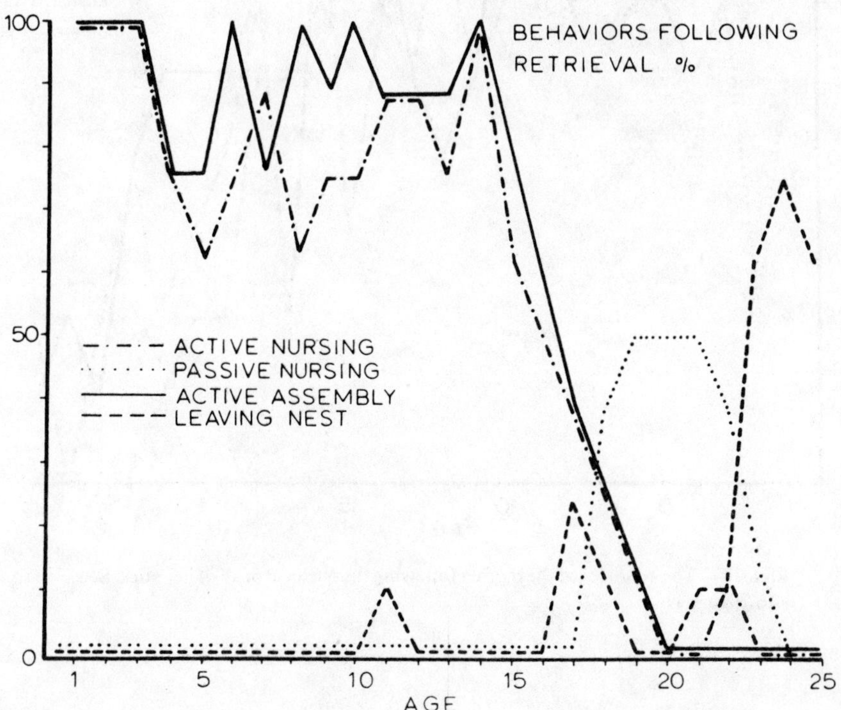

19. *Hovering Following Retrieval.* This is the same behavior as measure #11 but occurs in the nest after all of the pups have been retrieved. These data appear in Figure 12.

20. *Active Nursing Following Retrieval.* Active nursing was scored when the female actively kept the pups near her and continued to keep her nipples available to her pups. These data are shown in Figure 11.

21. *Passive Nursing Following Retrieval.* This behavior would be equivalent to pup initiated suckling. As can be seen in Figure 12, this behavior increased as the pups became older. They would often pursue the mother in an attempt to suckle.

22. *Nosing Following Retrieval.* This is the same behavior as measure #9 except that it occurs in the nest following the retrieval of all of the pups. These data are shown in Figure 12.

23. *Licking Following Retrieval.* This is the same behavior as measure #10. It occurs in the nest following the retrieval of all of the young. Figure 12 shows these data.

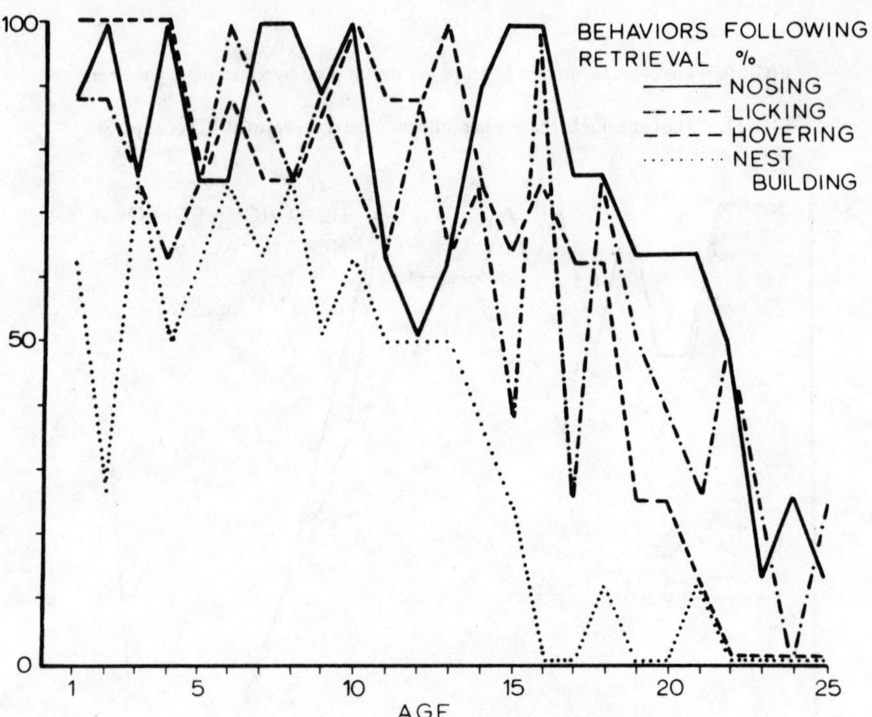

FIG. 12. The behavior of the mother following the retrieval of all of her pups. See also Figure 11.

24. *Nest Building Following Retrieval.* If the female engaged in nest building when she returned to the nest with the last pup to be retrieved, then this was recorded as Nest Building During Retrieval (#13). Nest Building Following Retrieval was seen only after the female had nursed the pups. It consisted of major modifications in the nest. These data are shown in Figure 12.

25. *Leaving the Nest Following Retrieval.* As the young became older the female would often leave the nest after she had retrieved the pups. While out of the nest she would engage in a variety of apparently nonmaternal activities. This behavior was recorded if the female was out of the nest for 4 or more minutes out of the 10-minute observation period. Short excursions of 15 seconds or less were not counted. The percentage of females leaving the nest following retrieval is shown in Figure 11.

26. *Mother Power.* This is a derived measure. It was calculated by: (Daily Average Weight of the Pup X Distance Carried On Retrieval)/Retrieval Time Excluding Maximum Scores. The distance carried was a constant. Figure 13 shows these data.

27. *Age of the Young.* Age was confounded with days since parturition because the maternal females were caring for their own litters. This is a normally confounded variable in Nature.

28. *Weight of the Young.* Weight was measured daily to the nearest one-tenth of a gram. Average weight per day is shown in Figure 14.

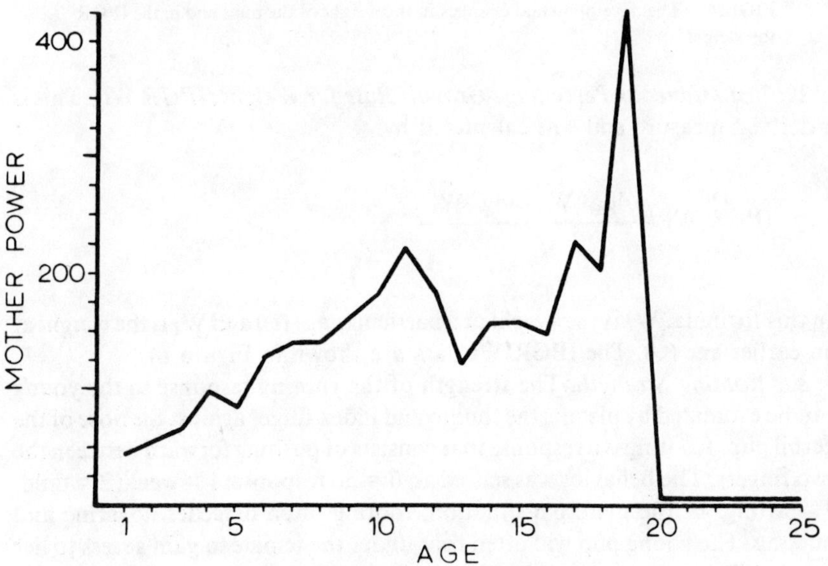

FIG. 13. The changes in Mother Power across the days of testing.

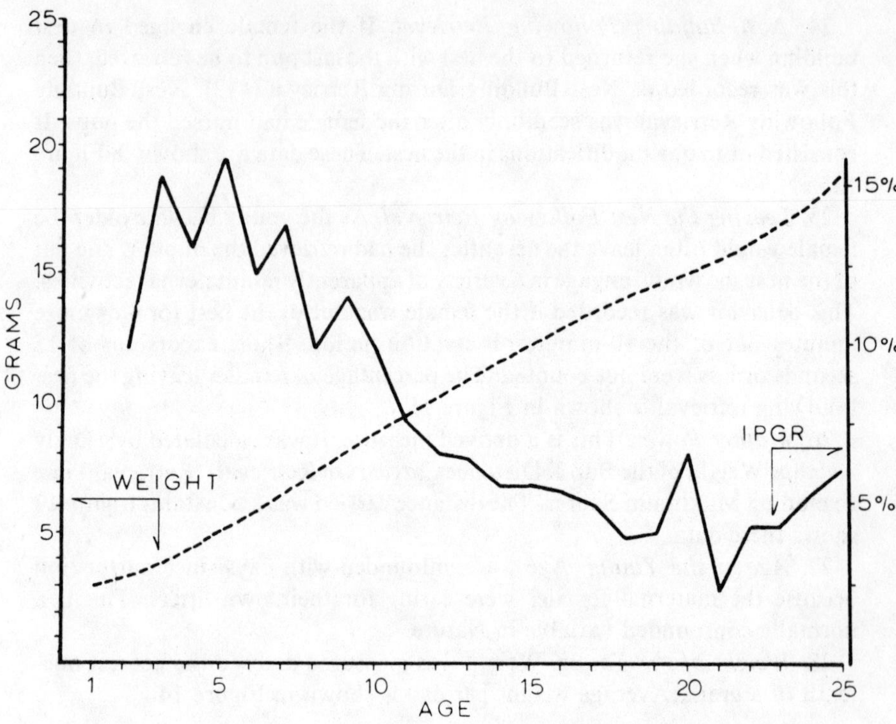

FIG. 14. The developmental changes in the weight of the pups and in the IPGR for weight.

29. *Instantaneous Percentage Growth Rate for Weight (IPGR Wt).* This is a derived measure and was calculated by:

$$\text{IPGR Wt} = \frac{\log_n W_2 - \log_n W_1}{t_2 - t_1}$$

In this formula, W_2 is the weight at a particular age (t_2) and W_1 is the weight at an earlier age (t_1). The IPGR Wt data are shown in Figure 14.

30. *Rooting Strength.* The strength of the rooting response to the young can be estimated by placing the thumb and index finger against the nose of the gerbil pup. Rooting is a response that consists of pushing forward between the two fingers. The behavior was scored as: 0 = no response; 1 = weak; 2 = mild; 3 = strong. In the maternal situation, rooting often precedes hovering and nursing. The young pup will often root under the female to gain access to her nipples. These data appear in Figure 15.

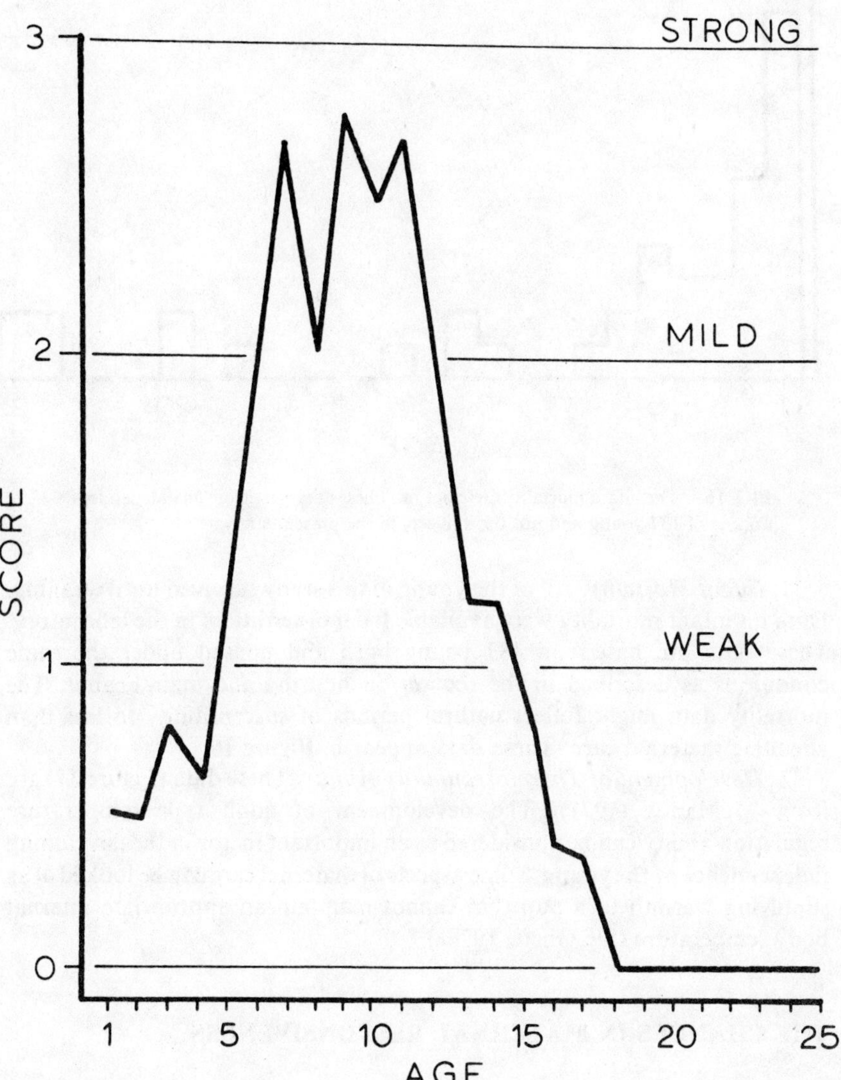

FIG. 15. The developmental changes in the strength of the rooting response.

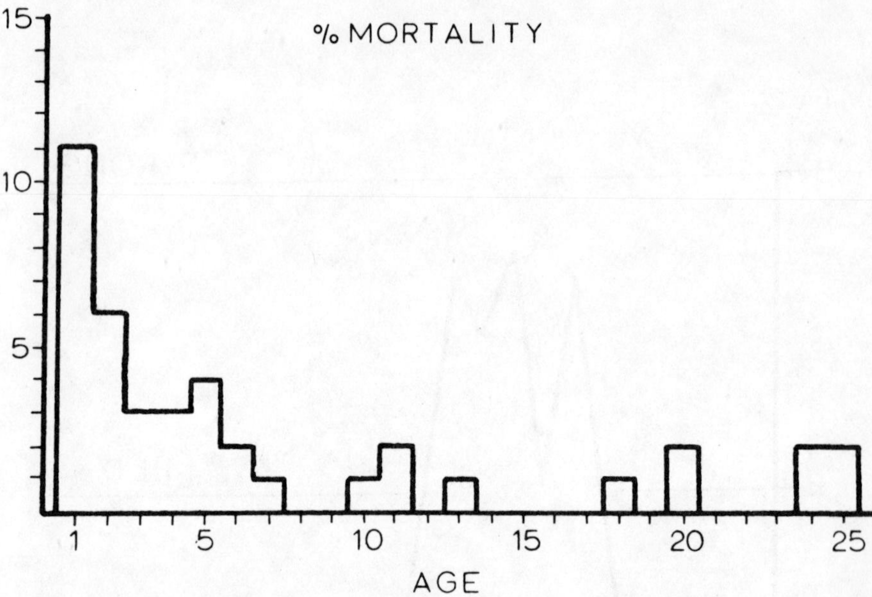

FIG. 16. The infant mortality distribution. These data were from an independent sample of 137 young and not the subjects in the present study.

31. *Infant Mortality*. All of the young in this study survived until weaning. Data on infant mortality were available from other litters in the laboratory. These data are based on 137 young born and housed under the same conditions as described in the section on housing and maintenance. The mortality data might reflect natural periods of susceptibility to less than adequate maternal care. These data appear in Figure 16.

32. *Development of Thermoregulatory Ability*. These data (Figure 17) are from McManus (1971). The development of adult type temperature regulation ability can be considered as an important factor in the developing independence of the young. Some aspects of maternal care can be looked at as supplying warmth to a pup that cannot maintain an appropriate internal body temperature (De Ghett, 1978a).

THE CHANGES IN MATERNAL RESPONSIVENESS

An examination of the graphs shows the kinds of changes in maternal responsiveness that occur in the Mongolian gerbil. For the first five days after birth between 90% and 100% of the females are nursing about the same

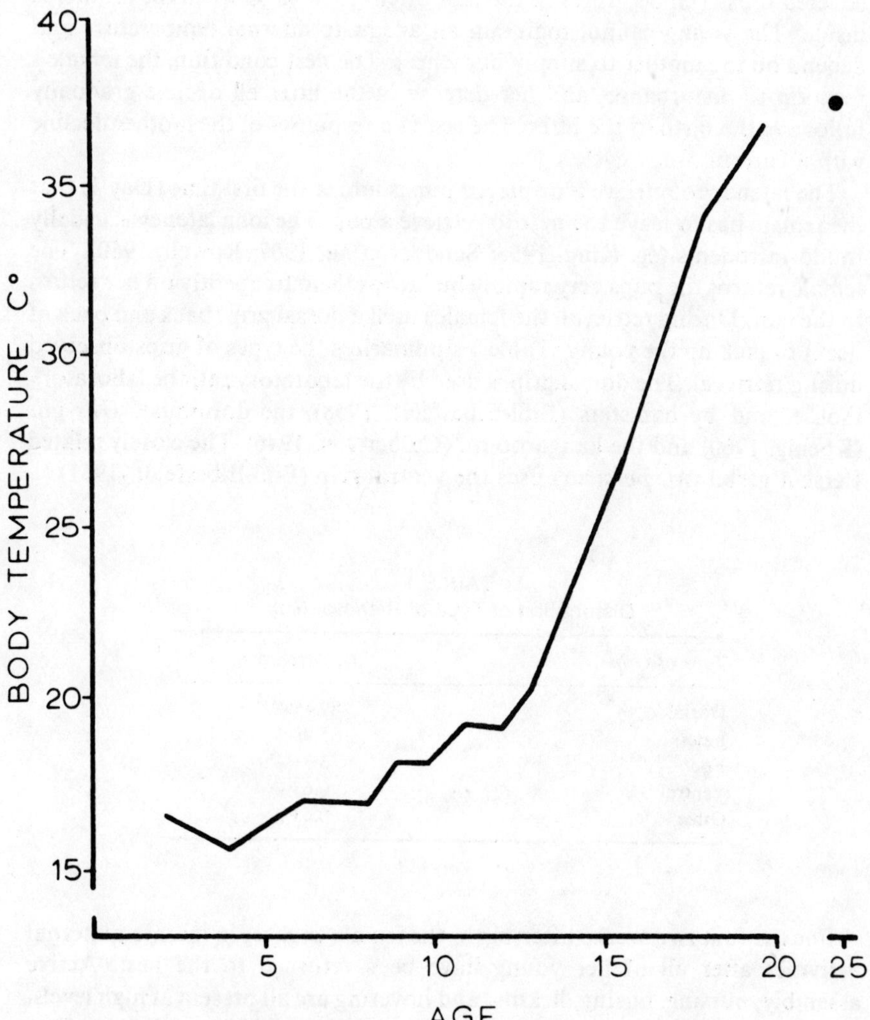

FIG. 17. The changes in the development of thermoregulatory ability. Redrawn from Mc Manus (1971). The body termperature represents the core body temperature following a 1-hour exposure to an ambient environment of 14°-15°C. The value at Day 25 is within the adult range. Reprinted with permission of the American Society of Mammalogists.

percentage of young immediately before testing. The mothers are nursing their young in well-formed nests with high sides. Many of the nests have covered tops. Temperatures in the nest often reach 40°C when the mother is inside. The young cannot maintain an adequate internal temperature and depend on the mother to supply body heat. The nest condition, the female's reaction to disturbance, and her defense of the litter all decline gradually following the birth of the litter. The last two responses of the mother decline with a curious 5-day cycle.

The latency to retrieve a displaced pup is longer the first time (Day 1) that the female has to leave the nest to retrieve a pup. The long latency is usually found in rodents (eg. King, 1958; Scudder et al., 1967; Rowell, 1960). The female returns the pups very rapidly but drops them frequently on her return to the nest. During retrieval, the females used a dorsal grip (back and back of neck) to pick up the young. Table 1 summarizes the types of grips observed during retrieval. The dorsal grip is used by the laboratory rat, the laboratory mouse, and by hamsters (Eibl-Eibesfeldt, 1958), the dormouse, *Glis glis* (Koenig, 1960) and the kangaroo rat (Culbertson, 1946). The closely related Persian gerbil (*M. persicus*) uses the ventral grip (Eibl-Eibesfeldt, 1951).

TABLE 1
Distribution of Type of Retrieval Grip

Type of Grip	*Occurrence*
Dorsal	89.45%
Lateral	5.98%
Foot	3.31%
Ventral	0.63%
Other	0.63%

For the first two weeks after birth, the female engages in intense maternal activities after all of her young have been returned to the nest. Active assembly, nursing, nosing, licking, and hovering are all present at high levels. Passive nursing is not seen until Day 18 and begins to decline following Day 21. At that time, more and more females begin to leave the nest and stay away from their young. The IPGR Wt function shows a marked degree of fluctuation at this time. This is caused by the shift onto solid food (Days 19 to 23) and a decline in the percentage of young suckling and females nursing. Weaning was complete by Day 24 for all litters. Some litters were weaned on Day 21.

HIERARCHICAL CLUSTER ANALYSIS OF THE MATERNAL BEHAVIORS

Hierarchical Cluster Analysis is a multivariate technique that can be useful for discovering patterns of associations that exist in large data sets (De Ghett, 1978b). The 32 measures in the present study produce 496 pairwize relationships. These are far too many to deal with in a meaningful fashion. Some of these 496 relations have higher associations than others. Hierarchical Cluster Analysis starts with the total pairwize set of relations, in this case correlation coefficients, and extracts clusters from this set. The clusters are nested into hierarchies at levels of similarity associated with the degrees of relationship that exist. The decision rule or clustering algorithm used in the present analysis was the Complete Linkage algorithm. This is a very strict clustering rule and tends to produce well-defined clusters or none at all.

In this study, clustering was based on the correlations between the 32 measures. Because correlation coefficients represent the starting point for clustering, the measures will be joined into clusters based on the way they covary. Measures that have similar profiles of change across the 25 days of testing will tend to cluster. Measures will also cluster that have an inverse relationship (a mirror image profile).

The results of the Hierarchical Cluster Analysis are depicted as a dendrogram in Figure 18. In the dendrogram, the nodal points (where the lines join) indicate the level of similarity between the two measures or the two clusters that are united. The similarity scale at the bottom of the dendrogram can be interpreted in the same fashion as an absolute value correlation coefficient. All measures or clusters will always unite at a similarity value of zero. The visual inspection of the dendrogram reveals that seven clusters exist. There are no formal criteria for defining a cluster. Some readers may see a different number of clusters than others.

Cluster I contains two measures; IPGR Wt (#29) and rate of ultrasonic vocalization (#6). This indicates that the highest rates of ultrasonic vocalization are associated with the highest rates of weight gain. The development of temperature regulation (#32) has often been considered as a causal factor in the ontogeny of ultrasound production (De Ghett, 1978a) yet it does not join this cluster. A possible link between the two measures of Cluster I might be energy expenditure. As more energy is shunted into tissue growth (high rate of weight gain) less might be available for use in generating heat within the body. This would cause a drop in internal body temperature probably several days after birth when the growth rate is high. Figure 17 on the development of thermoregulatory ability shows such a drop. The drop in

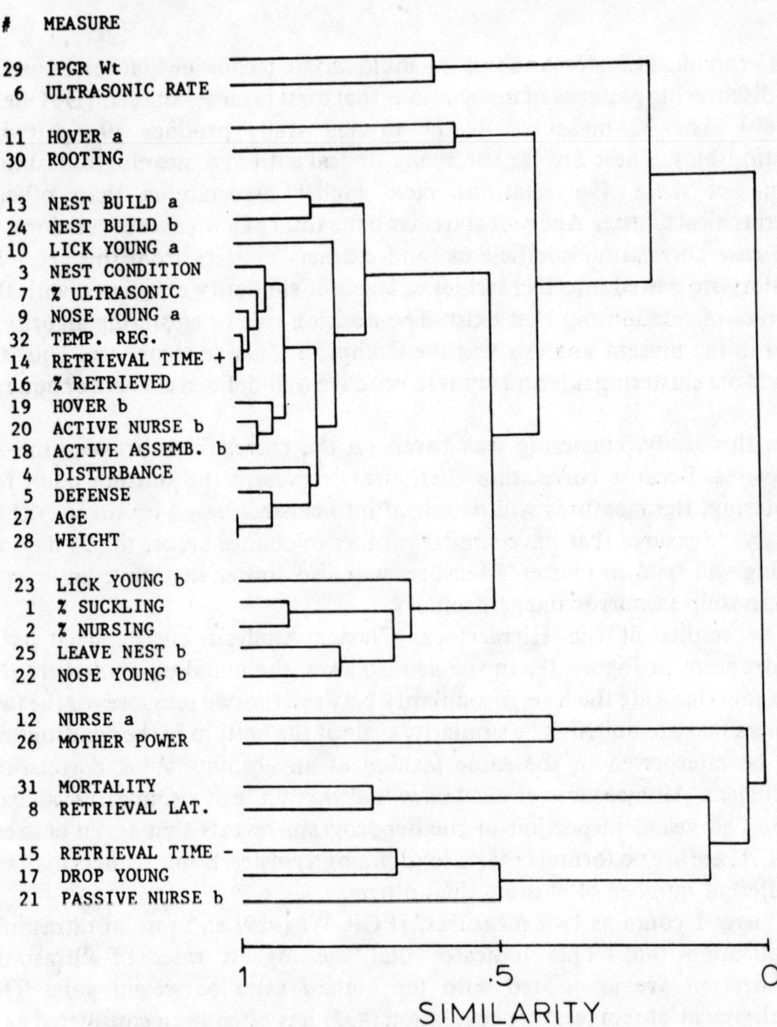

FIG. 18. The dendrogram showing the results of the Hierarchical Cluster Analysis (complete-linkage algorithm) of the 32 maternal measures. The numbers (#) before each measure correspond to the numbers in the text describing each measure.

core body temperature would then cause an increase in the rate of ultrasound production at about the same time. As can be seen by the above passage, cluster analysis can give a hint but not an answer.

Cluster II contains hovering during retrieval (#11) and rooting strength (#30). Rooting is strongest on Days 7 through 11 and hovering is most frequent on Day 7. As the mother approaches the young pup to be retrieved, the pup often roots under her. This is the same behavior that Rosenblatt (1976, page 347) calls "nuzzling." This might be interpreted as an attempt at suckling but note that nursing during retrieval (#12) does not join in this cluster. Rooting in this situation might be related to securing contact with a warm textured surface as suggested by Rosenblatt (1976).

Cluster III is a large supercluster containing 21 measures and could be considered as a core of maternal maintenance activities. Starting from the top of Cluster III we see that nest building during and following retrieval (#13 and #24) are joined indicating that these activities of the mother, although more extensive after the young are all in the nest, have the same profiles across the 25 days of observation. Licking the pups during retrieval (#10) is a single member subcluster and as such is difficult to interpret. Licking remains independent until after three other subclusters are united. Licking during retrieval is drawn into this large Cluster III because of the existence of other subclusters. The next subcluster contains five tightly linked behaviors: nest condition (#3); percentage of young emitting ultrasonic vocalizations (#7); nosing young during retrieval (#9); development of temperature regulation (#32); retrieval time including maximum scores (#14); and percentage of young retrieved (#16). These five behaviors unite at such a high level of similarity that they can be considered to have profiles that depict the same kinds of change. Retrieval time including the maximum scores for the failure to retrieve is certainly a reflection of the percentage of young retrieved for when a pup is not retrieved then that particular retrieval is given a maximum score of 60 seconds. As young gerbils become more efficient at temperature regulation they emit fewer ultrasounds. This has already been reported (De Ghett, 1978a). Vocalizing pups are retrieved more rapidly by the maternal female and an important component of retrieval is the initial contact between the mother and the pup. This initial contact is the nosing response of the mother. This is most certainly an olfactory investigation. Olfactory stimuli in addition to ultrasounds appear to be cues central to retrieval (Smotherman et al., 1974; Smotherman et al., in press). The nest is not only a physical factor around which maternal care is organized but it is also a tremendous insulating factor that slows the rate of heat loss in an ectothermic rodent pup.

The next subcluster contains measures that join at a high level of similarity: hovering following retrieval (#19); active nursing following retrieval (#20); and active assembly of the pups following retrieval (#18). When the maternal female returns to the nest following the retrieval of the last pup she gathers or assembles the pups about her and then hovers over them and begins to nurse them. As the young suckle, the female continues to assemble and reassemble the pups. Like the previous subcluster, this one has tremendous appeal.

The mother's reaction to disturbance (#4); defense of her litter (#5); the age of the young (#27); and the weight of the young (#26) comprise the next subcluster. The first two measures to join are age and weight. Following these are two classes of reaction by the maternal female: reaction to disturbance and to litter removal. Both reactions decline with the increasing age of the young and weight of the young.

Cluster IV contains five measures. The percentage of females nursing (#2) and the percentage of young suckling (#1) form a subcluster at a high level of similarity. These two measures provide different views of a central aspect of maternal care. Leaving the pups following retrieval (#25) and nosing the pups following retrieval (#22) are inversely related. Nosing is an integral part of nursing behavior. As nosing (#22), nursing (#2), and suckling (#1) decline with the approach of weaning, the female spends less time in the nest with her young. Licking following retrieval (#23) declines erratically during the 25 days of testing. Just as in licking during retrieval (#10), licking following retrieval (#23) remains independent of the cluster for sometime. But, licking in these two contexts is not similar enough to cluster together indicating a situation specific aspect to this behavior.

Cluster V contains nursing during retrieval (#12) and mother power (#26). Nursing during retrieval occurs infrequently and is related to mother power at a low level of similarity. Mother power may not be a meaningful measure because it is linked with an infrequently occuring behavior. However, it does join a measure and form a cluster. The Complete-Linkage algorithm does not force measures into clusters. In fact, this algorithm admits measures hesitantly because it is a strict algorithm. As a derived measure, mother power does not cluster with the measures used to construct it—retrieval time (#15) and weight (#28). It should be estimating the power expended or in common language the work involved in returning the young to the nest. The cluster is saying that the more the mother nurses the young before returning them to the nest, then the more effort it takes to return them.

Cluster VI contains mortality of the young (#31) and latency to retrieve (#8). The mortality data were not gathered from the subjects in this study. Its linkage with latency to retrieval indicates that the female is hesitant to leave the nest (long latency) during the time when the probability of infant mortality is high. At first glance this might seem to be a poorly adapted response. But, except for when the interfering hand of the ethologist removes them, young are normally in the nest during the first week after birth. They are seldom seen out of the nest. If the mother's behavior is tied to the nest then she will be with her young.

Cluster VII contains retrieval time excluding the maximum scores (#2), dropping the young during retrieval (#17), and passive nursing following retrieval (#21). The mothers dropped the young frequently during the first week after birth but this did not affect their retrieval time. The number of drops reaches a minimum on the 7th day and then begins to increase again. This increase during the 2nd week does appear to have a slight effect on retrieval time. The young are heavier, more active, and probably more difficult to hold on to. This causes more drops which in turn causes an increase in retrieval times. Passive nursing following retrieval increases dramatically prior to weaning. The young often appear to attack and corner the female in an attempt to suckle. From the female's point of view, the young are getting "difficult." This is consistent with the slightly longer retrieval times and the increase in the number of drops.

The results of the Hierarchical Cluster Analysis allow one to reach some overall conclusions. Each cluster could be considered as a system. Seven systems are then present. Two large conglomerates exist. Clusters I through IV remain totally independent of Clusters V through VII. Cluster V is virtually independent from Clusters VI and VII, and the same could be said about the relationship between Clusters VI and VII. Maternal behavior is not a unitary concept, but rather a complex web of interacting systems with some definite boundaries between the systems in the context of the present study. The complete integration of the maternal and the developmental measures indicates a dynamic interplay between the reactions of the normal female and the developmental status of the young. Those studies of maternal care that attempt to measure the changing responses of the mother with alien young of a constant age are removing an essential and natural feature of maternal responsivness. While the experimental designs might dictate the control of specific extraneous variables such as developing young, natural selection has molded an integrated set of behavior systems without examining the pages of a design text.

PRINCIPAL COMPONENTS ANALYSIS OF THE MATERNAL BEHAVIORS

Principal Components Analysis (PCA) is a multivariate technique that, like Hierarchical Cluster Analysis, is useful for identifying the structure that may exist in a large data set. For specific information on the application of PCA to ethological data see Dudziński and Norris (1970) and Frey (1978).

PCA extracts factors from the data set in a way that is similar to factor extraction in Factor Analysis. Traditionally, enough factors are extracted so that about 75% to 85% of the total variance is accounted for by the factors. In the PCA of the maternal beahaviors, three factors accounted for 81.3% of the total variance in the following manner: Factor I 64.8%, Factor II 9.1%, and Factor III 7.4%. The 32 measures and their rotated (Varimax rotation) factor loadings are shown in Table II. Also in Table II are the communalities (h^2). The communality of a measure is an index of the extent to which a particular measure is accounted for by the factors.

The factor loadings for Factors I and II were used as coordinates to plot the 32 measures in a two-dimensional space (Figure 19). Since three factors were extracted, the loading on the third factor can be used to move the point above

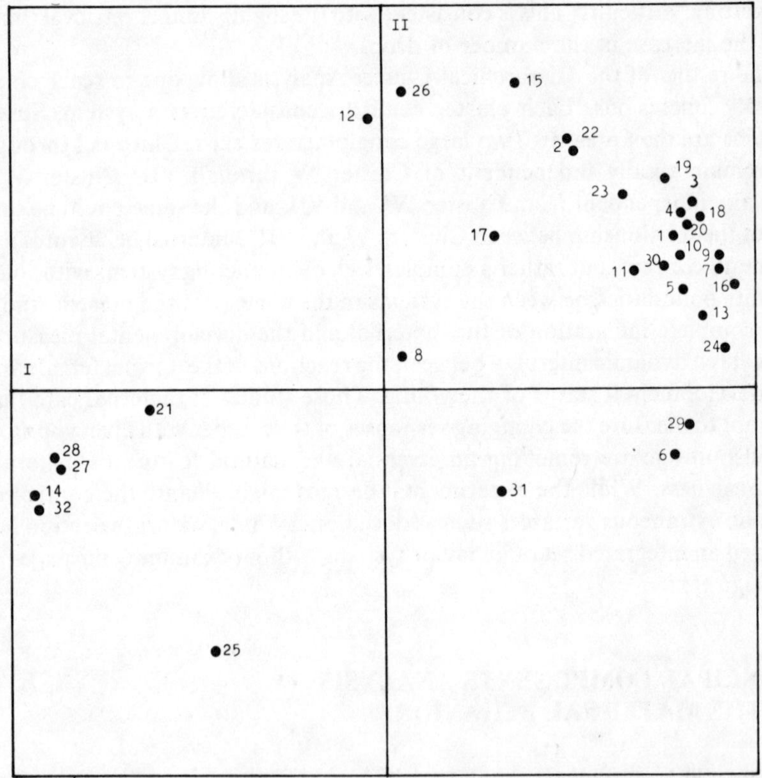

FIG. 19. The two-dimensional mapping of the 32 measures following a Principal Components Analysis (Varimax rotation). The numbers used to identify the points are the same as those used to identify the measures in the Hierarchical Cluster Analysis (Figure 18) and are the same as those used in the text. Factor I is the horizontal line and Factor II is the vertical line. See also Table II.

or below the page on an axis perpendicular to the page surface. It is difficult to portray the 32 points in a three-dimensional space. In Figure 20 the points are joined by lines that link the nearest neighbors as a function of the three-dimensional distances between points. Each point has another point that is its nearest neighbor. A line is used to connect one point with its nearest neighbor. When that second point has a nearest neighbor that is different from the first point, then the line progresses to a third point. At sometime in the progression a point has a nearest neighbor that brings the line back over the just connected path. The progression then stops. The result is a constellation of points. These constellations are shown in Figure 20. There are eight constellations indicated A through H.

In the previous section we examined the contents of the clusters that resulted from the application of Hierarchical Cluster Analysis. The contents

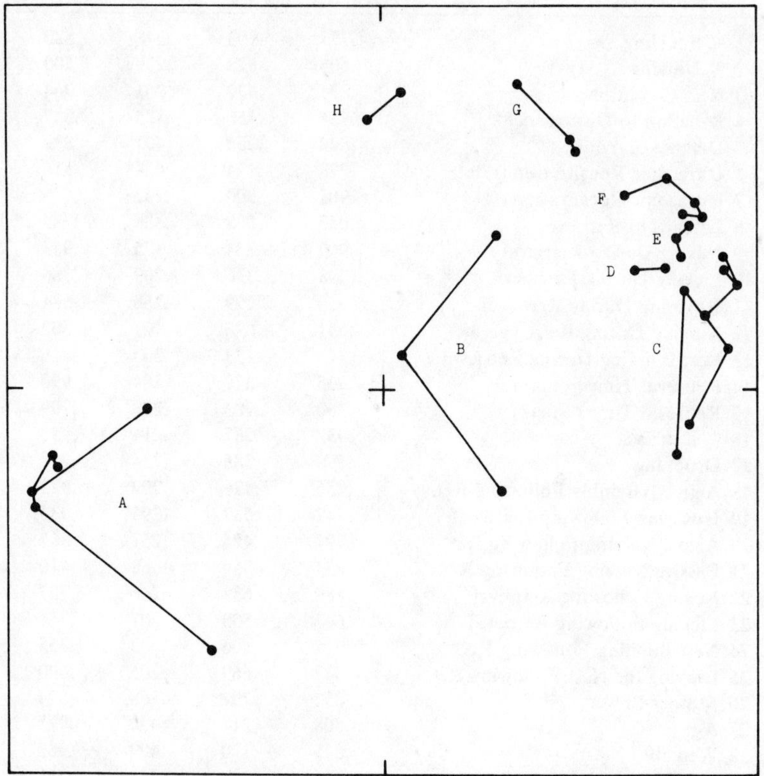

FIG. 20. The constellations resulting from the nearest neighbor joining of the points based on their three-dimensional distances. The arrangement of points is the same as in Figure 19.

of the clusters should bear some resemblance to the contents of the factors but not necessarily the constellations. Factor I of the PCA contains measures that are generally included in Clusters I through IV, the supercluster that is completely independent from the remaining supercluster. Different procedures for extracting factors and different clustering algorithms yield different amounts of correspondence between the contents of the factors and the contents of the clusters. The conclusion reached following the Hierarchical Cluster Analysis that maternal behavior is not a unitary concept is verified by the existence of more than a single factor in the PCA.

TABLE 2
Factor Loadings and Communalities (h^2) for the PCA

#	Measure	I	II	III	h^2
1	% Suckling	.777	.393	.248	.820
2	% Nursing	.505	.623	.239	.700
3	Nest Condition	.821	.472	.261	.964
4	Reaction to Disturbance	.784	.456	.185	.857
5	Defense of Young	.808	.255	.401	.879
6	Ultrasonic Vocalization (rate)	.778	–.174	.424	.816
7	Ultrasonic Vocalization (%)	.902	.300	.232	.958
8	Latency to Retrieve	.048	.088	.888	.799
9	Nosing During Retrieval	.900	.334	.175	.953
10	Licking During Retrieval	.798	.326	.209	.786
11	Hovering During Retrieval	.650	.299	–.268	.584
12	Nursing During Retrieval	–.031	.698	–.121	.502
13	Nest Building During Retrieval	.847	.173	.263	.816
14	Retrieval Time (+ max)	–.935	–.272	–.204	.990
15	Retrieval Time (– max)	.360	.783	.236	.799
16	% Retrieval	.932	.267	.214	.985
17	Dropping	.299	.385	.734	.777
18	Active Assembly Following Ret.	.836	.426	.209	.923
19	Hovering Following Retrieval	.747	.537	.295	.933
20	Active Nursing Following Ret.	.797	.425	.257	.882
21	Passive Nursing Following Ret.	–.634	–.060	–.068	.410
22	Nosing Following Retrieval	.489	.638	.246	.707
23	Licking Following Retrieval	.647	.500	.207	.711
24	Nest Building Following Ret.	.917	.106	.083	.858
25	Leaving the Nest Following Ret.	–.447	–.669	–.205	.690
26	Mother Power	.052	.707	–.268	.574
27	Age	–.868	–.214	–.420	.975
28	Weight	–.875	–.190	–.409	.968
29	IPGR Wt	.816	–.098	–.264	.745
30	Rooting	.750	.313	–.353	.785
31	Infant Mortality	.310	–.271	.840	.875
32	Thermoregulation	–.922	–.315	–.192	.987

The constellations reflect the factor loadings only in that the loadings were the coordinates used to map the points in the three-dimensional space. Nearest neighbors were not always measures that loaded high on the same factor. The constellations can be viewed as partitions of the total data set that cut through a three dimensional space.

Constellation A contains measures that reached high values or levels as weaning approached. While most of the measures used in the present study declined across the 25 days of observation, a few increased and nearly all of these are in Constellation A. Constellation B contains measures that are at high levels shortly after birth and then decline abruptly. Constellations C, D, E, and F contain measures that are generally high until the second week after birth and then decline. Constellation G contains measures that seem to remain at a constant level until weaning and then decline. Constellation H makes little sense from this temporal change analysis of the constellations. The contents of this constellation, mother power and nursing during retrieval were the entire contents of Cluster V in the Hierarchical Cluster Analysis and caused problems of interpretation in that analysis too. As a constellation it is located out of the sweep of constellations that move from the lower left to the upper right of Figure 19.

The multivariate analyses of the maternal behaviors yielded different pictures of the structure of this complex set of behavioral systems. The different pictures are like different views of the same object. As these pictures taken from different angles accumulate it will become possible to gain greater insight into the structure of the maternal behaviors and their interrelationships.

The behaviors of the maternal female occupy a central position in the early life of the Mongolian gerbil. The female appears to be tracking the response capabilities and survival requirements of her young. The nest deteriorates and is not repaired as vigorously as the young get older and are more capable of internal temperature regulation. As growth rates decline, less and less nursing activities are seen. As locomotor capabilities emerge and mature, retrieval occupies a less central position in the mother's activities. These changes in maternal responsiveness are not really that different from what has been found in other nonprecocial rodents. Immature rodents have similar survival needs: nutrition, protection from conspecifics and heterospecifics, warmth, and particular levels of early experience and stimulation. The actions of the maternal female provides a partial buffer between the immature young with its immature central nervous system and the effects of natural selection. The early experiences and early forms of stimulation during this period of protection provide an important input to the organizing central nervous system. As Mayr (1970) has said: "Parental care protects the young while they are acquiring all the learned information that they need to cope successfully with the challenges of the environment."

REFERENCES

Allen, G. M. *Natural History of Central Asia, Vol. XI: The Mammals of China and Mongolia*, Part 2. American Museum of Natural History, New York: (1940).

Bannikov, A. G. *Mammals of the Mongolian People's Republic*. U. S. S. R. Academy of Science, Moscow. Report #53 (1954).

Barfield, M. A. and Beeman, E. A. The oestrus cycle in the Mongolian gerbil, *Meriones unguiculatus. J. Reprod. Fertil. 17*, 247–251 (1968).

Culbertson, A. E. Observations on the natural history of the Fresno kangaroo rat. *J. Mammal. 27*, 189–203 (1946).

De Ghett, V. J. The behavioral and morphological development of the Mongolian gerbil (*Meriones unguiculatus*) from birth until thirty days of age. Ph.D. thesis, Bowling Green State University, 1972. (University Microfilms, Ann Arbor, Michigan #73-12002)

De Ghett, V. J. Developmental changes in the rate of ultrasonic vocalization in the Mongolian gerbil. *Dev. Psychobiol. 7*, 267–272 (1974).

De Ghett, V. J. The ontogeny of ultrasound production in rodents. In *The Development of Behavior: Comparative and Evolutionary Aspects*, G. M. Burghardt and M. Bekoff, eds. Garland Press, New York: (1978a).

De Ghett, V. J. Hierarchical cluster analysis. In *Quantitative Ethology*, P. Colgan, ed. Wiley Interscience, New York: (1978b).

Dewsbury, D. A. Patterns of copulatory behavior in male mammals. *Quart. Rev. Biol. 47*, 1–33 (1972).

Dudzinski, M. L. and Norris, J. M. Principal components anaysis as an aid for studying animal behavior. *Forma et Functio 2*, 101–109 (1970).

Eibl-Eibesfeldt, I. Gefangenschaftebeobachtungen an der persischen wustenmaus (*Meriones persicus persicus* Blanford): an beitrag zur vergleichenden ethologie der nager. *Zeitschrift fur Tierpsychologie, 8*, 400–423 (1951).

Eibl-Eibesfeldt, I. Das verhalten der nagetiere. *Handbuch der Zoologie, 8* (10), 6, 1–88 (1958).

Elwood, R. W. Paternal and maternal behavior in the Mongolian gerbil. *Anim. Behav. 23*, 766–772 (1975).

Elwood, R. W. Changes in the responses of male and female gerbil (*Meriones unguiculatus*) towards test pups during the pregnancy of the female. *Anim. Behav*. 25, 46–51 (1977).

Frey, D. F. Principal components analysis and factor analysis. In *Quantitative Ethology*, P. Colgan, ed. Wiley Interscience, New York: (1978).

Gulotta, E. F. *Meriones unguiculatus. Mammal. Spec.* 3, 1–5 (1971).

King, J. A. Maternal behavior and behavioral development in two species of *Peromyscus maniculatus. J. Mammal.* 39, 177–190 (1958).

Kuehn, R. E. and Zucker, I. Reproductive behavior of the Mongolian gerbil (*Meriones unguiculatus*). *J. Comp. Physiol. Psychol. 66*, 747–752 (1968).

Leont'ev, A. N. Kizucheniyu populyatsii mongol'skikh peschanok metodom mecheniya. *Izvest Irkutsk Nauchn-Issled Protivovhumnogo Inst Sibiri Dal Nogo Vost, 24*, 296–302 (1963). (Biological Abstracts, 1964, Abstr. #103056).

Marston, J. H. and Chang, M. C. The breeding, management and reproductive physiology of the Mongolian gerbil (*Meriones unguiculatus*). *Lab. Anim. Care 15*, 34–48 (1965).

Mayr, E. *Populations, Species, and Evolution*. Harvard University Press, Cambridge: (1970).

McManus, J. Early postnatal growth and development of temperature regulation in the Mongolian gerbil (*Meriones unguiculatus*). *J. Mammal. 52*, 782–792 (1971).

Meckley, P. E. and Ginther, O. J. Effects of litter and male on corpora lutea of the postpartum Mongolian gerbil. *J. Anim. Sci. 34*, 297–301 (1972).

Nakai, K., Nimura, I., Tamura, M., Shimizu, S., and Nishimura, H. Reproduction and postnatal development of the colony bred *Meriones unguiculatus kurauchii* Mori. *Bull. Exper. Anim.* (Japan), *9*, 157–159 (1960).

Naumov, N. P. and Lobachev, V. S. Ecology of desert rodents of the U. S. S. R. (Jerboas and Gerbils). In *Rodents in Desert Environments*, I. Prakash and P. K. Ghosh, eds. Junk, The Hague: (1975).

Norris, M. L. and Adams, C. E. Delayed implantation in the Mongolian gerbil (*Meriones unguiculatus*). *J. Reprod. Fertil.* 27, 486–487 (1971).

Rich, S. T. The Mongolian gerbil (*Meriones unguiculatus*) in research. *Lab. Anim. Care 18*, 235–243 (1968).

Roper, T. J. and Polioudakis, E. The behaviour of Mongolian gerbils in a semi-natural environment, with special reference to ventral marking, dominance and sociability. *Behaviour 61* (3–4) 207–237 (1977).

Rosenblatt, J. S. Stages in the early behavioural development of altricial young of selected species of non-primate mammals. In *Growing Points in Ethology*, P. P. G. Bateson and R. A. Hinde, eds. Cambridge University Press, Cambridge: (1976).

Rowell, T. E. On retrieving of young and other behaviour in the lactating golden hamster. *Proc. Zool. Soc. Lond. 135*, 265–282 (1960).

Scudder, C. L., Karczmar, A. G. and Lockett, L. Behavioral development studies on four genera and several strains of mice. *Anim. Behav. 15*, 353–363 (1967).

Smotherman, W. P., Bell, R. W., Hershberger, W. A., and Coover, G. D. Orientation to pup cues: Effects of maternal experiential history. *Anim. Behav. 26,* 265–273 (1978).

Smotherman, W. P., Bell, R. W., Starzec, J., Elias, J., and Zachman, T. A. Maternal responses to infant vocalizations and olfactory cues in rats and mice. *Behav. Biol. 12*, 55–66 (1974).

Tanimoto, K. Ecological studies on plague-carrying animals in Manchuria. *Zool. Mag.* (Tokyo), 55, 111–127 (1943).

Thiessen, D. and Yahr, P. *The gerbil in behavioral investigations: Mechanisms of territory and olfactory communication.* Austin: University of Texas Press, 1977.

Vick, L. H. and Banks, E. M. The estrus cycle and related behavior in the Mongolian gerbil (*Meriones unguiculatus* Milne-Edwards). *Comm. Behav. Biol. 3*, 117–124 (1969).

Maternal Influences and Early Behavior

4
Determinants of Maternal Aggression in Mice

Ronald Gandelman

It is well-known both through formal and informal observations that animals of a variety of species exhibit intra and interspecific aggressive behavior during the lactation phase of the reproductive cycle. Maternal or postpartum aggression has been reported in such diverse species as the rabbit (Mykytowycz, 1959), mouse (King, 1963), rat (Barnett, 1969), squirrel (Taylor, 1966), hamster (Wise, 1974), langur (Jay, 1963), cat (Schneirla et al., 1963), moose (Altman, 1963), chimpanzee (Chance and Jolly, 1970), and baboon (DeVore, 1963). Beach (1948) went so far as to suggest that such aggressive behavior is characteristic of all vertebrate mothers.

Maternal aggression serves one obvious function, that of protecting the young during the early and most vulnerable stage of development. In addition to a protective function, it has been suggested that maternal aggression contributes to population regulation (Rowley and Christian, 1976, 1977).

The reports of maternal aggression and its presumptive importance notwithstanding, scant attention has been paid to the behavior by laboratory researchers. Perhaps this occurred because postpartum aggression can be subsumed under the rubric of either maternal or aggressive behavior. As a result, researchers concentrating upon aggression tended not to study postpartum aggression because it is considered an aspect of maternal behavior while investigators focusing upon maternal behavior ignored it because it is an agonistic response. This confusion in classification has led to a number of over simplifications and misconceptions about the nature of particular behaviors. For example, it has been assumed that females will exhibit aggressive behavior only if exposed to testosterone during certain periods of development (Edwards, 1968). As Rowley and Christian (1976b) state, "It should be noted that females have often been excluded from behavioral studies as a general attitude has historically prevailed suggesting that maternal aggression is just an important exception to the general rule of female nonaggressiveness (Edwards, 1975)." As another example, it has been reported that maternal behavior can be induced in virgin female and male rats by exposing them to young continuously for about seven days (Rosenblatt, 1967). Fleming and Rosenblatt (1974), in comparing the maternal behavior of virgin females to that of lactating animals reported that the behavior of the virgins was similar in nearly all respects to that of the dams. This is an important observation because it suggests that the maintenance of maternal behavior is not under hormonal control. However, the authors did not determine whether exposure to young induces postpartum-like aggressive behavior. LeRoy and Krehbiel (1978) have reported that maternally sensitized virgin females and males failed to attack male intruders.

The paucity of information about maternal aggression, its rather obvious utility for species survival, and its ubiquity at the species level prompted the establishment of a research program the goal of which was an elucidation of the factors involved in the initiation of aggression in lactating animals. This chapter will summarize our findings. It is not meant to be a general survey of the research in maternal aggression for an excellent review can be found in Moyer (1974). Much of the research that will be reported was carried out in collaboration with Dr. Bruce Svare and supported by grants from the National Institutes of Health.

MATERNAL AGGRESSION AND INTERMALE AGGRESSION: A COMPARISON

The aggressive behavior of lactating mice differs markedly in certain respects from that normally exhibited by males and, for that matter, by testosterone-treated females, suggesting that maternal and intermale aggression may be controlled by different mechanisms. One such difference concerns behaviors which precede an actual biting attack. Rough-grooming and genital sniffing of the opponent and tail-rattling are exhibited by males just prior to an attack. It is not uncommon for these behaviors to account for more time than the fight itself. In contrast, these rather ritualized responses do not serve as a prelude to an aggressive encounter by lactating mice. Instead, the dam quickly initiates the fight by lunging at the opponent and biting at the neck and flank areas. Occasionally, short bursts of tail-rattling may be displayed by the female while attacking.

The absence in lactating mice of the stereotypic behaviors that are exhibited by males prior to an attack results in a very short latency to fight.

Lactating Rockland-Swiss albino mice[1] display a latency to attack of approximately 6 seconds whereas males generally begin to fight in about 150 seconds. Rowley and Christian (1976b), using descendents of wild-trapped *Peromyscus leucopus* reported no difference between lactating animals and males in the latency to aggress. (The range of latencies for both was about 4–340 seconds). In addition, significantly fewer lactating mice of strain C57BL and C3H display aggression as compared to mice of strain BALB, DBA, and HS (St. John and Corning, 1973). These data demonstrate strain differences in the propensity of lactating animals to fight as manifested in both the latency to attack and the actual appearance of an attack.

The intensity of the aggressive encounter differs between lactating and male mice. Basically, postpartum aggression appears to be much more intense than intermale aggression. Lactating animals spend considerably more time chasing and biting the opponent than do males. This difference may be due, partly, to the absence in females of ritualized behaviors during a fight. In particular, the 'submissive posture', standing on the hind paws and exposing the ventral surface, often exhibited by one member of a pair of males which appears to cause a temporary cessation of fighting on the part of the other member, does not alter the behavior of a lactating animal. For lack of a more insightful description, suffice it to say that the lactating female seems to be more ferocious than the male.

Another difference between the aggression of the male and the lactating female concerns the stimuli which elicit the behavior. It is well-established that olfactory cues exert a profound influence upon the aggressive behavior of male mice. These olfactory cues or pheromones determine, to a great extent, whether or not the male will initiate an attack. Specifically, an androgen-dependent aggression-promoting pheromone, emitted by mature males, triggers the initiation of an attack by another male (Mugford and Nowell, 1970). In contrast, mature females appear to release an ovarian-dependent aggression-inhibiting pheromone (Mugford and Nowell, 1971). The outcome of this differential sex-dependent emission of pheromonal stimuli is that males tend to attack males but not females. Lactating mice, however, attack males and females (Gandelman 1972; St. John and Corning, 1973). Thus, unlike the male, the behavior of the dam toward a conspecific is not determined by the sex of the opponent.

Rosenson and Asheroff (1975) reported that fewer gonadectomized animals of either sex were attacked by lactating animals as compared to intact

---

[1]Rockland-Swiss albino mice were derived from stock obtained from the late Dr. M. X. Zarrow. They have been maintained as an outbred strain in a closed colony. Rockland-Swiss mice were used in all of the research by us cited in this chapter.

animals. It is possible that ovarian and testicular steroid hormones act to produce a similar pheromone that facilitates maternal aggression toward males and females.

Although maternal aggression is not subject to the pheromonal constraints placed upon intermale aggression, it is obvious that it does occur in response to a particular environmental stimulus—the presence of another animal. What is it about that other animal that elicits an attack? We attempted to answer this by presenting lactating animals with mice of various ages (Svare and Gandelman, 1973). The results are summarized in Table 1. As can be seen, 20- and 14-day-old mice were attacked readily (and killed) whereas maternal behavior was displayed toward 1-day-olds. The dams were ambivalent toward 10-day-olds, displaying both aggression and maternal behavior. Generally, the adult would begin to retrieve the 10-day-old to the nest, stop and bite it, carry it a little further, bite it, lick it, and so forth. This finding led to a second question, namely, what is there about the 14-day-old that elicits attack? There are two major external morphological differences between 14- and 10-day-olds. One is that the 14-day-old is bigger. A second is that the 14-day-old has an adult-like coat of fur while the coat of the 10-day-old is still sparse. In an attempt to hold one of these factors constant while varying the other, lactating animals were presented with normal 14-day-olds and others that had had their fur removed. The results showed that few lactating animals (3 of 20) attacked the hairless 14-day-old mice, indicating, then, that fur may be one stimulus which elicits aggression. Thus, the young mouse stands more of a chance of being attacked by a lactating animal as it comes to resemble the adult. The 10-day-old may be perceived as being somewhat adult-like and somewhat infant-like, thereby eliciting both aggression and maternal behavior. Rowley and Christian (1977) reported that lactating *Peromyscus leucopus* attacked 19- to 23-day-old juveniles and that

TABLE 1
The Proportion of Lactating Mice that Aggressed Against, Ignored, Were Maternal Toward, and Were Ambivalent (Aggressive and Maternal) Towards a 20-, 14-, 10-, and a 1-Day Old Mouse Pup

	Age of Intruder (days)			
Behavior	20	14	10	1
Aggressive	15/20	15/20	1/20	0/20
Ignored	3/20	4/20	5/20	0/20
Ambivalent	2/20	1/20	11/20	0/20
Maternal	0/20	0/20	3/20	20/20

One pup was presented each day for four successive days. A total of 20 lactating mice were used (from Svare and Gandelman, 1973).

those that survived failed to reach sexual maturity. This propensity on the part of the lactating female to attack juveniles may serve to limit population growth.

In addition to the amount of fur, familiarity with the stimulus animal also modulates the display of postpartum aggression. Lactating animals rarely attacked an adult male that for seven days prior to testing resided in the cage of the dam and its young (Svare and Gandelman, 1973). The male was prevented from making physical contact with the dam and litter by placing it on the opposite side of a wire mesh partition. These data suggest that a novel cue is important for the elicitation of fighting behavior. The data of Lynds (1976) confirm this and show that the novel stimulus is an olfactory one. Wild lactating mice were tested for aggression against wild males coated with either urine of the test female, urine of other wild females, or water. Significantly more aggression was directed against males coated with urine from other females ("strange urine") than against males coated with the test female's own urine or water.

The conditions under which tests for fighting are conducted can further differentiate intermale from maternal aggression. St. John and Corning (1973) reported that males were equally likely to attack in the homecage and strange test cage whereas females attacked only about half as much in a strange cage. The authors stated:

> The relatively lower number of female attacks in the strange cage suggests that in nature the attack disposition of maternal females decreases rapidly with distance from the nest. Such a restriction of attack behavior would have considerable adaptive significance, since females would be less likely to initiate conflicts with dominant males on neutral grounds, where, other things being equal, one would expect the greater size and history of successful combat to favor the males (p. 639).

In short, there are a number of striking differences between the aggressive behavior displayed by males and that of lactating females. These differences involve the topography of the encounter, its intensity, and its eliciting stimuli. There is one other difference which, because of its obviousness, was not mentioned. Simply stated, postpartum aggression only occurs when the animal is lactating whereas intermale aggression occurs anytime subsequent to maturity. The following section deals with the relationship between lactation and aggression.

MATERNAL AGGRESSION AND LACTATION

Postpartum aggression is exhibited by the female between the birth and weaning of its young. Although Noirot (1969) reported that aggressive behavior in mice occurs during gestation, peaks toward the time of parturition, and then declines, neither St. John and Corning (1973) nor we (Svare and Gandelman, 1976a) have observed an increased frequency of fighting during pregnancy. In order to more precisely specify the relationship between lactation and aggression, fighting behavior was examined throughout the course of the 21-day lactation period (Svare and Gandelman, 1973). Animals were tested twice a day by placing either an adult male or female into their cages and recording the amount of time during the 3 minute session that the dam spent biting the stimulus animal. Aggression was highest between Day 3 and 7, declined between Day 8 and 14, and was lowest between Day 15 and 21.

Another experiment was performed to determine whether an animal would display maternal aggression across a number of lactation periods and the extent to which aggression is displayed (Svare and Gandelman, 1976a). Fifty

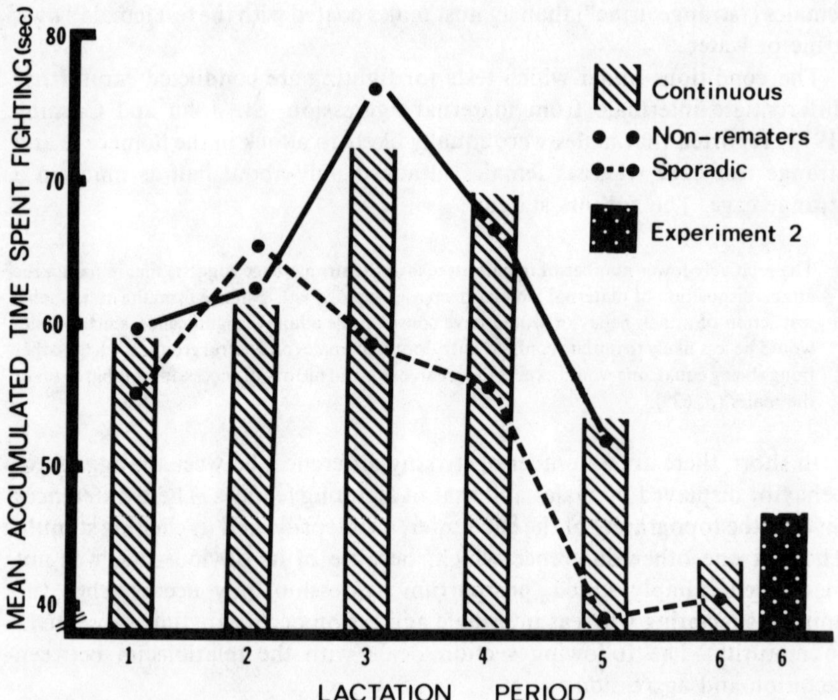

FIG. 1. Average accumulated time spent fighting on each lactation period. Most mice fought during every lactation (continuous) while some fought during some but not others (sporadic). Non-rematers did not complete 6 lactations but fought during every lactation period they did complete. The stippled bar depicts the data from mice that were tested for aggression only during the 6th lactation period. (From Svare and Gandelman, 1975).

nulliparous mice were tested for fighting on Day 6, 10, 14, and 18 of six successive pregnancies and lactation periods or until they ceased to remate. As expected, fighting did not occur during pregnancy but only during lactation. The results are depicted in Figure 1. Although most animals fought during every lactation period completed, some mice fought during some but not others. The amount of aggression was determined by assessing the amount of time spent biting and chasing the stimulus animal. Fighting increased across the first three lactations and declined thereafter to a point below initial levels. To determine whether the decline was due to the fighting experience obtained during previous lactations or whether it was due to something unrelated to experience, additional animals were tested for fighting during only their sixth lactation. Their results also are shown in Figure 1. It is clear that their level of aggression was similar to that of animals having been tested during the first 5 lactations.

We cannot as yet account for the changes in the amount of aggressive behavior over successive lactation periods. It may, perhaps, be related to litter size which increased across the first four reproductive cycles and declined thereafter. Furthermore, animals that exhibited high overall levels of aggression tended to produce more young than did animals displaying lower overall levels. This suggests either the existence of a biologically adaptive mechanism favoring increased fecundity of highly aggressive dams or that increased fecundity augments aggression.

The results of these experiments emphasize again the relationship between lactation and aggression. At this point we began what to us seemed the most important aspect of the research program, that of specifying the aspect of lactation that is related causally to fighting behavior. This is considered in the following section.

THE SUCKLING STIMULUS: A POSSIBLE MECHANISM

The term 'lactation' has been defined in two ways. Endocrinologists define it as the production and secretion of milk from the mammary glands while to others, most notably psychologists, it suggests the act of transmitting milk from the mother to the young, that is, nursing. Both definitions, one concerned with the physiological and the other with the behavioral component, are correct and important aspects of the phenomenon. In order to delineate the aspect of lactation that is related causally to aggression, various approaches were taken. One was to separate the young from the dam for various periods of time prior to the assessment of aggression (Gandelman, 1972). Lactating mice having previously displayed fighting behavior were retested after being separated from their young for either 1 or 5 hours on the

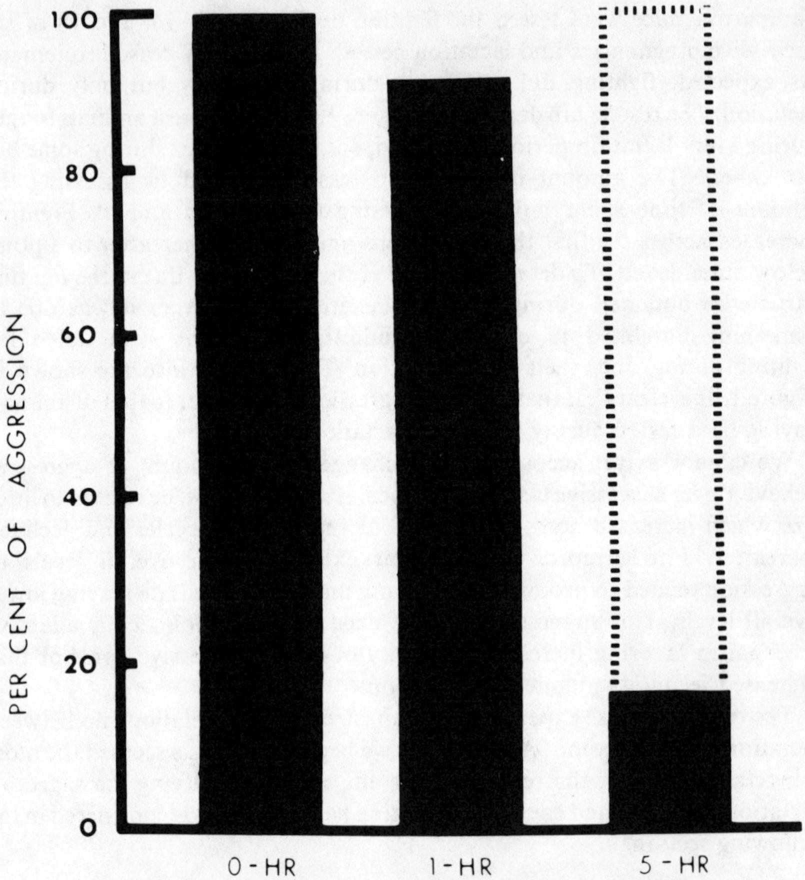

PER CENT OF AGGRESSION

100
80
60
40
20
0

0-HR 1-HR 5-HR

FIG. 2. Percentage of lactating mice that fought after their young had been removed either for 0, 1, or 5 hours on Postpartum Day 8. The hatched bar shows the data of other animals that were tested 5 minutes after their young were returned following 5 hours of separation. (After Gandelman, 1972).

eighth postpartum day. The results appear in Figure 2. It is obvious that 5 hours of separation led to a significant decline in the number of animals that fought. It also was found that aggressive behavior was restored in animals that had been separated from their young for 5 hours by replacing the offspring for as little as 5 minutes prior to the fighting test (Svare and Gandelman, 1973). Thus, removal of the suckling stimulus eliminates and restoration of the stimulus restores fighting behavior.

If suckling stimulation is a sufficient condition for the establishment of aggression, one should be able to advance the normal onset of aggressive behavior by inducing lactation and nursing prior to the time in which it normally occurs, that is, prior to parturition. Such a demonstration, in addition to implicating suckling stimulation, would mean that parturition is not necessary for the appearance of maternal aggression. Our first task, then, became one of inducing lactation prior to parturition. This was accomplished by hysterectomizing animals during gestation. Hysterectomy of mice from Day 12 of pregnancy onward induced lactation as assessed by weight gain of 1-day-old foster young (Gandelman and Svare, 1975). Lactation did not develop if hysterectomy was performed prior to the 12th day. This procedure, we believe, produces lactation by removing the placental source of luteotrophin, a substance that maintains the release of progesterone from the corpora lutea. Thus, removal of placental tissue causes a fall in the level of progesterone. Since progesterone putatively blocks lactation, hysterectomy will remove the block, permitting lactation to commence.

After having developed a procedure for advancing the onset of lactation, testing was carried out to discover whether aggression would be advanced as well (Gandelman and Svare, 1974). Immediately following hysterectomy on Day 14 of gestation, animals were given five 1-day-old foster young which were exchanged each day for another set of 1-day-olds in order to maintain constancy of the suckling stimulus. Lactation was assessed by weighing the young before and after their stay with the foster mother. Two days later the adult received the first of three daily tests for fighting. These data, along with those of control animals, are summarized in Table 2. It is clear that animals hysterectomized on Day 14 of pregnancy and given foster young displayed maternal aggression. Hysterectomy alone or pup-fostering alone were without effect.

In another experiment, groups of animals were hysterectomized on Days 10–15 of pregnancy. As in the previous experiment, all animals were given foster young and were tested for aggression. The data, given in Table 3, show

TABLE 2
The Number of 14-Day Pregnant Mice Hysterectomized and Presented with Young (HYST), Sham-Operated and Presented with Young (SHAM), Left Undisturbed and Allowed to Deliver (PART), and Hysterectomized (HYST-NP) that Lactated and Fought with Adult Male Mouse
(From Gandelman and Svare, 1974).

	Group			
	HYST	*SHAM*	*PART*	*HYST-NP*
Number lactating (n = 16)	15	0	16	—
Number fighting (n = 16)	10	1	8	0

TABLE 3
The Number of Mice that Lactated and Fought as a Function of the Day of Gestation on Which Hysterectomy was Performed. Fifteen Animals were Hysterectomized on each of the 6 Gestation Days (From Gandelman and Svare, 1974).

	Day of Hysterectomy					
	10	11	12	13	14	15
Number lactating	1	3	10	15	15	15
Number fighting	1	4	5	8	9	10
Number lactating and fighting	0	2	4	8	9	10

that fighting behavior was induced only if hysterectomy was performed at a time of gestation during which lactation could be established. The results of these lactation-advancement experiments supported the idea of a causal relationship between the stimulation arising from nursing and fighting. The following series of experiments was conducted to further substantiate this hypothesis.

Instead of establishing maternal aggression by manipulating the onset of lactation, the effect of removing suckling stimulation was assessed (Svare and Gandelman, 1976b). This was done by surgically excising the nipples (thelectomy) of the adult and presenting her with replete foster young. It must be noted that thelectomy does not interfere with the display of a variety of maternal activities such as pup-retrieval, anogenital licking, and the assumption of nursing postures over the young. The results are given in Table 4. It was found in the first experiment that thelectomy prior to mating caused a reduction in the number of postparturient animals displaying aggression (only 4 of 24 fought). A similar effect was produced when thelectomy was performed on the 18th day of pregnancy. What role does suckling stimulation play in the maintenance of fighting, that is, its role when animals already have received suckling stimulation from the young? This question was dealt with by thelectomizing animals at various times subsequent to parturition. Thelectomy on Postpartum Day 5 did not affect the percentage of animals that fought when tests were conducted on Postpartum Days 6–12. Similarly, thelectomy on Postpartum Day 5 was without effect when animals were tested on Days 12–16. However, removal of the suckling stimulus 24 hours following delivery significantly reduced the number of animals that fought when tests were begun on Day 2 postpartum.

These experiments show quite clearly that most animals must receive suckling stimulation for the first two to four days following delivery in order for postpartum aggression to be established. Aggression on Postpartum Day 5 and, presumably, onward can be maintained in the absence of stimulation

TABLE 4
The Results of 5 Experiments Describing the Behavior of Thelectomized Mice Fostered Young (Thel-P) and Sham Thelectomized Mice Fostered (Sham-P) and Not Fostered Young (Sham-NP) toward Adult Males. In Experiment 5 Thelectomy and the Fostering of Young Occurred either 24 (Thel-24-P) or 48 hr (Thel-48-P) following Parturition. Sham Operations were Performed 24 hr following Parturition (Sham-24-P) (from Svare and Gandelman, 1976b).

Experiment	*Time of Thelectomy*	*Group*	*Proportion and Percentage of Animals Fighting*	*Presence or Absence of Milk in Mammary Glands*
1	Prior to mating	Sham-P	17/24 (71%)	+
		Thel-P	4/24 (17%)	0
		Sham-NP	0/24 (0%)	0
2	Day 18 of Pregnancy	Sham-P	15/24 (63%)	+
		Thel-P	3/24 (13%)	0
3	Postpartum Day 5 (First test-Postpartum Day 6)	Sham-P	12/24 (50%)	+
		Thel-P	13/24 (54%)	0
4	Postpartum Day 5 (First test-Postpartum Day 12)	Sham-P	15/24 (63%)	+
		Thel-P	17/24 (71%)	0
5	Immediate post-partum interval	Sham-24-P	15/24 (63%)	+
		Thel-48-P	15/24 (63%)	0
		Thel-24-P	6/24 (25%)	0

from the young. This finding agrees with other data which show that maternal aggression can be maintained by nonsuckling stimulation from the young, that is, by stimulation other than tactile stimulation of the nipples. For example and as mentioned previously, as little as 5 minutes of exposure to young following 5 hours of separation from them reestablished fighting behavior (Svare and Gandelman, 1973). In a number of cases, however, adults that fought did not nurse during the 5-minute replacement period. Also, aggression can be maintained by placing young on the opposite side of a wire mesh partition in the cage of the dam (Svare and Gandelman, 1973). It is not as yet known what stimuli from the young maintain aggression. It has been reported that prolactin, a hormone essential for lactation, is released by the pituitary of the lactating rat in response to nontactile stimulation from the young (Grosvenor, 1965; Grosvenor et al., 1970). Specifically, it was shown that prolactin release occurs in response to the odor of young (Mena and Grosvenor, 1971). It is possible that a similar mechanism functions to maintain aggression in the absence of tactile stimulation from the offspring. Such a mechanism, however, would involve a hormone other than prolactin for we have found that the administration of the prolactin-releasing blocker ergocornine hydrogen maleate to lactating mice eliminates milk production but does not affect maternal aggression (unpublished observations). Interestingly, Wise and Pryor (1977) reported that ergocornine treatment significantly reduces the aggressive behavior of lactating hamsters, suggesting the existence of species differences in the maintenance of postpartum aggression.

As compelling as these data are in inferring a link between the receipt of suckling stimulation and the initiation of aggression, further testing seemed warranted owing to the potential import of these findings. Instead of eliminating aggression in the lactating animal and inducing fighting in the pregnant animal, a different tactic was chosen, that of establishing aggression in the nonpregnant, nonlactating mouse by exposure to the suckling stimulus. If suckling induces aggression, then the virgin female should fight if it receives an adequate amount of nipple stimulation. The first attempt at testing this consisted of presenting foster young to the virgin female. The young were left with the adult for 24 hours and were then exchanged for other nourished young. This procedure continued for 10 days. It should be noted that mice are spontaneously maternal, exhibiting pup-retrieval, anogenital licking, and nursing posturing regardless of reproductive state (c.f. Beniest-Noirot, 1958). The attempt failed. None of the animals attacked an intruder when tested every other day beginning on Day 11. In examining the females, it was noticed that the nipples were very small, precluding the foster young from attaching and sucking. Thus, it seemed likely that the adult did not receive nipple stimulation adequate for the establishment of aggression. This negative finding prompted still another approach.

Ovariectomized virgin females were administered a regimen of hormones which produces nipple growth (Svare and Gandelman, 1976c). The regimen consisted of 19 daily injections of .02 *u*g estradiol benzoate and 500 *u*g progesterone. (Table 5 shows the effect of this treatment as well as nipple growth normally seen in parturient mice). All animals were tested for aggression 24 hours after the final injection. Immediately following the aggression test, each animal was presented with five 3- to 8-day-old foster young. Another aggression test was given on the following day. After this test the young were removed and replaced by five replete young. This was necessary because the hormone treatment, although producing growth of mammary tissue and nipples, did not induce milk production. This procedure was continued for nine additional days or was terminated when an animal exhibited aggression on two successive days.

The results, given in Table 6, show that none of the animals fought when tested 24 hours following the last injection, prior to the presentation of young. However, 12 of 24 hormone-treated mice fought following the presentation of

TABLE 5
Average Length (mm) and Base Diameter of a Representative Nipple of Different Animals. Animals were either Mated (parturient), Ovariectomized and Hormonally Primed with Oestradiol Benzoate and Progesterone (OVX+OB+P), Ovariectomized and Treated with Oil (S-OVX+Oil). (from Svare and Gandelman, 1976c).

Group	*Average Length*	*Base Diameter*
Parturient	1.40 ± 0.05*†	0.66 ± 0.06*†
OVX+OB+P	0.99 ± 0.07	0.55 ± 0.14*
OVX+Oil	0.49 ± 0.08	0.43 ± 0.08
S-OVX+Oil	0.47 ± 0.13	0.41 ± 0.06

*Significantly different (Fisher's least significant difference test, $P < 0.05$) from OVX + Oil and S–OVX + Oil.
†Significantly different from OVX + OB + P.

young. Daily inspection of the hormone-treated animals after exposure to the young revealed red and distended nipples. Also, the nipples were large enough to permit the pups to attach themselves to them such that they could maintain contact with the adult when the latter was lifted by the tail.

Since fighting behavior was not exhibited prior to the presentation of young, it appears that the factor critical for the initiation of aggression was the receipt of suckling stimulation which was now adequate due to the increased size of the nipples. To corroborate this, ovariectomized virgins were administered the hormone regimen and were thelectomized prior to the presentation of young. The results of this experiment are given in Table 6 and reveal that hormone-treated thelectomized animals typically do not display aggression.

DISCUSSION

We feel that the data demonstrate that suckling stimulation is a necessary and sufficient stimulus for the initiation of maternal aggressive behavior. At this time we only can speculate as to the mechanism by which suckling stimulation produces its rather dramatic effect. One possibility is that the neural signals arising in response to the suckling stimulus impinge upon an area of the central nervous system involved in agonistic display.

For many years investigators have been interested in specifying the areas of the brain involved in the milk-letdown reflex. To that end, data have been obtained which show that certain areas receive afferent input from the

TABLE 6

Experiment 1: aggressive behavior of RS female mice that were either mated (parturient), ovariectomized and primed with oestradiol benzoate and progesterone to induce nipple growth (OVX+OB+P), ovariectomized and treated with oil (OVX+Oil), or sham ovariectomized and given oil (S-OVX+Oil). Aggressive behavior was scored before exposure to pups (on the last day of hormone or oil treatment or on day 19 of gestation) and on each succeeding day for 10 d after presentation of foster young or until fights were displayed on 2 successive days. Experiment 2: aggressive behavior of RS females that were mated and either thelectomized (parturient-THEL) or sham thelectomized on day 19 of pregnancy (parturient-S-Thel) and of ovariectomized hormone-treated mice either thelectomized (OVX+OB+P-THEL) or sham thelectomized (OVX+OB+P-S-THEL) on the day after the last hormone injections. (from Svare and Gandelman, 1976c).

Group	*n*	*No. Fighting Before Presenting Foster Young*	*Proportion (and %) of Animals Fighting After Pup Exposure*	*Latency to Begin Fighting After Pup Exposure (d)*	*Average No. of Fights*†*
Experiment 1					
Parturient	22	0	12/22 (54)	1.8 ± 0.8	—
OVX+OB+P	24	0	12/24 (50)	1.3 ± 0.6	—
OVX+Oil	20	0	1/20 (05)	1.0	—
S-OVX+Oil	19	0	1/19 (05)	2.0	—
Experiment 2					
Parturient-THEL	20	0	4/20 (20)	1.3 ± 0.8	9.8 ± 0.4
Parturient-S-THEL	20	0	13/20 (65)	1.6 ± 1.1	8.6 ± 2.1
OVX+OB+P-THEL	20	0	2/20 (10)	2.5 ± 1.5	8.0 ± 1.0
OVX+OB+P-S-THEL	20	0	12/20 (60)	2.1 ± 2.4	8.2 ± 2.5

*Animals in experiment 1 were killed after they fought in two successive tests.

†Animals in experiment 2 were given 10 aggression tests. The data are derived from only the animals that fought.

nipples. The data can be summarized as follows: 1) Afferent signals from the nipples travel along the dorsal roots of the spinal cord (Eayrs and Baddeley, 1956; Mena and Beyer, 1963). 2) The input reaches the brainstem and from there the hypothalamus (Anderson, 1951; Cross, 1961). 3) The periventricular-diencephalic region of the hypothalamus has been implicated as the location through which pass afferent signals from the nipples. Lincoln and Wakerley (1974, 1975), using electrophysiological recording techniques in the lactating rat, reported an activation of supraoptic and paraventricular cells as a consequence of suckling stimulation. The hypothalamus, therefore, receives neural input from the nipples which in turn affects pituitary functioning.

The hypothalamus also has been implicated in the mediation of agonistic behavior (c.f. Panksepp and Trowill, 1969; Chi and Flynn, 1971; Woodworth, 1971). It is possible that afferent signals arising from the nipples in response to the suckling stimulus, in addition to triggering the milk-letdown reflex, eventuate into the activation of hypothalamic neurons involved in the display of aggressive behavior.

Another possibility is that stimulation of the nipples by nursing young is aversive and that the adult actually is displaying what Moyer (1968) has termed "irritable aggression." According to Moyer, irritability and, thus, the tendency to aggress can be instigated by any stressor. Also, irritable aggression is nonspecific in nature, that is, it is constrained less by the stimulus characteristics of the opponent than are other forms of aggression. This somewhat characterizes maternal aggression in that the dam will attack males and females, adults and juveniles, and even members of other species. (We have observed lactating mice to attack adult rats). Thus, it is possible that nursing itself is stressful, evoking aggression from the parturient animal.

It is apparent that much more needs to be learned concerning the relationship between suckling stimulation and aggression. One major issue concerns whether and to what extent the findings obtained from mice generalize to other species. One thing, however, is certain. For the mouse, suckling not only serves to transmit nutrients from the mother to its young, but also drastically alters the relationship between the dam and other members of its species and, for that matter, members of other species. It is hoped that the research thus far conducted will serve as an impetus for future investigation both by researchers concerned with maternal behavior and those focusing upon agonistic behavior.

ACKNOWLEDGMENTS

The writing of this chapter was supported by Grant HD-06863 from NICHD, NIH by Grant MH-28660 from NIH and by Grant BNS-07347 from NSF. Thanks are extended to Dr. June M. Reinisch for insightful comments on earlier versions of the manuscript.

REFERENCES

Altman, M. In *Maternal Behavior in Mammals*. H. L. Rheingold, ed. John Wiley and Son, New York (1963).

Anderson, B. The effect and localization of electrical stimulation of certain parts of the brain stem in sheep and goats. *Acta Physiol. Scand. 23*, 8–11 (1951).

Barnett, S. A., In *Aggressive Behavior*. S. Garattini and E. B. Sigg, eds. John Wiley and Son, New York (1969).

Beach, F. A. *Hormones and Behavior*. Hoeber, New York (1948).

Beniest-Noirot, E. Analyse du comportement dit "maternal" chez la souris. *Mong. Francaises de Psychol.* Paris No. 1 (1958).

Chance, N., and Jolly, C. *Social Groups of Monkeys, Apes, and Man*. E. P. Dutton, New York (1970).

Chi, C. C., and Flynn, J. P. Neural pathways associated with hypothalamically elicited attack behavior in cats. *Science 171*, 703–706 (1971).

Cross, B. A. In *Oxytocin*. R. Calderjera and R. Barcia, eds. Pergamon Press, London (1961).

DeVore, I. In *Maternal Behavior in Mammals*. H. L. Rheingold, ed. John Wiley & Sons, Inc., New York 305–335 (1963).

Eayrs, J. T., and Baddeley, R. M. Neural pathways in lactation. *J. Anat. 90*, 161–172 (1956).

Edwards, D. A. Mice: Fighting by neonatally androgenized females. *Science 161*, 1027–1028 (1968).

Edwards, D. A. Neural and endocrine control of aggressive behavior. In *Hormonal Correlates of Behavior*, Vol. I, R. L. Sprott and B. E. Eleftherious, eds. Plenum Press, New York (1975), pp. 276–303.

Fleming, A. S., and Rosenblatt, J. S. Maternal behavior in the virgin and lactating rat. *J. Comp. Physiol. Psychol. 86*, 957–972 (1974).

Gandelman, R. Mice: Postpartum aggression elicited by the presence of an intruder. *Horm. Behav. 3*, 23 (1972).

Gandelman, R. and Svare, B. Mice: Pregnancy termination, lactation, and aggression. *Horm. Behav. 5*, 397–405 (1974).

Gandelman, R. and Svare, B. Lactation following hysterectomy of pregnant mice. *Biol. Reprod. 12*, 360–367 (1975).

Grosvenor, C. E. Evidence that exteroceptive stimuli can release prolactin from the pituitary gland of the lactating rat. *Endocrinology 76*, 340–342 (1965).

Grosvenor, C. E., Maiweg, H., and Mena, F. A study of factors involved in the development of the exteroceptive release of prolactin in the lactating rat. *Horm. Behav. 1*, 111–120 (1970).

Jay, P. In *Maternal Behavior in Mammals*, H. L. Rheingold, ed. John Wiley & Sons, Inc., New York (1963).

King, J. A. In *Maternal Behavior in Mammals*, H. L. Rheingold, ed. John Wiley & Sons, Inc., New York 58–93, 282–304 (1963).

LeRoy, L. M. and Krehbiel, D. A. Variations in maternal behavior in the rat as a function of sex and gonadal state. *Horm. Behav. II*, 232–247 (1978).

Lincoln, D. W. and Wakerley, J. B. Electrophysiological evidence for the activation of supraoptic neurons during the release of oxytocin. *J. Physiol. 242*, 533–554 (1974).

Lincoln, D. W. and Wakerley, J. B. Factors governing the periodic activation of supraoptic and paraventricular neurosecretory cells during suckling in the rat. *J. Physiol. 250*, 443–461 (1975).

Lynds, P. G. Olfactory control of aggression in lactating female housemice. *Physiol. Behav. 17*, 157–159 (1976).

Mena, F. and Beyer, C. Effect of high spinal section on established lactation in the rabbit. *Amer. J. Physiol. 205*, 313–319 (1963).

Mena, F. and Grosvenor, C. E. Release of prolactin in rats by exteroceptive stimulation: Sensory stimuli involved. *Horm. Behav. 2*, 107–116 (1971).

Moyer, K. E. Kinds of aggression and their physiological basis. *Commun. Behav. Biol. 2*, 65–87 (1968).

Moyer, K. E. Sex differences in aggression. In *Sex Differences in Behavior*, R. C. Friedman, R. M. Richart, and R. L. Vande Wiele, eds. John Wiley & Sons, Inc., New York (1974), pp. 335–372.

Mugford, R. A., and Nowell, N. W. Pheromones and their effect on aggression in mice. *Nature 226*, 967–968 (1970).

Mugford, R. A., and Nowell, N. W. Endocrine control over production and activity of the anti-aggression pheromone from female mice. *J. Endocrinol. 49*, 225–232 (1971).

Mykytowycz, R. Social behaviour of an experimental colony of wild rabbits, *Oryctolagus cuniculus. C.S.I.R.O. Wildlife Research 4*, 1–13 (1959).

Noirot, E. Interactions between reproductive and territorial behaviour in female mice. *Int. Mental Health Res. Newslett. 11*, 10–11 (1969).

Panksepp, J., and Trowill, J. A. Electrically induced affective attack from the hypothalamus of the albino rat. *Psychon. Sci. 16*, 118–119 (1969).

Rosenblatt, J. S. Nonhormonal basis of maternal behavior in the rat. *Science 156*, 1512–1514 (1967).

Rosenson, L. M. and Asheroff, A. K. Maternal aggression in CD-1 mice: Influence of the hormonal condition of the intruder. *Behav. Biol. 15*, 219–224 (1975).

Rowley, M. H. and Christian, J. J. Interspecific aggression between *Peromyscus* and *Microtus* females: A possible factor in competitive exclusion. *Behav. Biol. 16*, 521–525 (1976a).

Rowley, M. H. and Christian, J. J. Intraspecific aggression of *Peromyscus leucopus. Behav. Biol. 17*, 249–253 (1976b).

Rowley, M. H. and Christian, J. J. Competition between lactating *Peromyscus leucopus* and juvenile *Microtus pennsylvanicus. Behav. Biol. 20*, 70–80 (1977).

Schneirla, T. C. Rosenblatt, J. S., and Tobach, E. In *Maternal Behavior in Mammals*, H. L. Rheingold, ed., John Wiley & Sons, Inc., New York 122–168 (1963).

St. John, R. D. and Corning, P. A. Maternal aggression in mice. *Behav. Biol. 9*, 635–639 (1973).

Svare, B. and Gandelman, R. Postpartum aggression in mice: Experiential and environmental factors. *Horm. Behav.* 4, 323–334 (1973).

Svare, B. and Gandelman, R. A longitudinal analysis of maternal aggression in Rockland-Swiss albino mice. *Devel. Psychobiol. 9*, 437–446 (1976a).

Svare, B. and Gandelman, R. Postpartum aggression in mice: The influence of suckling stimulation. *Horm. Behav. 7*, 407–416 (1976b).

Svare, B., and Gandelman, R. Suckling stimulation induces aggression in virgin female mice. *Nature 260*, 606–608 (1976c).

Taylor, J. C. In *Play, Exploration, and Territory in Mammals*, P. A. Jewell and C. Loizos, eds. Academic Press, New York 229–235 (1966).

Wise, D. A. Aggression in the female golden hamster: Effects of reproductive state and social isolation. *Horm. Behav. 5*, 235–250 (1974).

Wise, D. A., and Pryor, T. L. Effects of ergocornine and prolactin on aggression in the postpartum golden hamster. *Horm. Behav. 8*, 30–39 (1977).

Woodworth, C. H. Attack elicited in rats by electrical stimulation of the lateral hypothalamus. *Physiol. Behav. 6*, 345–353 (1971).

Maternal Influences and Early Behavior

5 Ultrasonic Behavior and Mother-Infant Interactions in Rodents

Jane C. Smith

Gillian D. Sales

In all mammals the relationship between the mother and her young is vital for the successful physical and behavioral development of the young. In rodents, as in other mammals, the initiation and maintenance of this relationship depends on communication between the mother and young and this may be through visual, auditory, thermal, tactile or olfactory cues.

In altricial rodents the pups are immobile for the first few days after birth and the mother must approach her young to give them maternal care. As the young develop they become progressively more active and approach responses may be made by both mother and pups. During the last stage of development the pups readily approach the mother to nurse but she begins to reject them until they become independent.

Of prime importance in the development of many young rodents is access to the mother, not only for food, but also for warmth. The majority of rodent species are poikilothermic at birth and until homeothermy is fully developed the pups rely on the warmth of the mother's body and the thermal insulation of the nest and siblings to maintain their body temperature. Among murid and cricetid species the pups vary in their degree of physical growth and their sensory and motor development at birth. This affects the relative importance of mother-infant relationships in the various species. For example, the house mouse (*Mus musculus*) is altricial and is born without fur, unable to crawl, to thermoregulate, or to see or hear. The eyes open at about 13 days and the development of homeothermy begins on about Day 6–7 but it is not complete until about 20 days (Okon, 1970a) although the young are weaned at about 18 days in the wild (Southern, 1964). Some other species such as the

Mongolian gerbil (*Meriones unguiculatus*) and the woodmouse (*Apodemus sylvaticus*) develop rather more slowly than the house mouse; the eyes open at 19–20 days and 16–18 days respectively, the development of homeothermy begins on about Day 6 but is not completed until about 24 days (McManus, 1971; Okon, 1972). Gerbils leave the nest at about 20 days and woodmice become independent at about 21 days (Southern, 1964). On the other hand some other species in these groups are more precocial, for example the spiny mouse (*Acomys cahirinus*) which has fur at birth and the pups walk and open their eyes on the first day. The pups leave the nest at about six days after birth (Dieterlen, 1961) and presumably thermoregulation is similarly advanced.

In many myomorph rodent species then, separation of very young pups from the mother will result in a loss of warmth by the pups and if the separation involves displacement of the pups from the nest, it may also result in changes in their olfactory and tactile environment. During prolonged separation the pups may also suffer increased hunger. Perhaps the most obvious response of murid and cricetid rodent pups to separation from the mother is the production of loud and persistent ultrasonic cries. These calls are also produced in response to rough handling and to lack of familiar olfactory cues. Although other stimuli from the pups are by no means thought to be unimportant in the mother-infant relationship, it is likely that the ultrasonic cries from the pups play a major part in eliciting and maintaining maternal behavior, particularly searching or approaching responses during the period when the pups' motor abilities are poor.

THE ULTRASONIC CRIES OF PUPS

Structure

The structure of the ultrasonic calls of laboratory rats and mice has been studied in some detail, while more superficial studies have been made on other species. These show that there are certain differences between the calls of infant murid and cricetid rodents. Most of the calls of murids are comparatively long, up to 200 ms, and are relatively stereotyped in structure, consisting of a single frequency component that shows a gradual onset and cessation with little frequency or amplitude modulation (e.g. Noirot and Pye, 1969; Bell et al., 1972; Sales and Smith, 1978) (Fig. 1a). Exceptions to this are some of the calls of spiny mice (Sewell, 1969) and the calls of hopping mice, *Notomys* spp. (Watts, 1975) and other Australian murid rodents which consist of a fundamental and one or more harmonic components (Fig. 1b). Some of the calls of infant house mice also differ from the basic pattern in containing frequency jumps of up to 36 kHz (Fig. 1c). A summary of pulse

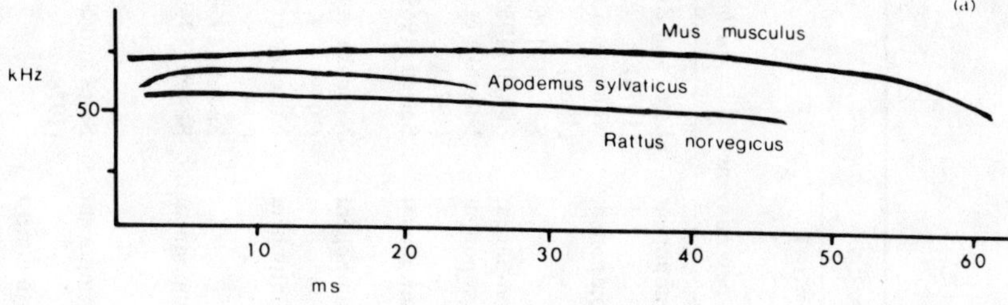

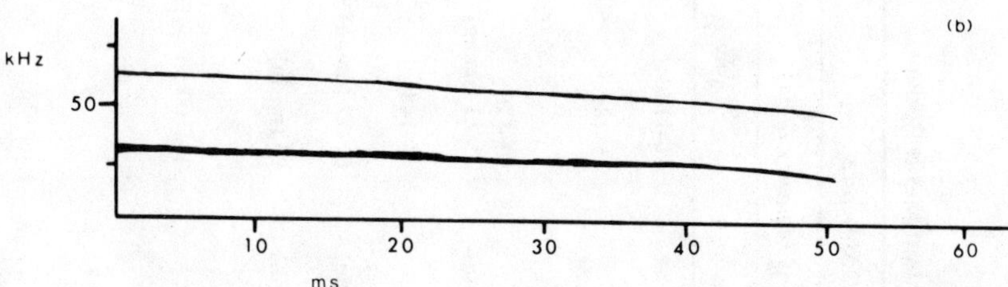

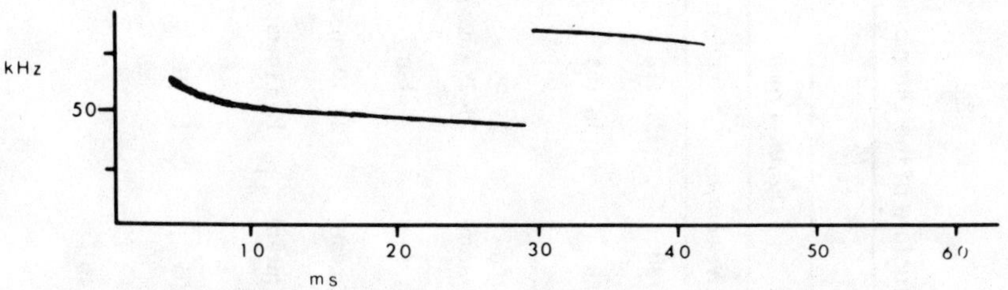

FIG. 1. Sonagrams of typical calls of newborn murid rodents: a) calls produced by house mouse, *Mus musculus*; woodmouse, *Apodemus sylvaticus*; and Norway rat, *Rattus norvegicus*, pups showing drifts in frequency, b) call produced by a 1 day old spiny mouse *Acomys cahirinus* showing a fundamental and one harmonic component, c) call produced by a 4 day old albino laboratory house mouse showing a frequency step upwards.

parameters for the pups of various species is given in Tables 1 and 2. These show that there is considerable overlap in the total ranges of pulse frequency and duration among the different murid and cricetid species.

Although there appear to be no exclusively species-specific frequency bands, a more thorough survey is required to reveal the extent of differences between the calls of various species. Detailed studies have already indicated

TABLE 1
Structure of the Ultrasonic Calls of Infant Murid Rodents.

	Animals		Call Structure					
			Duration (ms)		Frequency (kHz)			
Species	*Day Eyes Open*	*Day Isol. Calls Cease*	*Newborn*	*Older*	*Newborn*	*Older*	*Frequency Patterns*	*Author*
Mus musculus (wild)	13	13	15–180	21–112	35–90	42–118	single component	Sales and Smith (1978)
M. musculus (EN*)	13	13	8–140	30–105	40–120	45–148	single component	Noirot and Pye (1969)
								Sewell (1969)
M. musculus (C_3H)	13	13	30–100	25–95	60–85	50–120	single component	Sewell (1969)
	13		48 (mean)	25–38 (mean)	78 (mean)	75–81 (mean)	single component	Nitschke et al (1972)
M. musculus (C_3H × EN)	13	13	23–136	25–130	45–116	38–148	single component	Sewell (1969)
M. musculus (BALB)	13		48 (mean)	24–40 (mean)	69 (mean)	69–77 (mean)	single component	Nitschke et al (1972)
M. musculus (C57)	13		20 (mean)	12.5 (mean)	78 (mean)	80 (mean)	single component	Nitschke et al (1972)
M. minutoides					70–90			Sewell (1969)
Rattus norvegicus albino Wistar	15–16	16	2–205	1–170	35–112	30–100	single component	Sewell (1969)
R. exulans	12–14		3–140		35–80		single component	Sales and Smith (1978)
R. villosissimus					30 or wideband		single component or harmonic series	Watts (in litt.)

Arvicanthis niloticus	6–7		30–50	15–30	60–90	65–80	single component	Sales and Smith (1978)
Apodemus sylvaticus	16–18	19	5–145	3–200	35–100	38–117	single component	Sewell (1969)
								Sales and Smitn (1978)
A. flavicollis			10–170		50–92		single component	Sales and Smith (1978)
		13						Zippelius (1974)
Acomys cahirinus	1	6	100–200	2–70	30–50	50–95	fundamental often + 1 h.†	Sewell (1969)
Praomys natalensis					60–90			Sewell (1969)
Thamnomys sp.			60–150	5–30	35–60	30–80	single component	Sewell (1969)
Pseudomys australis		7	50–150		24–40	28–40	many h.	Watts (1976)
	14–18							Smith et al (1972)
Notomys alexis		14	10–100		35–55		many h.	Watts (1975)
	19–21							Happold (1976)
N. cervinus		10	30–100		30–40		wideband	Watts (1975)
	17–28							Smith et al. (1972)
N. mitchelii		14	20–90		22–40		many h.	Watts (1975)
	18–23							Smith et al. (1972)
N. fuscus		7	10–40		35–70		many h.	Watts (1975)

*EN mice—albino mice from E. Noirot's colony.
†h—harmonic component.

TABLE 2
Structure of the Ultrasonic Calls of Infant Cricetid Rodents.

	Animals		Call Structure					
			Duration (ms)		Frequency (kHz)			
Species	*Day Eyes Open*	*Day Isol. Calls Cease*	*Newborn*	*Older*	*Newborn*	*Older*	*Frequency Patterns*	*Author*
Clethrionomys glareolus	13–14	10–12	3–100	3–30	20–55	60–110	single component or fundamental + 1 h.*	Sewell (1969)
Microtus agrestis	11		5–120	3–30	20–125	20–110	single component or fundamental + 1 h.	Sewell (1969) Smith (unpub.)
M. arvalis		16	25–60		35–46			Zippelius (1974)
M. arvalis orcadensis	11		1†) 27–135		20–72		single component or fundamental + 1 h.	Smith (unpub.)
			2) 33–52		12–72		multicomponent	
M. pennsylvanicus			79 (mean)		39 (mean fundamental)		single component or fundamental + 1 h.	Colvin (1973)
M. montanus			74 (mean)		39 (mean fundamental)		single component or fundamental + 1 h.	Colvin (1973)
	8–10	15	30 (mean)					de Ghett (1977)
M. californicus			71 (mean)		40 (mean fundamental)		single component or fundamental + 1 h.	Colvin (1973)
M. longicaudus			77 (mean)		41 (mean fundamental)		single component or fundamental + 1 h.	Colvin (1973)
M. ochrogaster			121 (mean)		32 (mean fundamental)		single component or fundamental + 1 h.	Colvin (1973)
Mesocricetus auratus	16–17	1) 18	2–180	2–50	28–55	50–80	single component	Sewell (1969)
		2) 18	60–200	34–200	20–55	30–60	several components	
		3)	30–200	5–200	10–60	up to 80	wideband	
		3) 9						Okon (1971b)

Meriones	18	1) 18–20	5–150	3–30	45–80	50–130	single component	Sewell (1969)
shawi		2)		80–200		5–148	fundamental	
							+ many h.	
M.	19–21	1) 23	5–200	25–150	37–80	37–75	single component	Sewell (1969)
unguiculatus		2)	80–200		6–70		fundamental	Smith (1974)
			few		few		+ many h.	
Calomys	8	1) 9	3–40	20–65	60–140	55–140	single component	Smith (1974)
callosus		2) 5	15–200		8–72		fundamental	
							+ many h.	
Gerbillus	24–25	1)		5–200		50–70	single component	Sewell (1969)
sp.		2)		5–200		48–85	fundamental	
							+ many h.	
		3)		25–200		up to 60	wideband	
Peromyscus	12–13	1) 17	15–20	2–20	60–115	60–90	single component	Smith (1974)
maniculatus		2) 12–13	30–200		8–70		fundamental	Hart and King
							+ many h.	(1966)
								Smith (1974)
Lagurus			15–70		40–65		single component	Sales and Pye
lagurus								(1974)
Dicrostonyx		11–16	100–800		17–44		single component	Brooks and
groenlandiculus								Banks (1973)
Sigmodon					25–60			Brown (1971)
hispidus								
Phodopus	12		2–160		35–79		single component	Smith (unpub.)
sungorus							fundamental + 1 h.	
Cricetulus			40–60		30–117		fundamental + 1 h.	Smith (unpub.)
griseus								

*h—harmonic component

†number denote different pulse types

differences in the ultrasonic calls produced by pups from various strains within single species. For example Nitschke and his colleagues (1972) studied the calls emitted by three strains of laboratory mice; C_3H/HeJ, BALB/cJ and $C_{57}BL$/6J. They reported that at room temperature pups of the C_3H and BALB strains produce longer and somewhat louder calls than comparably aged pups of the C_{57} strain; the C_3H and C_{57} strains both produce calls with a higher mean peak frequency than similarly aged BALB pups. In addition the rate of calling also varies between strains, but in a complex way that changes with age.

Strain differences have also been reported in the calls of laboratory rats. Donovan (personal communication) found that pups of the albino Wistar strain produce calls at a greater intensity and rate than hooded Lister pups, while Nitschke et al. (1975) reported that when exposed to cold (2–3°C) Wistar/Furth rat pups call at a greater rate than Sprague-Dawley pups. In addition the Sprague-Dawley pups emit calls that are shorter and have a higher mean peak frequency than Wistar/Furth pups.

The calls of newborn cricetid rodents show a greater variety of structure both within and between species than do murids. Like murids, many cricetid species such as the voles, *Clethrionomys glareolus* and *Microtus* spp. (Sewell, 1969; Colvin, 1973; Smith, unpub.) and collared lemmings, *Dicrostonyx groenlandicus* (Brooks and Banks, 1973), produce purely ultrasonic calls from birth; but these are generally lower in frequency than those of murid rodents and often consist of more than one harmonic component (Table 2). Some cricetid species such as Mongolian gerbils and deermice (*Peromyscus maniculatus*) produce both narrowband, single component, purely ultrasonic calls and broadband calls which are often at around the upper limit of human hearing and are thus partly audible. These broadband calls generally consist of one or more series of harmonics (Fig. 2a), otherwise, like the calls of young murids they show a gradual onset and cessation and little frequency or amplitude modulation. Golden hamster pups are unusual as, in addition to purely ultrasonic calls with a single component, they produce narrowband ultrasonic calls that show marked amplitude modulation and also very wideband calls with no clear harmonic structure, again with rapid amplitude modulation (Fig. 2b and c). In species with more than one type of call the purely ultrasonic calls are detected mainly from older pups, especially during handling (see below).

In all species, murid and cricetid, the simple and relatively stereotyped call structure changes as the pups develop and become more independent. The calls of older pups show a greater variety of frequency patterns such as rapid changes, sweeps and fluctuations in frequency (Fig. 3) and generally become shorter and have a greater bandwidth with the increasing age of the pups (Sales and Smith, 1978). However in some species such as rats and gerbils, older pups also produce some very long calls which may either be of almost

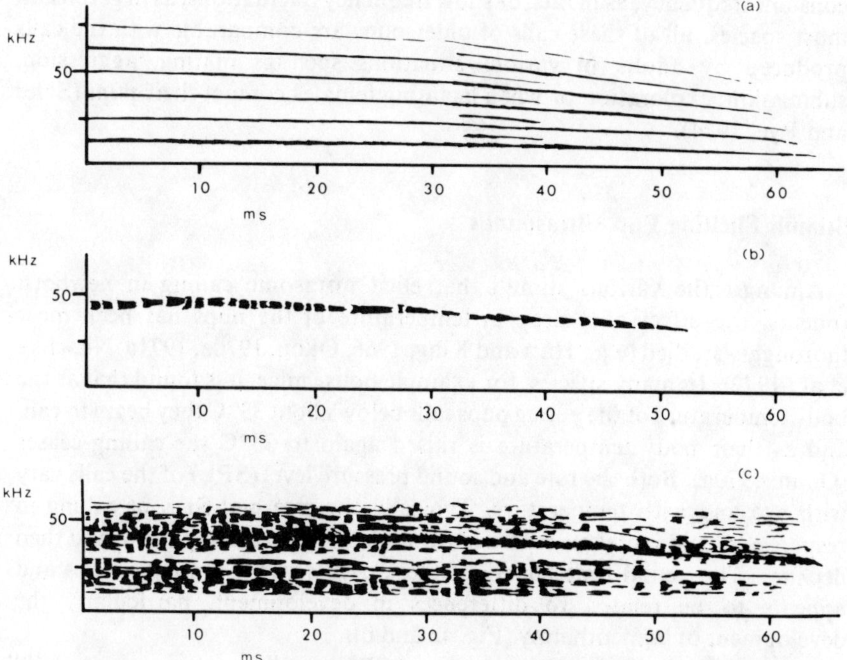

FIG. 2. Sonagrams of typical calls of newborn cricetid rodents: a) broadband call produced by a 5 day old Mongolian gerbil *Meriones unguiculatus* that extends from the audible to the ultrasonic range and shows two series of harmonic components, one appearing for only a short part of the call, b) narrowband purely ultrasonic call produced by a 1 day old golden hamster, *Mesocricetus auratus* showing rapid amplitude modulation, c) wide-band call produced by a 3 day old golden hamster showing many harmonically unrelated components and amplitude modulation.

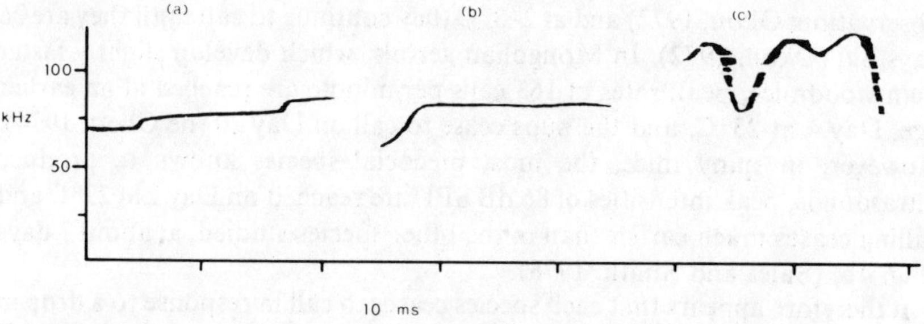

FIG. 3. Sonagrams of the calls of some older rodents: a) part of a call emitted by a 52 day old gerbil, *Meriones shawi* showing rapid frequency changes, b) short call produced by a 17 day old African forest mouse *Thamnomys* showing an initial frequency sweep upwards, c) part of a train of calls produced by a 19 day old *Apodemus sylvaticus* showing frequency fluctuations.

constant frequency, as in rats, or show frequency fluctuations, as in gerbils. In most species, all of these calls of older pups are comparable with the calls produced by adults in various situations such as mating, aggression, submission, exploration or when lactating females contact their pups (Sales and Pye, 1974).

Stimuli Eliciting Pup Ultrasounds

Amongst the various stimuli that elicit ultrasonic calling in newborn rodents, the effect of a drop in temperature of the pups has been most thoroughly studied (e.g., Hart and King, 1966; Okon, 1970a, 1971a; Nitschke et al., 1972). In many species, for example house mice, it is found that as the body temperature of thc young pups falls below about 33°C they begin to call, and as their body temperature is raised again to 33°C the calling ceases (Okon, 1970a). Both the rate and sound pressure level (SPL) of the calls vary with age and with temperature. Typically the rate and SPL of calling in response to cold increases with age from birth to a peak or plateau and then declines. The actual time course of these events varies among species and appears to be related to differences in development, particularly the development of homeothermy (Fig. 4a and b).

In wild house mice, both the rate and SPL of calling in response to mild cold stress (22° C) reach maximal values of about 200 calls per minute and 75 dB SPL (re 2×10^{-4} μbar RMS) between Days 6 and 13 after birth, and calling ceases after about 13 days at this temperature, but continues until 19–20 days in pups exposed to 2–3° C. Infant woodmice, which are slower to develop thermoregulation, produce more and louder calls than house mice. At 22° C maximum levels of 250 calls per minute (Sales and Smith, 1978) and 96 dB SPL (Okon, 1972) are reached on Days 14 and 7–13, respectively. Pups continue to call at this temperature until they are 23–24 days old (personal observation; Okon, 1972) and at 2–3° C they continue to call until they are 26 days old (Okon, 1972). In Mongolian gerbils, which develop slightly faster than woodmice, peak rates of 163 calls per minute are reached at an earlier age, Day 4 at 23° C, and the pups cease to call on Day 20 (de Ghett, 1974). However, in spiny mice, the most precocial species known to produce ultrasounds, peak intensities of 86 dB SPL are reached on Day 2 at 22° C and calling ceases much earlier than in the other species studied, at about 7 days (Fig. 4b) (Sales and Smith, 1978).

It therefore appears that each species ceases to call in response to a drop in ambient temperature when thermoregulation is achieved. For house mice, and probably for the other species too, the ultrasonic responses to cold can be related to three phases in development (Okon, 1970a). During the first five days after birth, house mouse pups are poikilothermic; when exposed to cold

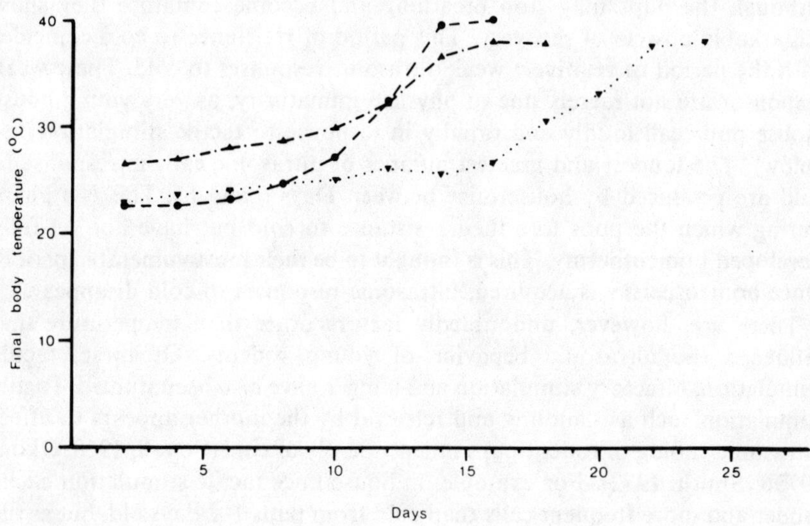

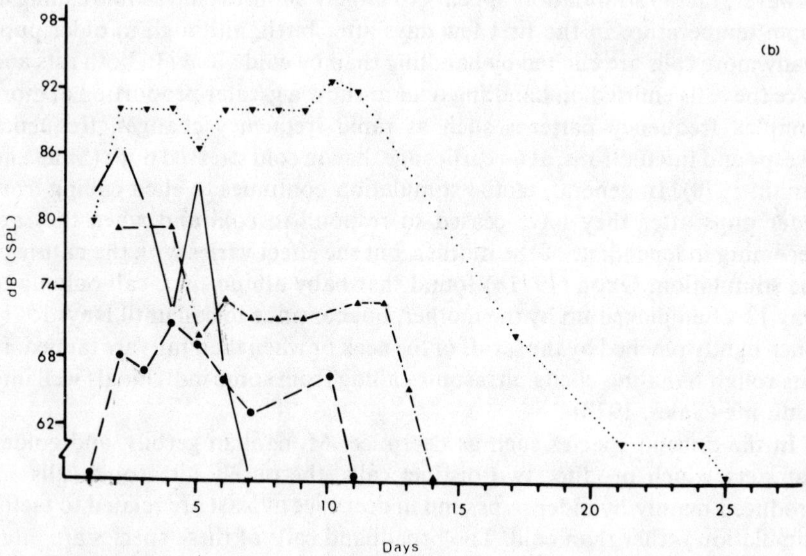

FIG. 4. Development of temperature regulation and changes in ultrasonic calling with age in some myomorph rodents: a) final body temperature of pups after 1 hour exposure at 22°C (redrawn after Okon, 1970a, 1971b, 1972), b) SPL of calls emitted by pups exposed to 22°C for up to 10 minutes. For a) and b) ●— —●*Clethrionomys glareolus*, bank voles; ▲— . —▲, EN strain of albino laboratory house mice; ▼. . . ▼, *Apodemus sylvaticus*, woodmice; □——□ *Acomys cahirinus*, spiny mice.

their body temperature quickly drops to near ambient temperature, but although the pups may stop breathing and become comatose they show remarkable powers of recovery. This period of resistance to cold coincides with the period of relatively weak ultrasonic responses to cold. These weak responses are not merely due to physical immaturity, as very young house mouse pups call loudly and rapidly in response to tactile stimulation (see below). The loudest and greatest number of ultrasonic calls in response to cold are produced by house mice between Days 6 and 13. This is a phase during which the pups lose their resistance to cold but have not yet fully developed homeothermy. This is thought to be their most vulnerable period. Once homeothermy is acquired, ultrasonic responses to cold disappear.

There are, however, undoubtedly factors other than temperature that influence the ultrasonic behavior of young rodents. Of these, tactile stimulation, olfactory stimulation and hunger have also been studied. Tactile stimulation such as handling and retrieval by the mother appears to affect ultrasonic calling in rodent pups independently of cold (Sewell, 1968; Okon, 1970b; Smith, 1972). For example, in house mice tactile stimulation elicits louder and more frequent calls than cold from pups 1–2 days old, but as the pups become older handling elicits fewer and lower intensity calls. In rats, however, tactile stimulation appears to largely suppress ultrasonic calling at room temperature in the first few days after birth, although in older pups many more calls are elicited by handling than by cold alone. In both rats and mice the calls emitted on handling tend to show a greater proportion of more complex frequency patterns such as rapid frequency changes, frequency sweeps and fluctuations, at an earlier age than in cold stressed pups (Sales and Smith, 1978). In general, tactile stimulation continues to elicit calling from older pups after they have ceased to respond to cold and when they are becoming independent of the mother, but the effect varies with the nature of the stimulation. Okon (1971b) found that baby albino mice call only up to Day 12 when picked up by the mother, but continue to call until Days 15–17 when lightly pinched by the scruff of the neck or when their tails are tapped. In rats rough handling elicits ultrasonic calling from some individuals well into adult life (Sales, 1972).

In the cricetid species such as deermice, Mongolian gerbils, and golden hamsters which produce two distinct calls, the purely ultrasonic calls are produced mainly by older pups, and in deermice at least are related to tactile stimulation rather than cold. The broadband calls of these species are more typical of very young cold-stressed pups (Okon, 1971b; Smith, 1972). The different effects of tactile stimulation on rodent calls, thus, appear to be rather complex and have yet to be fully evaluated. One of the problems is the difficulty of adequately defining and controlling a tactile stimulus; another is separating it from the effects of other stimuli such as cold.

Other factors affecting the ultrasonic behavior of rodent pups, such as olfactory stimulation and hunger, have been studied only briefly. Oswalt and Meier (1975) found that rat pups will call in response to lack of familiar olfactory stimuli normally associated with the nest and that they will call less when they can smell their home bedding. Olton (personal communication) is gathering data that suggest that the ultrasonic response of T.O. Swiss laboratory house mice to cold is enhanced by hunger, especially when the pups are 13–18 days old.

The ultrasonic calls of very young rodents thus appear to be a response to stimuli associated with the prolonged absence of the mother from the nest, or their own absence, perhaps by wandering or scattering by the mother. The calls of older pups, those approaching independence, appear to be produced more in response to tactile stimuli and are probably related to the onset of social responses and adult behavior.

THE ROLE OF ULTRASOUNDS IN MOTHER-INFANT INTERACTIONS

Ultrasounds as Communication Signals

Ever since the ultrasonic calls of young rodents were first discovered (Zippelius and Schleidt, 1956), it has been assumed that they are distress calls and that they affect maternal behavior, particularly by initiating retrieving and by directing the mother to displaced pups. For such communication to occur, the mother or other recipient must be able to detect the calls. In addition the effectiveness of the calls as communication signals, their directionality and the range over which detection is possible, will be determined by the physical characteristics of the calls.

In many murid and cricetid species there is good evidence that the adults can hear the calls of their young and other conspecifics. Early studies indicated high frequency hearing in laboratory rats (Gourevitch and Hack, 1966), laboratory house mice (Berlin, 1963) and a variety of other species (Schleidt, 1952; Ralls, 1967). More recently, Brown (1973a, b) studied the neural responses to sounds at the cochlea and at the inferior colliculus in 10 species of murid and cricetid rodents. She found that each species had two peaks of sensitivity: one at or below 20 kHz and another one in the ultrasonic range (Fig. 5a). The upper peak of sensitivity corresponded approximately to the frequencies most readily detected from the young. Behavioral studies on the house mouse (Ehret, 1974) show a similar bimodal hearing curve (Fig. 5b).

The structure of the ultrasonic calls of infant rodents has been described above: in most species the calls of newborn pups are generally longer, of

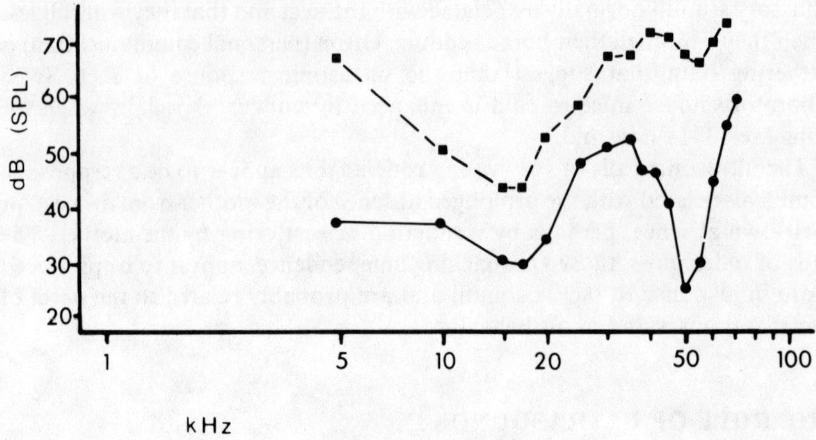

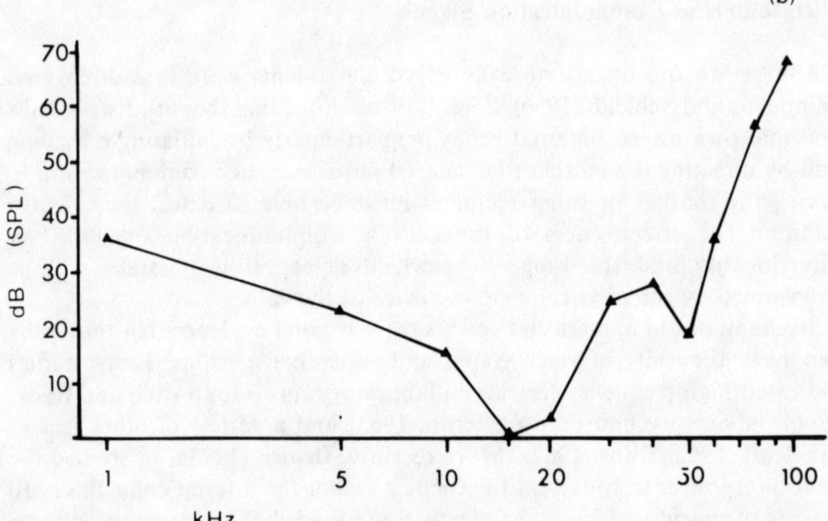

FIG. 5. Auditory response curves of *Mus musculus*, house mice: a) ■— —■ cochlear microphonic responses of an individual, ●——● gross evoked responses of the inferior colliculus of an individual (redrawn after Brown, 1971a), b) behavioral response curve (redrawn after Ehret, 1974).

narrower bandwidth, and show more gradual changes in frequency and amplitude than those of older pups. Since abrupt changes of frequency or amplitude, short pulse duration and wide bandwidth all increase the ease with which signals can be localised (Marler, 1957; Sales and Pye, 1974), it would appear that the calls of newborn pups would be more difficult to localise than those of older pups. In addition, the short wavelengths of such high frequency calls (6.8–4.8 mm at 50–70 kHz) means that they would be reflected by similarly small objects such as blades of grass and so scattered, and also would be absorbed more rapidly in air than lower frequency sounds (Sales and Pye, 1974). Although precise measurements have not yet been made, it appears that rodent pup ultrasounds would not be easily localisable, or even detectable, at great distance through grass. But it is not known how well ultrasounds might be transmitted through a burrow, where relatively smooth walls could reflect the sounds. These arguments mainly apply to the single component high frequency ultrasounds of murids. The lower frequency multicomponent calls of some cricetid rodents may be much easier to localise and would probably travel further.

It will only be possible to predict the useful range and normal function of infant ultrasonic cries, when it is known from the ecology and behavior of each species exactly when and where the newborn pups call in the wild. Most murid and cricetid species live in holes or burrows (Walker et al., 1968) and it seems unlikely that newborn pups of such species would stray or be scattered out of the burrow. The calls then may serve merely to attract the mother back to the burrow from nearby, or back to the nest from within the burrow system. The actual location of the burrow and nest would be familiar to her. Another possibility is that the calls may affect the female in a more non-specific way, perhaps by maintaining a high level of maternal behavior by priming or through an arousal effect. In either case the calls need not be localized.

If infant rodent calls are used only for short-range communication, this may account for their lack of specific distinctiveness, since such calls could only be used between animals brought together by other means (Marler and Hamilton, 1966). Mother rodents generally show a strong attachment to the nest site, thus specificity in the responses between mother and young may be ensured without the necessity for coding it in the ultrasonic calls of the pups.

Poorly localisable short-range calls would have the advantage of not advertising the position of a burrow to predators. It is known that cats and many other carnivores can hear ultrasounds (Evans, 1968; Peterson et al., 1969), although many of the natural predators of rodents such as weasels and stoats have not yet been studied. It appears, however, that owls are unable to detect sounds above 20 kHz and locate their prey from the lower frequency rustling sounds produced during the movement of the prey (Payne, 1971).

Experimental Evidence for Effects on Mothers and Other Adults

Despite the restrictions on the use of ultrasonic calls as communication signals, there is good evidence that the calls of pups do affect rodent maternal behavior, at least at close range. Early studies on laboratory house mice (Noirot, 1964a, b) showed that external stimuli from pups would elicit maternal responses such as retrieving, nest building, licking and covering the pups, from virgin females and even from males. Thus the post-parturitional hormonal state did not appear to be essential for the expression of maternal behavior patterns in house mice. Furthermore, Noirot (1964c) found that 5-minute exposure to a live 1-day-old baby house mouse pup, which is normally a strong stimulus for eliciting maternal behavior, would later enhance the maternal responses shown by virgin female and male house mice towards weak stimuli for maternal behavior, such as a drowned day-old house mouse pup or a live baby rat. This effect, which could last up to eight days, Noirot termed "priming" and she showed that it was not consequent on the animals retrieving the live pup during the initial exposure.

In order to establish which stimuli from live pups are involved in priming, Noirot (1969a) primed naive virgin female and male house mice with day-old pups hidden in metal boxes with small perforations. It was considered that the boxes would allow the passage of olfactory and auditory stimuli from the pups but not allow visual or tactile contact. After exposure to this stimulus, the animals were tested for maternal behavior towards a weak stimulus as before, and it was found that maternal behavior was still enhanced, compared with controls which had no previous experience with any pup cues. In a third experiment, Noirot (1970) exposed two separate groups of naive virgin female house mice to 4- to 6-day-old pups hidden either in perforated metal boxes or in closed metal boxes. The closed boxes were supposed to abolish olfactory stimuli but allow auditory stimuli from the pups. However, it is not certain how good the separation was. After 20-minute exposure to the priming stimuli and 1½ hours interval the females were tested with live 1- to 2-day-old house mice. Females of both groups spent a similar amount of time sniffing and licking the test pups but those exposed to pups in closed boxes performed slightly more nest building. Since the test pup was a very strong stimulus for retrieving, this behavior was not studied.

These techniques were not very powerful, as it was not possible to test single cues from live pups. However, in 1970, Sewell used replayed tape recordings of the ultrasonic calls of a 5-day-old litter of woodmice to investigate the responses of lactating females on the nest to auditory cues alone. This technique clearly separated auditory cues from all others. On 38 of 56 presentations of the prerecorded ultrasounds, the lactating females left their nest within 30 seconds, often with pups still attached to their nipples, and went to a loudspeaker 15 cm away. Control sounds elicited only three departures from the nest in 54 presentations. This experiment showed that ultrasonic calls of pups alone can elicit the approach behavior of lactating woodmice and can be localized over at least 15 cm.

Similar tape-recorder playback experiments have now been carried out on several other species. Smith (1975), using similar apparatus to that of Sewell, obtained a high level of response to prerecorded pup calls from lactating deermice. Both the partly audible and the purely ultrasonic cries of young deermice effectively elicited directed approach behavior over 15 cm. Allin and Banks (1972) obtained less definite responses from lactating albino Wistar rats presented with a recording of a 9-day-old rat pup, but 20 out of 40 females left the nest box at least once in response to the sounds and on most presentations females orientated correctly towards the sound source.

Colvin (1973) used real pups to study the effects of conspecific pup ultrasounds on the behavior of adults of three species of *Microtus: M. montanus, M. californicus* and *M. pennsylvanicus,* with other cues adequately controlled. The subjects were males and females which were the parents of pups less than 10 days old; each male was housed with his mate and her offspring. Each animal was tested in a Y-maze; the arms contained screens behind which were placed either quiet pups (olfactory cues), calling pups (ultrasonic and olfactory cues) or no pups (control condition). In all three species calling pups elicited more directed responses than quiet pups, over a distance of 62.5 cm. From the structure of the ultrasounds of neonatal *Microtus,* Colvin also suggested that the calls are likely to be short-range communication signals.

Smotherman and his colleagues (1974) made a similar comparison of the effects of olfactory and auditory cues from pups on the behavior of Long-Evans laboratory rats and C57 BL/10 laboratory house mice. They used chilled pups which had passed into cold coma as an olfactory stimulus; previously handled pups as an ultrasonic + olfactory stimulus; tape-recorded pup ultrasounds as an ultrasound only stimulus and an empty maze arm as a no stimulus condition. Various paired combinations of these were presented in the two arms of a Y-maze, of which the home cage of the test animal formed a start box. Both lactating Long-Evans rats and lactating C57/BL10 house mice showed a significant preference for handled pups when these were paired with any other stimulus. Rats, but not house mice, showed a significant preference for a loudspeaker relaying pup ultrasounds when this was paired with a chilled pup; but both rats and house mice showed random choice when presented with tape-recorded ultrasounds versus an empty maze arm. It was concluded that ultrasounds alone were not sufficient for choice behavior, although they appeared to give directional cues when olfactory stimuli were present in the other arm of the maze. Although there is general agreement that laboratory rats are not very responsive to replayed pup ultrasounds alone (Allin and Banks, 1972; Smith, unpublished observations), Smith (1974) found that T.O. Swiss mice do respond to replayed pup calls, although the response is not so strong as that of woodmice or deermice. It is not clear why T.O. Swiss mice should differ from the C57BL/10 strain in this respect.

More recently Smith (1976) has investigated the effectiveness of differently structured ultrasounds in eliciting approach responses from T.O. Swiss house mice. Lactating females, primed females, (with Day 4–5 young), naive females, primed males and naive males were tested individually in a small choice chamber for approach responses to an electronically generated model of the calls of a newborn mouse (Fig. 6). Priming increased the responsiveness of both males and females, while lactating females and primed females made more approach responses than other mice. Primed females were then tested with five different electronically generated ultrasonic signals. More approach responses were made to the 65–45 kHz, 80 ms pulse shown in Figure 6, than to similar pulses of 75–55 kHz or 55–35 kHz. An 80 ms pulse of constant frequency, 65 kHz, elicited more approaches than a similar 15 ms pulse. The responses of wild house mice were comparable to those of laboratory animals.

These experiments indicate that, although the mice did not respond exclusively to one particular ultrasonic pulse type, they showed a preference for the model pulse which was most like the calls of the very young (Fig. 6). Departures from this structure lessened the attractiveness of the pulse.

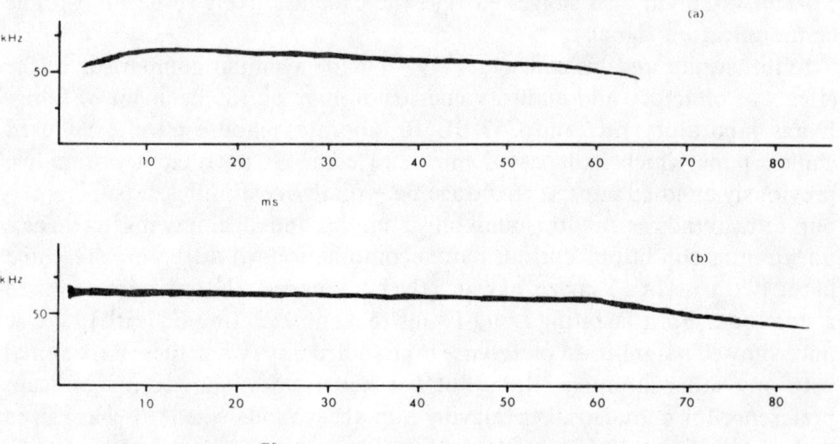

FIG. 6. a) Sonagram of typical call emitted by 1 day old T.O. Swiss laboratory house mouse, b) electronically generated ultrasonic signal used to investigate adult mouse behavior (redrawn after Smith, 1976).

Further experiments of this sort should reveal exactly which features of infant rodent ultrasounds are attractive to adults.

Most studies have concentrated on the role of pup ultrasounds in eliciting approach responses from adults. But pup ultrasounds may also affect other aspects of maternal behavior such as nest building (Noirot, 1974). It has also been suggested that whereas the calls of isolated pups may promote maternal behavior, the calls produced by pups during manipulation and retrieving may serve to inhibit ongoing behavior and particularly maternal aggression, which is very high after birth (Noirot, 1966).

Unfortunately, the evidence for the effects of ultrasound from pups on maternal nest building is more difficult to interpret than that for approach responses, since no experiments have yet been carried out using tape-recorder playback of infant ultrasounds alone, but instead have used rather complex stimuli involving live pups. Noirot (1974) measured the weight, style, and position of the nests built by virgin female laboratory house mice in large cages containing a small cage with either a mother house mouse and her litter (Experimental group E), or a virgin female house mouse (Control group C). In some litters (Experimental group EC), the mother and nest were removed from the small cage for 10 minutes each day to expose the test animals to the ultrasounds from cold pups. In other litters (Experimental tactile group ET), the pups were removed from the nest and replaced individually by rolling them on their backs into the nest, to expose the test animals to ultrasounds from handled pups.

It was found that animals in groups EC or ET built nests nearer the small cage than animals in group C. Animals in group EC built heavier nests than those in groups ET or C. Group ET females appeared to build lighter nests and to bite the straw into smaller pieces than the females in other groups. It was concluded that ultrasounds from cooled pups (group EC) promoted building of heavier nests and that ultrasounds from handled pups (group ET) inhibited nest building but promoted straw biting. However, although the test animals could not touch the litters, cues from the pups other than ultrasounds, cues from the mother, as well as disturbance by the experimenter, were present in the experimental, but not the control groups. It is not certain, therefore, to what extent the results can be explained in terms of ultrasounds alone.

Evidence for the inhibitory effect of ultrasounds on maternal behavior, particularly aggression, is largely circumstantial. Noirot (1966) observed that virgin female mice were often rather rough during their first attempts to retrieve pups and that the pups produced many ultrasounds when the females picked them up. Often the females would then drop the pup and engage in another activity such as nest building. This was thought to be due to the inhibitory effect of the ultrasounds produced during tactile stimulation.

Noirot (1969b) also found that fidget mice, a deaf mutant strain, would often eat their pups as well as the placenta and umbilical cord after birth; possibly because they could not hear the cries of the pups, which may normally act as a signal to stop eating.

However it is now possible to cite equally strong evidence that the ultrasounds of handled pups may have a positive effect on maternal behavior. In the sound replay experiments, Smotherman and his colleagues (1974) found that recently handled house mouse and rat pups were very strong stimuli for adult approach responses. Similarly Colvin (1973) found that short-tailed vole pups suspended by the tail elicited adult approach and Smith (1975) found that both of the types of call produced by deermouse pups elicited approach from adults. Also, in the nest building experiment described above (Noirot, 1974), the ultrasounds from both cold and handled pups caused test females to build their nests close to the litter.

Thus the suggestion made in early studies, that there are two distinct types of ultrasonic call in rodent pups, one produced by cooled pups and the other produced by handled pups, each with a separate function, may be an oversimplification. Apart from the lack of conclusive functional evidence, there appears to be no clear cut difference in the structure of ultrasounds from handled and isolated pups (Sales and Smith, 1978). Although at any particular age, handled pups produce a greater proportion of calls with complex frequency patterns than do isolated pups; similar complex patterns can be detected from slightly older isolated pups (see above.). There are differences in intensity and rate of the calls emitted in response to handling and isolation on any one day, but these differences change with age and vary between species (Sales and Smith, 1978).

Bell (1974) has proposed that ultrasounds from young and adult rodents should not be classified according to the stimuli that elicit them (e.g., isolation or handling calls) or according to their supposed functions (e.g., aggressive or submissive calls). He suggests that the ultrasonic calls of rodent pups merely reflect a state of arousal in the emitter due to stressful stimulation (cold, handling, or electric shock); and that the occurrence and acoustical properties of the signals may be related to the degree of arousal of the emitter and may induce a similar state of arousal in nearby animals. The behavioral response of the recipient would depend on interaction between the state of arousal produced and such factors as internal state, previous experience, as well as other external stimuli.

Another possible role for infant rodent ultrasounds in mother-infant interactions is in mediating the "early experience" phenomena through their action on maternal behavior (Bell et al., 1974). The effects of infantile stimulation upon subsequent development in mammals, especially rodents, has been reviewed by several authors (e.g., Levine, 1962; Russell, 1971). The evidence indicates that early treatments such as cooling, handling and electric shock all can affect rodent growth, physiology and behavior. Stressed pups show faster growth and when adult show lower physiological responses to mild stress and less emotionality compared with controls. However it is not yet known how these effects are brought about. One theory is that stress changes the stimulus characteristics of the pups which alters maternal behavior towards them; the changed maternal behavior in turn producing the typical early experience effects in the pups (e.g., Bell et al., 1971). Bell and his colleagues (1974) suggested that ultrasounds from pups could be the main stimulus for mediating these effects. In common with other workers they found that different forms and degrees of stress (handling, mild cold stress and severe cold stress) elicited different patterns of ultrasonic response in rat pups. These in turn were thought to elicit different maternal responses: mild cold stressed pups elicited more maternal care than pups subjected to the other treatments (Bell et al., 1974).

Smotherman and his colleagues (1977) have recently shown that mother rats' corticosterone level changes according to the experimental treatment of their pups. Fourteen-day-old pups were removed from their mothers and were either picked up by hand and placed in a wire basket for two minutes (handled pups) or shocked (0.4 mA, 90 s) and then placed in a wire basket for two minutes (shocked pups). Litters were then returned to their mothers, but remained in the baskets to prevent tactile contact. Twenty minutes later, blood samples were collected from the mothers. Mothers of both groups showed a higher corticosterone level than control mothers which were sampled without interference with the pups; but shocked pups elicited a higher corticosterone response than handled pups. The authors suggest that ultrasounds from the handled or shocked pups may have been responsible for eliciting the corticosterone response, although they did not monitor these during the experiment. However, Zarrow and his coworkers (1972) have shown that the corticosterone response of lactating rats on reunion with the pups after a 3-hour separation is abolished by olfactory bulbectomy. So perhaps ultrasonic stimuli merely enhance what is primarily an olfactory effect.

Thus, apart from their involvement in eliciting approach responses from adults, it is still unclear to what extent ultrasounds from pups, especially in species other than house mice and rats, affect maternal behavior, either directly or in a nonspecific way. Other stimuli from pups, especially olfactory cues, play an important part (e.g., Zarrow et al., 1972; Smotherman et al., 1974) and the hormonal state of the animal and previous experience, in priming for example, also affect maternal behavior. It must be remembered that the relative importance of different factors in mother-infant interactions probably varies among the different rodent species, so it can be misleading to generalise.

MATERNAL STIMULI AND INFANT RESPONSES

In the previous section the part played by ultrasonic signals from rodent pups in mother-infant relationships was considered. However, as indicated earlier, this relationship is two-way: the pups may also respond to signals from the mother.

Sewell (1969; Sales, 1972) first detected ultrasounds from mother rodents after she had removed litters from lactating spiny mice. The females ran in and out of the nest box and sniffed round their cages, producing many ultrasonic calls. These were similar to the calls of the young; most showed slow drifts of frequency; but some shorter calls had step-like frequency changes. Sewell later made similar observations on lactating woodmice and bank voles, and Okon (1971b) found that this behavior sometimes occurred in lactating albino EN house mice, especially if the pups were returned and subsequently withdrawn a second time. All these calls appeared to be similar to those of the young and were of low SPL (Table 3).

More recently Smith (1974) has detected pulses from lactating females of several more myomorph species, when their pups were removed and then replaced. The calls were generally tape-recorded, and the maternal calls were found to be much softer, usually shorter and had more complex frequency structure than those of newborn pups, the structure of which was already known. It was therefore possible to distinguish the maternal calls from those of the newborn young, both from the recordings and when using an ultrasound detector. However, in order to confirm that the females were indeed calling, some were tested with a freshly killed 9-day-old rat pup (barbiturate overdose) which obviously could not call. Similar responses were obtained from these females as from those tested with live pups. Sounds also have been recorded from virgin female and male house mice tested with live mouse pups placed in their cages or presented with a freshly killed 9-day-old rat pup. Similarly, ultrasounds have been detected from virgin female house mice when they were investigating a loudspeaker that had previously been relaying pup ultrasounds. The calls elicited in all these studies are summarized in Table 3.

On the basis of her results, Sales (1972) and Sales and Pye (1974) suggested that the pulses of lactating females might either be warning signals or might elicit searching behavior in other adults and thus increase the chances of lost young being found. She considered that it was unlikely that the function of

TABLE 3
Ultrasonic Calls Elicited from Adult Rodents after Association with Stimuli from Pups

Species	*Subject*	*Stimulus*	*Pulse Parameters* *Duration (ms)*	*Frequency (kHz)*	*Bandwidth (kHz)*	*Pulse Pattern**	*Comments*
spiny mice	lact. ♀	pups removed	1) 80–120	25–35	2–5	s.f.d. steps	Sales (1972)
			2) 80	50–60	3–25		
wood-mice	lact. ♀	pups removed	10–40	60–82	5–12	s.f.d, r.f.c.	Sales (1972) and unpub.
bank voles	lact. ♀	pups removed	220–50	12–25	1–5	fundamental, often + 1.h.	Sales (1972)
house mice	lact. ♀ EN†	pups removed + replaced	30–110	60–80		s.f.d., steps	Okon (1971b)
house mice	lact. ♀ T.O. Swiss	pups removed + replaced	30–80	60–100	7–37	steps, s.f.d., f.f.	Smith (1974)
house mice	lact. ♀ T.O. Swiss	dead d. 9 rat		65			bat-detector only Smith (1974)
house mice	virgin ♀ T.O. Swiss	live mouse pup	27–76	64–99	8–32	steps, s.f.d., f.f.	Smith (1974)

(continued)

TABLE 3 *(continued)*

Species	Subject	Stimulus	Pulse Parameters: Duration (ms)	Frequency (kHz)	Bandwidth (kHz)	Pulse Pattern*	Comments
house mice	virgin ♀ T.O. Swiss	after sound replay	26–70	65–110	4–45	steps, s.f.d.	Smith (1974)
house mice	male T.O. Swiss	live mouse pup	26–73	60–100	7–35	steps, r.f.c., s.f.d.	Smith (1974)
house mice	wild virgin ♀	live mouse pup		65			bat-detector only Smith (1974)
deer-mice	lact. ♀	pups removed + replaced	2–22	43–94	1–20	v. short, or long + f.f.	v. low SPL Smith (1974)
Wistar rats	lact. ♀	pups removed + replaced	15–57	45–81	4–23	trains, s.f.d., long + f.f.	Smith (1974)
Wistar rats	lact. ♀	dead d. 9 rat	20–65	47–83	6–25	trains, s.f.d., long + f.f.	Smith (1974)
gerbils	lact. ♀	pups removed + replaced	12–36	28–42	5–7	upsweeps	Smith (1974)
gerbils	lact. ♀	dead d. 9 rat	13–109	29–43	2–11	upsweeps, long + f.f.	Smith (1974)

*s.f.d.—slow frequency drift; r.f.c.—rapid frequency change; f.f.—frequency fluctuations; h—harmonic component.
†albino from E. Noirot's colony.

such calls was communication with newborn young since house mice, at least, do not show physiological or behavioral responses to sound until 9–14 days after birth (Alford and Ruben, 1963; Ehret, 1976). In spiny mouse pups however, hearing probably develops much sooner than this and it seems possible that they might be able to hear the maternal calls. A further possible explanation for maternal calls was suggested by Okon (1971b), who thought that they might be the females' aggressive response to the removal of the young.

Smith (1974) suggested that the calls she obtained under wider conditions than those of Sewell or Okon (i.e., when animals were contacting a dead pup, replaced young or a loudspeaker), might be investigation calls, or could promote amicable contact, especially with older pups. In Mongolian gerbils, similar calls were detected during the initial stages of heterosexual encounters and in all species the calls appear to be similar to those produced by older pups, which perhaps have a similar function (Smith, 1974). "Maternal" calls at audible frequencies have been described for at least two species of the more precocial caviomorph rodents: the guinea-pig, *Cavia porcellus* (Berryman, *in litt.*) and the green acouchi, *Myoprocta pratti* (Kleiman, 1972). A "purr" was described in each case. In the green acouchi, as the neonates followed the mother more when she purred, it was suggested that this call was a contact call designed to keep the young informed of the whereabouts of the mother. The ultrasonic calls of lactating myomorph rodents could have a similar function during the period when the pups are active and likely to stray but are not ready for complete independence. Their hearing would be developed at this stage, and in both rats and house mice there is a marked increase in sensitivity to ultrasonic frequencies between Days 13 and 18 (Crowley and Hepp-Reymond, 1966; Ehret, 1976). Further work is clearly necessary in this aspect of the role of ultrasounds in mother-infant relationships.

It is now known that lactating Wistar laboratory rats (Leon and Moltz, 1971; Leon, 1974), Sprague-Dawley laboratory rats (Holinka and Carlson, 1976), spiny mice (Porter and Doane, 1976) and CD-1 laboratory house mice (Breen and Leshner, 1977) produce a 'maternal pheromone': an odor which is attractive to pups. In Wistar rats, the emission of the pheromone begins on Day 14, the day on which the pups also begin to respond to it, and lasts until Day 27 postpartum, by which time the pups no longer respond (Leon and Moltz, 1971). This period between Days 14–27 is thought to coincide with the period during which the pups begin to leave the nest, but before they become independent. In spiny mice (Porter and Doane, 1976) both the emission of the pheromone and the response of the pups appear to start immediately after birth, which is presumably correlated with the advanced development of this species. The maternal pheromone would therefore appear to act in a similar way to that suggested for maternal ultrasounds.

It is obvious that communication between mother and infant rodents is complex and involves a two-way exchange of a variety of stimuli. However, the widespread occurrence of ultrasonic calling among infant murid and cricetid rodents and the special sensitivity of the auditory system of adults to ultrasonic frequencies, suggests that the calls play a significant part in mother-infant relationships in these animals. Experimental work has established the role of the infant calls in eliciting and possibly in directing searching behavior in adults and has indicated that they may also enhance the general responsiveness of mothers towards their pups, either through a direct effect on the arousal system or through the endocrine system. In this way the calls could increase maternal responsiveness towards other stimuli from the pups, for example olfactory cues. In addition, cues from the mother may affect the behavior of older pups, although the extent to which ultrasounds are involved is not yet known. Clearly further work is required to establish the roles of the various stimuli, including ultrasounds, in mother-infant interactions.

ACKNOWLEDGMENTS

This work was carried out at King's College and at Queen Mary College London. GDS was supported by grants from the Delegacy of King's College (Layton Award), the Science Research Council and The Royal Commission for the Exhibition of 1851; JCS was supported by the Delegacy of King's College (Harold Row Studentship), the Science Research Council and the Ministry of Agriculture, Fisheries and Food as Senior Research Fellow.

We are grateful to Professor D. R. Arthur of King's College and Professor N. B. Marshall of Queen Mary College for providing facilities and also to Professor J. D. Pye for the use of equipment as well as for much advice and helpful criticism during the course of the work.

The comparative nature of the study would not have been possible without the help and co-operation of many people who made animals available to us.

Permission for the publication of illustrations has been granted by: A. M. Brown and *Nature*, MacMillan (Journals) Ltd. London (Fig. 5a); G. Ehret and *Die Naturwissenschaften*, Springer-Verlag, Heidelberg (Fig. 5b); J. D. Pye and Chapman & Hall, London (Fig. 5a); E. E. Okon and *J. Zoology*, London (Fig. 4a); *J. Comp. Physiol. Psychol.* (Fig. 6).

REFERENCES

Alford, B. R. and Ruben, R. J. Physiological, behavioural and anatomical correlates of the development of hearing in the mouse. *Ann. Otol. Rhinol.* (St. Louis) *72*, 237–247 (1963).

Allin, J. T. and Banks, E. M. Functional aspects of ultrasound production by infant albino rats (*Rattus norvegicus*). *Anim. Behav. 20*, 175–185 (1972).

Bell, R. W. Ultrasounds in small rodents: Arousal-produced and arousal-producing. *Devel. Psychobiol. 7*, 39–42 (1974).

Bell, R. W., Nitschke, W., Bell, N. J., and Zachman, T. A. Early experience, ultrasonic vocalizations, and maternal responsiveness in rats. *Devel. Psychobiol. 7*, 235–242 (1974).

Bell, R. W., Nitschke, W., Gorry, T. H. and Zachman, T. A. Infantile stimulation and ultrasonic signaling: a possible mediator of the early handling phenomena. *Devel. Psychobiol. 4*, 181–191 (1971).

Bell, R. W., Nitschke, W. and Zachman, T. A. Ultrasounds in three inbred strains of young mice. *Behav. Biol. 7*, 805–814 (1972).

Berlin, C. I. Hearing in mice via GSR audiometry. *J. Speech Hear. Res. 6*, 359–368 (1963).

Breen, M. F. and Leshner, A. I. Maternal pheromone: a demonstration of its existence in the mouse (*Mus musculus*). *Physiol. Behav. 18*, 527–529 (1977).

Brooks, R. J. and Banks, E. M. Behavioural biology of the collared lemming (*Dicrostonyx groenlandicus* Traill): An analysis of acoustic communication. *Anim. Behav. Monogr.* 6, Part 1 (1973).

Brown, A. M. Auditory responses to high frequencies in small mammals. Ph.D. thesis Univ. of London (1971).

Brown, A. M. High frequency peaks in the cochlear microphonic response of rodents. *J. Comp. Physiol. 83*, 377–392 (1973a).

Brown, A. M. High levels of responsiveness from the inferior colliculus of rodents at ultrasonic frequencies. *J. Comp. Physiol. 83*, 393–406 (1973b).

Colvin, M. A. Analysis of acoustic structure and function in ultrasounds of neonatal *Microtus. Behaviour 44*, 234–263 (1973).

Crowley, D. E., and Hepp-Raymond, M. C. Development of cochlear functions in the ear of the infant rat. *J. Comp. Physiol. Psychol. 62*, 427–432 (1966).

de Ghett, V. J. Developmental changes in the rat of ultrasonic vocalization in the Mongolian gerbil. *Devel. Psychobiol. 7*, 267–272 (1974).

de Ghett, V. J. The ontogeny of ultrasonic vocalization in *Microtus montanus. Behaviour 60*, 115–121 (1977).

Dieterlen, V. F. Bieträge zur biologie der Stachelmaus, *Acomys cahirinus dimidiatus* Cretzshmar. *Zietschrift Saugetierk 26*, 1–13 (1961).

Ehret, G. Age-dependent hearing loss in normal hearing mice. *Die Naturwissenschaften 11*, 506 (1974).

Ehret, G. Development of absolute auditory thresholds in the house mouse (*Mus musculus*). *J. Am. Aud. Soc. 1*, 179–184 (1976).

Evans, E. F. Cortical representation, in: *Hearing mechanisms in Vertebrates*. A.V.S. de Reuck and J. Knight, eds. Ciba Symposium. Churchill, London. (1968).

Gourevitch, G. and Hack, M. H. Audibility in the rat. *J. Comp. Physiol. Psychol. 62*, 289–291 (1966).

Happold, M. Reproductive biology and developments in the conilurine rodents (Muridae) of Australia. *Austr. J. Zool. 24*, 19–26 (1976).

Hart, F. M. and King, J. A. Distress vocalizations of young in two subspecies of *Peromyscus maniculatus. J. Mammal. 47*, 287–293 (1966).

Holinka, C. F., and Carlson, A. D. Pup attraction to lactating Sprague-Dawley rats. *Behav. Biol. 16*, 489–505 (1976).

Kleiman, D. G. Maternal behaviour of the green acouchi (*Myoprocta pratti*, Pocock), a South American caviomorph rodent. *Behaviour 43*, 48–84 (1972).

Leon, M. Maternal pheromone. *Physiol. Behav. 13*, 441–453 (1974).

Leon, M. and Moltz, H. Maternal pheromone: discrimination by preweaning albino rats. *Physiol. Behav. 7*, 265–267 (1971).

Levine, S. Effects of infantile experience on adult behavior, in *Experimental foundations of Clinical psychology*, A. J. Bachrach, ed. Basic Books, New York. (1962).

Marler, P. Specific distinctiveness in the communication signals of birds. *Behaviour 11*, 13–39 (1957).

Marler, P. and Hamilton, W. J. *Mechanisms of Animal Behavior*. John Wiley & Sons, Inc., New York (1966).

McManus, J. J. Early postnatal growth and the development of temperature regulation in the Mongolian gerbil, *Meriones unguiculatus. J. Mammal. 52*, 782–792 (1971).

Nitschke, W., Bell, R. W., and Zachman, T. Distress vocalizations of young in three inbred strains of mice. *Devel. Psychobiol. 5*, 363–370 (1972).

Nitschke, W., Bell, R. W., Bell, N. J., and Zachman, T. The ontogeny of ultrasounds in two strains of *Rattus norvegicus. Experimental Aging Res. 1*, 229–242 (1975).

Noirot, E. Changes in the responsiveness to young in the adult mouse. I. The problematical effect of hormones. *Anim. Behav. 12*, 52–58 (1964a).

Noirot, E. Changes in responsiveness to young in the adult mouse. II. The effect of external stimuli. *J. Comp. Physiol. Psychol. 57*, 97–99 (1964b).

Noirot, E. Changes in responsiveness to young in the adult mouse. IV. The effect of an initial contact with a strong stimulus. *Anim. Behav. 12*, 442–445 (1964c).

Noirot, E. Ultrasons et comportements maternals chez les petits rongeurs. *Annls. Soc. r. Zool. Belg. 95*, 47–56 (1966).

Noirot, E. Changes in responsiveness to young in the adult mouse: V. Priming. *Anim. Behav. 17*, 542–546 (1969a).

Noirot, E. Interactions between reproductive and territorial behaviour in female mice. *International Mental health research newsletter 11*, 10–11 (1969b).

Noirot, E. Selective priming of maternal responses by auditory and olfactory cues from mouse pups. *Devel. Psychobiol. 2*, 273–276 (1970).

Noirot, E. Nest-building by the virgin female mouse exposed to ultrasound from inaccessible pups. *Anim. Behav. 22*, 410–420 (1974).

Noirot, E. and Pye, D. Sound analysis of ultrasonic distress calls of mouse pups as a function of their age. *Anim. Behav. 17*, 340–349 (1969).

Okon, E. E. The effect of environmental temperature on the production of ultrasounds by isolated non-handled albino mouse pups. *J. Zool., Lond. 162*, 71–83 (1970a).

Okon, E. E. The ultrasonic responses of albino mouse pups to tactile stimuli. *J. Zool., Lond. 162*, 485–492 (1970b).

Okon, E. E. The temperature relations of vocalization in infant golden hamsters and Wistar rats. *J. Zool., Lond. 164*, 227–237 (1971a).

Okon, E. E. Motivation for the production of ultrasounds in infant rodents. Ph.D. thesis, Univ. of London (1971b).

Okon, E. E. Factors affecting ultrasound production in infant rodents. *J. Zool., Lond. 168*, 139–148 (1972).

Oswalt, G. L. and Meier, G. W. Olfactory thermal and tactual influences on infantile ultrasonic vocalizations in rats. *Devel. Psychobiol. 8*, 129–135 (1975).

Payne, R. S. Acoustic location of prey by barn owls (*Tyto alba*). *J. Exp. Biol. 54*, 535–573 (1971).

Peterson, E. A., Heaton, W. C. and Wruble, S. Levels of auditory response in fissipede carnivores. *J. Mammal. 50*, 566–578 (1969).

Porter, R. H. and Doane, H. M. Maternal pheromone in the spiny mouse (*Acomys cahirinus*). *Physiol. Behav. 16*, 75–78 (1976).

Ralls, K. Auditory sensitivity in mice, *Peromyscus* and *Mus musculus. Anim. Behav. 15*, 123–128 (1967).

Russell, P. A. 'Infantile stimulation' in rodents: a consideration of possible mechanisms. *Psychol. Bull. 75*, 192–202 (1971).

Sales, G. D. Ultrasound and mating behaviour in rodents with some observations on other behavioural situations. *J. Zool., Lond. 168*, 149–164 (1972).

Sales, G. D. and Pye, J. D. *Ultrasonic Communication by Animals*, Chapman and Hall, London (1974).

Sales, G. D. and Smith, J. C. Comparative studies of the ultrasonic calls of infant murid rodents. *Devel. Psychobiol. 11,* 595–619 (1978).

Schleidt, W. M. Reactionen auf töne hoher Frequenz bei Nagern. *Naturwissenschaften 39*, 69–70. (1952).

Sewell, G. D. Ultrasound in rodents. *Nature 217*, 682–683 (1968).

Sewell, G. D. Ultrasound in small mammals. Ph.D. thesis, Univ. of London. (1969).

Sewell, G. D. Ultrasonic communication in rodents. *Nature 227*, 410 (1970).

Smith, J. C. Sound production by infant *Peromyscus maniculatus* (Rodentia : Myomorpha). *J. Zool., Lond. 168*, 369–379 (1972).

Smith, J. C. Sound communication in some myomorph rodents with special reference to adult-infant relationships. Ph.D. thesis, Univ. of London (1974).

Smith, J. C. Sound communication in rodents, in *Sound Reception in Mammals.* R. J. Bench, A. Pye and J. D. Pye, eds. *Symp. Zool. Soc. Lond. 37*, 317–330 (1975).

Smith, J. C. Responses of adult mice to models of infant calls. *J. Comp. Physiol. Psychol. 90*, 1105–1115 (1976).

Smith, J. R., Watts, C. H. S. and Crichton, E. G. Reproduction in the Australian desert rodents *Notomys alexis* and *Pseudomys australis* (Muridae). *Aust. Mammal. 1*, 1–7 (1972).

Smotherman, W. P., Bell, R. W., Starzec, J., Elias, J. and Zachman, T. A. Maternal responses to infant vocalizations and olfactory cues in rats and mice. *Behav. Biol. 12*, 55–66 (1974).

Smotherman, W. P., Wiener, S. G., Mendoza, S. P., and Levine, S. Maternal pituitary-adrenal responsiveness as a function of differential treatment of rat pups. *Devel. Psychobiol. 10*, 113–122 (1977).

Southern, H. N. *Handbook of British Mammals.* Blackwell Scientific Publications, Oxford (1964).

Walker, E. P., Warnick, F., Hamlet, S. E., Lange, K. I., Davis, M. A., Uible, H. E. and Wright, P. F. *Mammals of the World* 2nd Edition revised by J. L. Paradiso, The Johns Hopkins Press, Baltimore (1968).

Watts, C. H. S. Vocalizations of Australian hopping mice (Rodentia : *Notomys*). *J. Zool. Lond., 177*, 247–263 (1975).

Watts, C. H. S. Vocalizations of the plains rat *Pseudomys australis* Gray (Rodentia : Muridae). *Austr. J. Zool. 24*, 95–103 (1976).

Zarrow, M. X., Schlein, P. A., Denenberg, V. H., and Cohen, H. A. Sustained corticosterone release in lactating rats following olfactory stimulation from the pups. *Endocrinology 91*, 191–196 (1972).

Zippelius, H-M. Ultraschall-laute nestjunger mause, *Behaviour 49*, 197–204 (1974).

Zippelius, H-M. and Schleidt, W. M. Ultraschall-laute bei jungen mausen. *Naturwissenschaften 43*, 502 (1956).

Maternal Influences and Early Behavior

6 Pheromonal Control of Maternal Behavior

Howard Moltz
Sarah J. Kilpatrick

MATERNAL PHEROMONE: INTRODUCTION

The word *pheromone* derives from the Greek, and literally means "carrier of excitation." Such carriers of excitation have been found both in insects and mammals and, at each phyletic level, have been observed to exert not only physiological but behavioral effects as well. It is not our intention, however, to catalogue these diverse effects, nor indeed to discuss any but a single pheromone. That pheromone was discovered in our laboratory in 1971 while studying maternal behavior in the rat. What was discovered was that the lactating female emits a chemical substance that is carried in her feces and that strongly attracts young. The initial study on which this conclusion is based (Leon and Moltz, 1971) can be described briefly as follows.

A discrimination apparatus, pictured in Figure 1, was designed to permit approach across an open field from a start box to either of two goal boxes. A female that had been lactating for 16 days (16-day lactating female), a nulliparous female, or no stimulus animal at all were presented in the goal boxes in different paired combinations. Opaque plexiglass separated these boxes from the rest of the apparatus so that their contents were not visible from the open field. The pups, however, could enter either goal box by going over a small cliff. Forced air was introduced into each goal compartment from a central valve, to pass from there up through the cliff opening to the open area of the apparatus and then to the start box.

When 16-day-old young were given a choice between their own 16-day lactating mother and a nulliparous female, they chose their own mother

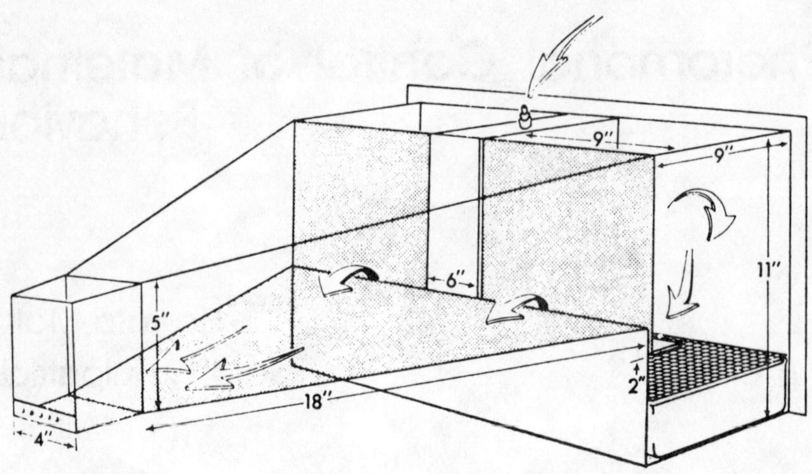

FIG. 1. Olfactory discrimination apparatus. Arrows indicate direction of airflow. Dimensions are shown.

overwhelmingly. And when a strange 16-day lactating female rather than the mother herself was opposed to a nulliparious female, 16-day-old young again chose the lactating female, indicating that each mother does not emit a unique odor, one to which only her litter will respond.

To demonstrate that the prefεrence was odor-based and not, in fact, grounded in other cues issuing from the goal compartments, two additional conditions were employed. In the first, a strange 16-day lactating female and a nulliparous female were placed individually in the goal compartments for 3 hours and then removed. The pups were tested immediately afterwards, being required, of course to choose between the now soiled but otherwise empty compartments. In the second condition, a nulliparous female and a 16-day lactating female were present in the goal compartments but with the direction of the airflow reversed through the central valve, which is to say that the air within the goal compartments was made to flow away from rather than towards the pups. The data obtained under each of these conditions indicated clearly that preference for the lactating female was indeed odor-based.

It might be well at this point to mention that, although the phenomenon just described was initially discovered in the Wistar rat, other investigators subsequently found a similar odor-based attractant in the Charles River (Gregory and Pfaff, 1971) and the Sprague-Dawley (Holinka and Carlson, 1976) strains. Indeed, a maternal pheromone appears also to be present in other rodent species such as the house mouse (*Mus musculus*) (Breen and Leshner, 1977) and the spiny mouse (*Acomys cahirinus*) (Porter and Ruttle, 1975; Porter and Doane, 1976).

The purpose of our next study (Leon and Moltz, 1972) was to determine just when, during the postpartum episode, this maternal pheromone characteristically appears and for how many days thereafter it is effectively emitted. Correlatively, we also wanted to determine when the young first begin to respond to the pheromone and the age range over which they subsequently maintain such responding.

Accordingly, we took our olfactory discrimination apparatus and tested young of different chronological ages against mothers of different lactational ages. What we found was a striking synchrony in the development and dissolution of what we have come to call "the pheromonal bond." On the one hand, this synchrony is expressed in the fact that the pheromone is first released by the mother at about 14 days postpartum, a time coincident with the age at which the young first become responsive to the pheromone. On the other hand, it is seen in the fact that at about 27 days postpartum the mother ceases to release the pheromone, which corresponds, in turn, to the age at which the young cease to be attracted to this pheromone.

As the next step in studying the maternal pheromone, we undertook to investigate whether the synchrony between emission and attraction is governed by the stimulus characteristics of the young. Two main findings emerged. First, pheromonal emission was clearly inhibited when our lactating females were made to experience only neonatal pups, that is, pups which, through litter substitution, were not permitted to advance beyond Day 1 of age (Moltz and Leon, 1973). And second, pheromonal emission was just as clearly prolonged by repeated substitution of young between 16 and 21 days of age, beginning as soon as the female's own litter reached 21 days of age (Moltz et al., 1974). Under the latter condition, some of our females continued to release the pheromone for more than 100 days. It appears then, that pheromonal emission is indeed governed by the stimulus characteristics of the young and not by some endogenous condition of the postparturient female which mediates release at 14 days and cessation of release at 27 days.

PROLACTIN AND THE MATERNAL PHEROMONE

But what of the physiological mechanisms governing this pup-controlled maternal pheromone? We speculated (Leon and Moltz, 1973) that one such mechanism might be hormonal in nature, since the period immediately preceding initiation of emission is a period of high endocrine output during which ovarian and adrenal steroids are actively discharged, as is prolactin from the adenohypophysis. Prolactin, in particular, seemed promising as a governing agent, for not only is prolactin characteristically present at high titers throughout the first half of the postpartum period (Amenomori et al.,

1970) but it is released in response to pup stimulation (Grosvenor, 1965; Moltz et al., 1969; Sar and Meites, 1969), stimulation evidently essential for pheromonal emission. Accordingly, the role of prolactin was investigated along with the role of ovarian and adrenal steroids. To this end, one group of puerperal females was ovariectomized, a second adrenalectomized, and a third subjected to the combined operation. The more likely possibility that prolactin alone might be critical for pheromonal emission was explored through the use of the drug ergocornine, a drug that acts as a dopamine analogue to inhibit the release of hypophyseal prolactin in vivo.

Our data confirmed the importance of prolactin for the emission of the pheromone. As the accompanying table shows, ergocornine inhibited the pheromone, while prolactin replacement restored the pheromone. Removal of adrenal and ovarian hormones, on the other hand, had no effect at all on the release of the attractant.

TABLE 1
Choice Behavior of 16-Day-Old Young to Females Lactating for 21 Days

	Number Choosing Lactating Females	*Number Choosing Nulliparous Females*	*No Choice*	*Significance*
Intact Control	110	4	6	<0.001
Ergocornine	53	65	7	>0.05
Ergocornine and Prolactin	88	13	19	<0.001
Adrenalectomized	101	17	2	<0.001
Ovariectomized	106	8	6	<0.001
Adrenalectomized-Ovariectomized	82	24	14	<0.01
Adrenalectomized-Ovariectomized and Prolactin	95	8	17	<0.001

CONCAVEATION AND THE MATERNAL PHEROMONE

Yet to be mentioned is the fact that many nulliparous females and adult males also behave maternally. In other words, it is not uncommon to find that such animals will build a nest, lick, retrieve and even crouch in a nursing posture when housed continuously with young, a procedure known as concaveation (Wiesner and Sheard, 1933). Of such concaveated animals, one might ask not only whether they release the pheromone, but as in the case of the lactating female, whether they do so only during a specific period of the maternal episode. Additionally, the question might be raised as to whether, for the pheromone to be emitted at all, maternal behavior must first be displayed or whether mere association with young is sufficient. A recent study from our laboratory was concerned with just these questions (Leidahl and Moltz, 1975).

The subjects used were nulliparous females and adult males, all born in the authors' laboratory. Each was transferred to a specially-designed maternity cage and each, after a period of habituation, was given nesting material and 4–6 foster pups, approximately 24 hours old. These pups were allowed to remain in the cage until the following day at which time a new litter of the same age was substituted.

This procedure of replacing one 24-hour-old litter with another continued until the day a given animal started to behave maternally. Thereafter it was proffered fresh litters that advanced commensurately in age, such that on Day 2 of maternal behavior it was caring for young 2 days of age and on Day 3, for young 3 days of age, and so on.

Temporally yoked to half of these experimental females were females that showed no maternal behavior whatsoever, despite their having been housed with foster young for the same length of time and under the same conditions. Such females also received pups of advancing age beginning at exactly the same time as their respective experimental twins. For reasons that will become apparent, the same control-yoking procedure proved superfluous in the case of males displaying maternal behavior. Thus, a total of three groups was formed: concaveated-maternal females, concaveated-nonmaternal females, and concaveated-maternal males. Testing for the presence of the pheromone was carried out in our olfactory discrimination apparatus using pups 16 days of age. The tests were begun 16 days from the onset of maternal behavior or, in the case of nonmaternal females, 16 days from the time their foster young began to advance in age. Each animal was tested against a nonconcaveated female of comparable age.

Our data yielded unequivocal evidence of pheromonal emission in the concaveated-maternal female insofar as such females were chosen overwhelmingly when tested against their non-concaveated test partners. Evidence was also obtained concerning the importance of maternal behavior as a precondition for pheromonal emission. This is illustrated in Figure 2 which compares the percentage of test choices received by concaveated-maternal females when paired with non-concaveated animals and the percentage of choices received by their nonmaternal counterparts when they, in turn, were similarly paired.

The males presented a picture entirely different from the females in that the males, even when showing full maternal behavior, failed to emit the pheromone. Indeed, at none of the test points that we explored, did the

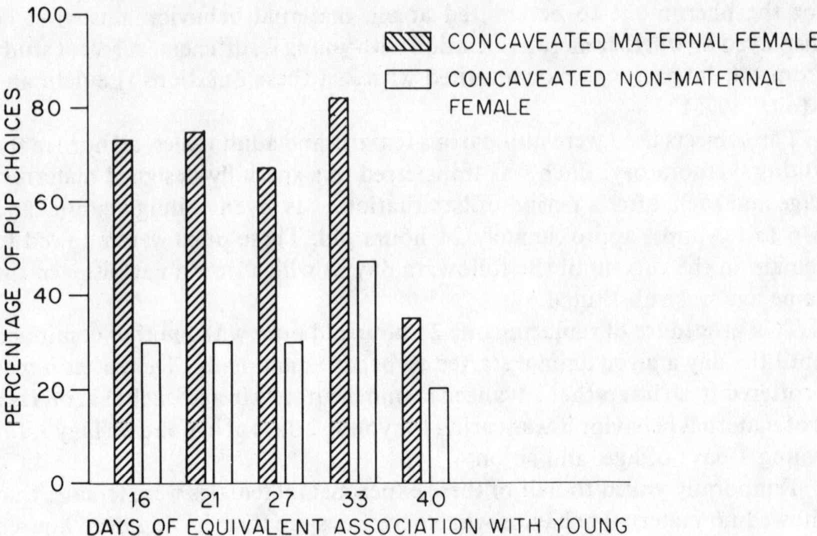

FIG. 2. Percentage of pup choices received by concaveated-maternal females as compared with that received by concaveated-nonmaternal females when each in turn was tested against a nonconcaveated animal.

number of choices received by such maternally-behaving males exceed chance expectancy.

Several conclusions clearly emerge from the study just discussed. First, nulliparous females can emit the pheromone, and in fact they do so for a somewhat longer period than postparturient females which usually cease releasing the attractant when their young reach 27 days of age. Second, pheromonal emission on the part of the nulliparous female requires the display of maternal behavior. The nulliparous female that fails to behave maternally, fails to attract young. Finally, males, even when showing the full range of maternal behavior—and in a manner indistinguishable from maternal, nulliparous females—do not emit the pherome. Obviously, these data raise several questions.

First, is the question of whether the attractant released by the maternally-behaving nulliparous female is identical with that released by the maternally-behaving lactating female. If it is—if on all comparisons the two prove to be the same—then we would have the opportunity to test an hypothesis recently advanced (Leon, 1974) concerning food intake as it relates to pheromonal emission.

And second, is the question of why the maternally-behaving male failed to show evidence of the pheromone. Was it because he failed to synthesize sufficient amounts of prolactin, a hormone essential for pheromonal emission? Or is it that the androgen of our intact males somehow interfered with the pheromone, or that an androgen metabolite, perhaps present in the feces, somehow masked the odor of the pheromone?

To answer the question of pheromonal identity, we undertook to compare the attractiveness of the pheromone emitted by the lactating female with that emitted by the maternally-behaving nulliparous female. Here, we used (Leidahl and Moltz, 1977) pups 16 days of age, selected because such pups are known to respond strongly to the pheromone emitted by the lactating female. The question, of course, was would they respond as strongly to the pheromone of the maternally behaving nulliparous female? The data left little doubt that they would: on all comparisons our standard 16-day-old young were as attracted to the nulliparous female that had been behaving maternally for 21 days as they were to the lactating female that had been behaving maternally for the same period of time. Also, as might be expected, the pups are equally attracted to the fecal material of the two females. Finally, they ceased being attracted to the nulliparous female after she was injected with ergocornine, just as, previously, they had ceased being attracted to the lactating female following the same treatment.

But of course tests of relative attractiveness do not establish chemical identity. To establish such identity, the pheromone derived from the lactating female would have to be matched in molecular structure with that derived from the nulliparous female. At the time, however, we could not even guess as to what the chemical structure of the maternal pheromone might be. Nonetheless, armed with behavioral data indicating that the "nulliparous pheromone" is identical with the "lactating pheromone," we decided (Leidahl and Moltz, 1977) to test the hypothesis that hyperphagia is a precondition for pheromonal emission. As already indicated, this hypothesis was first advanced by Leon (1974) and it can be stated briefly as follows. The increased food intake accompanying lactation results in a greater-than-normal excretion of fecal material derived from the distal end of the cecum. It is this material that contains the pheromone (in contrast to that derived from the proximal end of the cecum) and is preferentially eaten in the usual practice of coprophagia. When food-intake is normal, all feces containing the pheromone are consumed. However, when the female overeats, as she does when lactating, she produces more than she can consume. What remains, serves as an attractant to young and is thus identified as containing the pheromone.

This is an interesting hypothesis, one we undertook to test by monitoring the food-intake of our maternally-behaving nulliparous females for a period of some 20 days after the introduction of young. Not only did we fail to observe an increase in food intake, but in comparison with nonconcaveated females of comparable age and weight, our maternally-behaving nulliparae actually ate less. Evidently, lactation-induced hyperphagia is not a prerequisite for pheromonal emission.

BILE, PROLACTIN AND THE EMISSION OF THE MATERNAL PHEROMONE

We also addressed the second question above, namely, why maternally-behaving males fail to give evidence of the pheromone (Moltz and Leidahl, 1977). Knowing that high titers of prolactin are essential for pheromonal emission, we thought that perhaps the failure of the male to release the attractant was due to his failure to synthesize such titers. Data reported by Nicoll and Swearingen (1970), showing that the male has a significantly lower prolactin turnover rate than the female would be consonant with this suggestion. Accordingly, we took both intact and castrated males and injected them daily with either 25 or 50 I.U. of prolactin, beginning on the first day of maternal behavior. The injections continued for a full 24 days during which time they were tested repeatedly for pheromonal emission using standard 16-day-old young. Not a single male showed evidence of the pheromone.

We then thought that perhaps the failure of our maternally-behaving males to release the pheromone was due to lack of estrogen. Thus, we undertook the daily injections of both estradiol benzoate (5 *u*g) and prolactin, beginning on the first day of maternal behavior. Once again, not a single male gave evidence of the pheromone. It was at this point that we turned away from the idea of a simple endocrine insufficiency and sought instead to explain the male's failure to emit the pheromone by reference to events within the liver. What led us to focus on the liver can be described briefly as follows.

We know from the work of Leon (1974) that the pheromone is not the product of some anal gland but instead is the product of the cecum. We knew also from the work of Posner and his colleagues (Posner et al., 1974a, 1975; Posner et al., 1974b) and from the work of Costlow et al. (1975) that prolactin induces its own receptors in the liver and that the male characteristically shows a lower level of such receptor-induction than the female. Thinking, then, of some prolactin-hepatic interaction as underlying the synthesis of the pheromone, we decided to collect bile from pheromone-emitting females for injection directly into the ceca of adult males. If our speculations regarding the liver are correct, then such males might be expected to show evidence of the pheromone.

For the purpose of cecal injection, we collected bile by cannulating the bile ducts of three groups of females: (a) those that had been lactating for 21 days and consequently were actively emitting the pheromone (21-day bile); (b) those that had also been with their litters for 21 days, but which, since Day 10, had been receiving daily injections of ergocornine, and so because of prolactin inhibition, were not emitting the pheromone (21-day bile + Ergo); and (c) those females that had been lactating for only five days, and so had not yet begun to emit the pheromone (5-day bile).

Three groups of intact males, never before in contact with young, each received, intracecally, 2 ml of bile twice daily for a period of six days. Beginning on Day 3, and continuing until three days after the last injection, every male was tested for the pheromone in our olfactory-discrimination apparatus, using standard 16-day-old young.

By the fourth day of injection, those males receiving 21-day bile were selected overwhelmingly in preference to noninjected males (Fig. 3). Moreover, they continued to be preferred until the day after the injections ceased, at which time the choices became random (Table 2).

To obtain additional evidence that males receiving 21-day bile were actively emitting the pheromone, we tested their feces against the feces of females that had been lactating for 21 days. Such females, of course, strongly emit the pheromone, and so the question was whether the feces of 21-day bile-injected males would be comparable in attractiveness to the feces of 21-day lactating females. In all respects they were. Indeed, (Fig.4) it was only after the injections ceased that the feces of the lactating female came to be preferred over the feces of males injected with 21-day bile (Moltz and Leidahl, 1977).

In contrast to males receiving 21-day bile, those receiving either 5-day bile or 21-day bile + Ergo were not chosen significantly over their noninjected test partners. It is obvious that not all bile injected into the cecum results in pheromonal release.

However, the groups just mentioned were designed to serve as more than controls for the effects of bile injection. They go further to support the following conclusions: (a) when prolactin is inhibited, bile loses the capacity to induce release of the pheromone (21-day bile + Ergo); and (b) five days of lactation are not sufficient to alter bile so as to make it pheromone-inducing (5-day bile). The latter is particularly interesting, since the female that has been lactating for five days has high levels of prolactin; in fact she has had such levels since the time of parturition (Amenomori et al., 1970). How long prolactin must remain elevated before bile is appropriately altered can be inferred from the fact that the lactating female, as well as the concaveated female, does not begin to emit the pheromone until she has been with the young for about 14 days. What may well be occurring during this 14-day period is the formation of new prolactin binding-sites in the liver (Costlow et al., 1975). We can conceive of the resultant uptake in prolactin as bringing

TABLE 2

Response of 16-Day-Old Pups to Males Injected with 21-Day Bile vs. Non-Injected Males

Days of Injections	*Numbers Choosing Males Injected with 21-Day Bile*	*Number Choosing Non-Injected Males*	*No Choice*	*Statistical Significance**
3	25	12	11	n.s.
4	34	9	5	$p < 0.001$
5	34	10	4	$p < 0.001$
6	31	12	5	$p < 0.001$
Days Post-Injection				
1	30	12	6	$p < 0.001$
2	20	18	10	n.s.
3	18	16	14	n.s.

*Chi-square test was used.

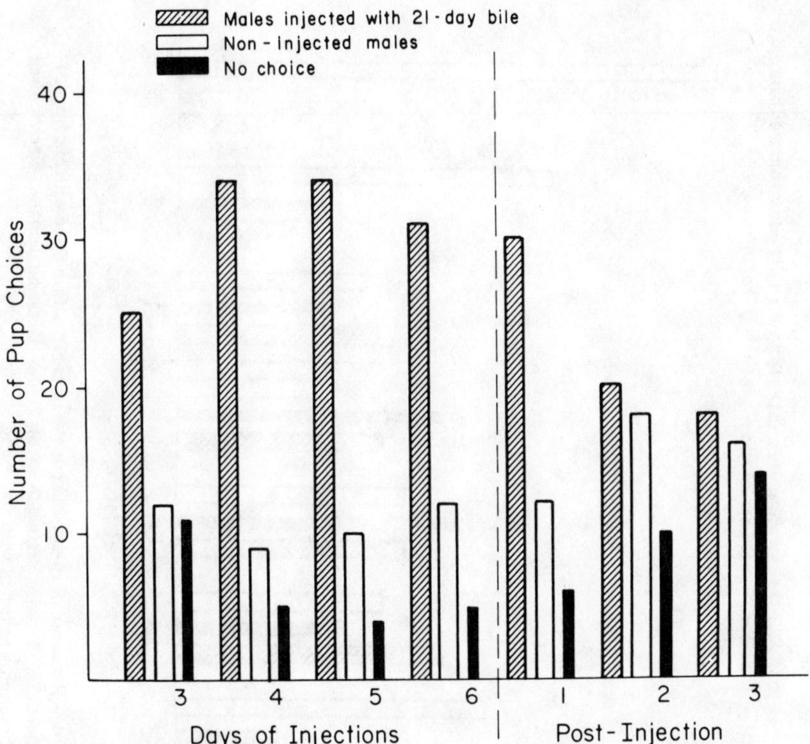

FIG. 3. Response of 16-day-old pups to males injected with bile from 21-day lactating females versus noninjected males. Each paired combination was tested with six young.

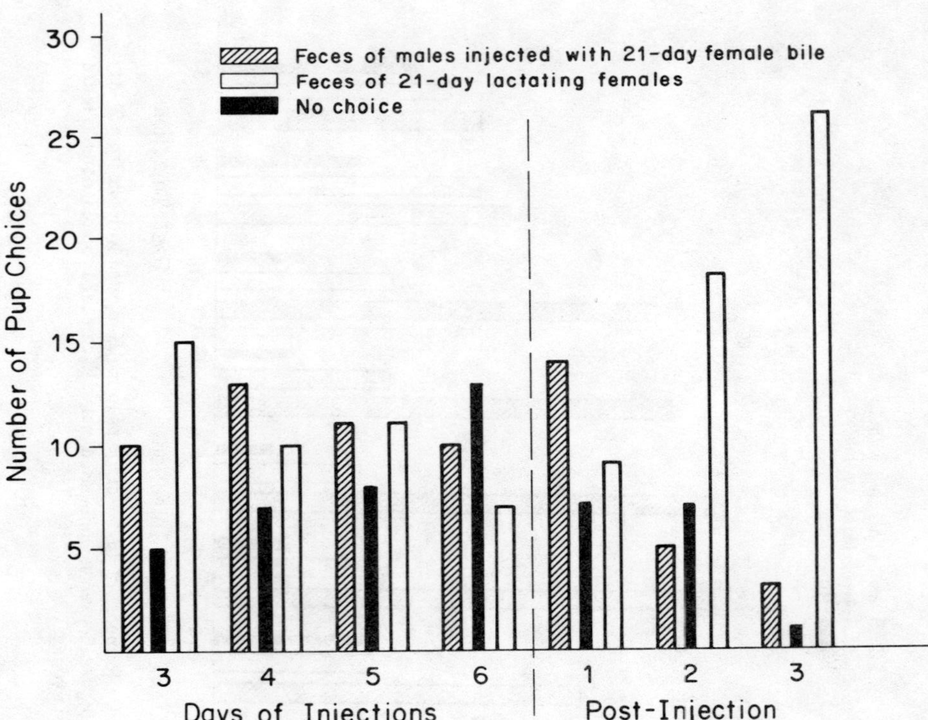

FIG. 4. Response of 16-day-old pups to feces of males injected with bile from 21-day lactating females versus feces of 21-day lactating females. Each paired combination was tested with six young.

about either an increase in total bile-acid concentration or a change in the ratio of one primary bile acid to another[1]. Through either avenue, the chemistry of the cecum may be altered such that fecal material comes to contain the pheromone. That the male, as mentioned earlier, characteristically forms fewer hepatic prolactin receptors than the female would explain why the male, although capable of releasing the pheromone in response to injected bile, cannot do so endogenously.

SEX DIFFERENCES AND PROLACTIN BINDING

Before turning to the question of how bile-acid composition in the female might be changed through the progressive uptake of prolactin by the liver, it would be instructive to explore further the apparent sex difference in prolactin binding. Kelly et al. (1974) have shown that in the female the number of hepatic binding sites recognizing prolactin increases dramatically at about the time of puberty. In contrast, no such increase is correlated with the attainment of puberty in the male and so in the male the number of binding sites thereafter remains relatively scant. We believe that this difference in liver development is "programmed" neonatally by androgen, which acts to restrict the number of prolactin receptors that can be formed. The result is that the male, having been exposed to androgen early in ontogeny, comes to develop a liver incapable of accumulating enough binding sites, and hence enough prolactin, to mediate pheromonal emission. (The parallel to the work of Denef and De Moor, 1970, 1972, on the sexual differentiation of steroid metabolizing enzymes in rat liver is obvious.)

We are aware of the work of Gustafsson and Stenberg (1974) and of Aragona et al. (1976), and so we appreciate the possibility that if the liver is in fact "programmed" neonatally with respect to prolactin, the responsible agent may not be of gonadal origin at all. Rather, the hypophysis alone may be responsible for the development of our hypothesized hepatic-binding. However, the results we have obtained thus far, while they do not rule out the involvement of the hypophysis, at least implicate the gonads. Specifically, each of several males that we castrated neonatally was found to emit the pheromone after behaving maternally for 16 days during adulthood. Neonatally-androgenized females that also behaved maternally as adults

[1]The first of these alternatives now appears unlikely. Since the present chapter was written, it has been shown that the overall concentration of bile acids in bile does not change significantly from the non-pregnant to the lactating state (Klaasen and Strom, *Drug Metabolism and Disposition 6,* 120–124, 1978) or throughout the course of lactation itself (Kilpatrick and Moltz, unpublished data).

failed entirely to show evidence of the attractant (Kilpatrick and Moltz, unpublished data).

THE POSSIBLE IDENTITY OF THE MATERNAL PHEROMONE

The results of our work thus far raise the following questions. First, how does prolactin, once it is bound, mediate pheromonal emission? And second, what changes does it bring in hepatic functioning to make fecal material strongly attractive to young? Before attempting an answer, we must first state a fact about the pheromone we have not mentioned, namely, that it is present in the ceca of all adult animals (Leon, 1974; Moltz and Leidahl, unpublished data). This has been established by taking material directly from the ceca of virgin females and adult males and demonstrating that it strongly attracts 16-day-old young. That such young are not attracted to the anal excreta of these same adult animals suggests that, although the pheromone may always be present in the cecum, it most often fails to survive passage through the colon. The question then becomes: what is it that is lost in the colon and how does increased prolactin binding protect against such loss? We think the answer involves bile-acid production.

Primary bile acids are synthesized by the liver, the major acids being cholic acid and chenodeoxycholic acid. (What other primary bile acids are found in the rat, such as α- and β- muricholic acid, are considered "minor constituents" of bile [Haslewood, 1964]). Conjugation by peptide linkage occurs with taurine and glycine, respectively, to yield the corresponding tauro- and glycoacids. These conjugated acids enter the small intestine where, at the terminal ileum, they are largely absorbed into the enterohepatic circulation. What fraction escapes into the cecum (4–5%) is deconjugated and dehydroxylated by enteric microflora to form the secondary bile salts, deoxycholic acid from cholic acid and lithocholic acid from chenodeoxycholic acid (Bergstrom and Norman, 1953; Gustafsson et al., 1957; Norman and Sjovall, 1958a). (Following customary practice, the terms "bile salt" and "bile acid" will be used interchangeably.)

There is now an appreciation of the fact that not only the small but the large intestine as well contributes to enterohepatic circulation. Weiner and Lack (1968), for example, estimate that, in the 200 g rat, a total of 5 mg per day of the secondary bile acids enter the portal system through passive diffusion from the cecum and colon. But of course the individual bile acids are not equally diffusable, since they are not equally polar nor equally soluble. Thus, lithocholic acid, being of low polarity and low solubility, is poorly reabsorbed from the large intestine. As a consequence, lithocholic acid and its metabolites comprise more than 50% of the bile acids most often found in anal excreta (Gustafsson and Norman, 1962; Norman and Sjovall, 1960). Deoxycholic acid, in contrast, is readily reabsorbed so that little is typically contained in the feces (Heaton, 1972; Lindstedt and Samuelsson, 1959; Mekhjian and Phillips, 1970; Norman and Sjovall, 1958b; Olivecrona and Sjovall, 1959).

We are suggesting (a) that the pheromone is deoxycholic acid or some derivate of deoxycholic acid, and (b) that it appears in anal excreta when sufficient quantities are synthesized to overcome colonic reabsorption[2]. Furthermore, we are suggesting that titers of circulating prolactin, by progressively increasing the number of hepatic receptor sites, change bile-salt production. We conceive of this change as occurring prior to pheromonal emission and as involving either an increase in total bile-acid concentration or an increase in the ratio of cholic to chenodeoxycholic acid.[3] Through either avenue, greater-than-normal amounts of deoxycholic acid would be synthesized in the cecum, enabling an increased fraction to show up in the anal excreta. Several experiments are currently underway in the authors' laboratory to assess the involvement of deoxycholic acid in pheromonal emission.

RESPONSIVENESS TO THE PHEROMONE ON THE PART OF THE YOUNG

Up to this point we have dealt only with the pheromonal emission of the adult, paying no attention to the pheromonal responsiveness of the young. But of course the two interact, and that interaction shows both a striking synchrony and an equally striking asynchrony. On the one hand, as we have already mentioned, emission and responsiveness are characteristically linked together in time, so that beginning at 14 days postpartum (or 14 days from the start of maternal behavior in the nulliparous female) there is a progression in which the pheromone first appears and then disappears while, simultaneously, it is first responded to and then ignored. On the other hand, this manifest synchrony between mother and young is paralleled by a dramatic asynchrony. Specifically, while pheromonal release on the part of the mother is sensitive to the character of the young, pheromonal responsiveness on the part of the young is altogether insensitive to the character of the mother

[2]We no longer conceive of the pheromone as being deoxycholic acid, and deoxycholic acid alone. Rather, we now hold the view that the pheromone is constituted by a number of different compounds which have deoxycholic acid as an essential moiety.

[3]Cf. Footnote 1.

(Moltz et al., 1974). Thus while we were able to prolong the mother's emission of the pheromone by successive substitution of foster litters, we could not prolong the young's attraction to the pheromone by successive substitution of foster mothers.

Although conclusive tests of adaptive function—at least with respect to the pheromone—can be conducted only outside the laboratory, nonetheless it is of interest to speculate about the natural situation and about the value of having the young terminate their responsiveness to the pheromone at 27 days.

Consider that in the burrow system rats of all ages and both sexes are invariably present and that several females at different stages of lactation are probably nursing litters (Calhoun, 1962), with some emitting the pheromone. To have adult animals, or even post-weaning young, respond to the pheromone—to have them in other words intrude into the litter situation and thereby disrupt maternal behavior—would be maladaptive indeed. Something must occur to ensure that attraction to the pheromone does not continue beyond 27 days, the time of weaning. Just what that "something" is has not been determined, although we can advance two hypotheses. The first concerns the enteric microflora of the weanling, the second, its bile-acid profile.

The small intestine has a relatively low concentration of bacteria, while in the cecum and colon bacterial density often reaches as high as 10^{10} organisms per gram of intestinal contents (Kellogg, 1973). These bacteria not only degrade primary bile salts, they also digest organic compounds not attacked by digestive enzymes. Moreover, evidence is emerging to show that in some species these same microorganisms exert a protective effect against high tissue accumulation of cholesterol (Danielsson, 1963; Kellogg, 1973).

We do not know precisely when during development the rat establishes the enteric microfloral profile of the adult. Nor do we know how it does so. Perhaps one way in which the preweanling rodent attains full colonization of its cecum and colon is through the ingestion of fecal material from the mother. If that is so, then it is possible that the consumption of this fecal material—material that we know the young consumes (Leon, 1974)—occurs in response to a specific hunger.

It is of interest that the young first become attracted to pheromone-containing feces at about the time they begin to eat "adult food" (laboratory pellets). If at that time they have not established their full microfloral profile, then perhaps some ingredient of the adult food remains incompletely digested, creating a particular nutritional deficit or, as we prefer to call it, a "specific hunger." One way to promote complete digestion, and therefore alleviate the hunger, would be to ingest the missing bacteria through the feces of the mother. Such "supplementary" feeding would be necessary, of course, only until the pup itself established the needed microorganisms. Once that occurred, it would no longer be dependent on maternal feces as a digestive aid. Perhaps it is at this time that the pup stops responding to the maternal pheromone as such.

One question that might be raised in relation to the hypothesis just presented is the question of why the adult microfloral population is not established at the very first ingestion of the maternal feces. This may be because the infantile gut is not competent to support the needed bacteria and, until it becomes so, these bacteria must repeatedly be "restocked" through supplementary feeding. Or it may be that the infantile gut contains certain other bacteria hostile to those the pup needs.

There is, as we have already mentioned, a second hypothesis that might be advanced to explain why pups stop responding to the pheromone when they reach 27 days of age. Here we have reference to bile-acids and to a condition known as endotoxic shock.

It has long been known that the young of many mammalian species are susceptible to dyspepsic colitis induced by *Escherichia coli* "and perhaps other gram negative organisms" (Bertok, 1977). These bacteria, normally inhabiting the intestinal tract and entirely harmless to the adult, produce endotoxins that, in the young, can result in enterotoxemia. Resistance to enterotoxemia is conferred by certain bile acids, particularly deoxycholic acid (Bertok, 1977; Rudbach et al., 1966). When present, deoxycholic acid fragments endotoxin molecules through detergent action, rendering such molecules harmless. However, as is sometimes the case in the young animal, if deoxycholic acid is not present, or if it is present only in suboptimal concentrations, these endotoxins enter the systemic circulation unaltered, and produce enterotoxemia.

What we are suggesting here is perhaps obvious and concerns both pheromonal responsiveness and the cessation of pheromonal responsiveness. Specifically, our second hypothesis is that the young rat, attracted to pheromone-containing maternal feces, ingests these feces and, in so doing, consumes enough deoxycholic acid to alleviate its own acholic condition. The adaptive advantage that presumably derives from the behavior and, of course, from the ensuing change in bile composition is protection against endotoxic shock. On this basis, we might expect that the young rat will continue to respond to the pheromone until it develops the bile-acid profile of the adult or, in other words, until it acquires its own cholic immunity. This presumably occurs at about 27 days of age.

There is yet a third hypothesis to explain why, at 27 days, the weanling stops responding to the pheromone. This hypothesis belongs to Leon (Leon, 1975; Leon and Behse, 1977), and is compelling in its simplicity. Briefly stated, Leon maintains that at 27 days of age the young rat characteristically develops an adult-like odor. The pup is familiar with this odor because it matches that of the mother, first because the pup has been sharing the mother's diet (laboratory pellets) and second because the pup has been ingesting the end-product of that diet, the mother's feces. It is at the point of self-recognition that the pup stops responding to the pheromone, since there is no longer any "need" for him to do so. He now carries her familiar odor which, as part of his immediate environment, reduces novelty and hence the fear that novelty brings. The pup, in other words, comes to provide for himself what the mother had provided, namely a frequently-experienced and thus reassuring ambience.

We cannot choose among the three hypotheses just presented. There is simply not enough evidence to determine whether the 27-day-old pup, in ceasing to respond to the pheromone, does so because it has finally alleviated a "specific hunger," has developed the cholic-acid profile of the adult, or has established a familiar olfactory environment of its own. Obviously, there is a great deal of research to be done.

REFERENCES

Amenomori, Y., Chen, C. L., and Meites, J. Serum prolactin levels in rats during different reproductive states. *Endocrinology 70,* 506–510 (1970).

Aragona, C., Bohnet, H. G., and Friesen, H. G. Prolactin binding sites in the male rat liver following castration. *Endocrinology 99,* 1017–1022 (1976).

Bergstrom, S. and Norman, A. Metabolic products of cholesterol in bile and feces of rats. *Proc. Soc. Exp. Biol. Med. 83,* 71–74 (1953).

Bertok, L. Physico-chemical defense of vertebrate organisms: the role of bile acids in defense against bacterial endotoxins. *Perspectives in Biology and Medicine 21,* 70–76 (1977).

Breen, M. F. and Leshner, A. I. Maternal pheromone: a demonstration of its existence in the mouse (*Mus musculus*). *Physiol. Behav. 18,* 527–529 (1977).

Calhoun, F. B. *The Ecology and Sociology of the Norway Rat,* U.S. Public Health Service, Bethesda (1962).

Costlow, M. E., Buschow, R. A., and McGuire, W. L. Prolactin stimulation of prolactin receptors in rat liver. *Life Sci. 17,* 1457–1466 (1975).

Danielsson, H. Present status of research on catabolism and excretion of cholesterol. *Adv. Lipid Res. 1,* 335–385 (1963).

Denef, C. and De Moor, P. Sexual differentiation in the liver metabolism of steroid hormones organized by testosterone at birth. *Ann. Endocr. 31,* 785–788 (1970).

Denef, C. and De Moor, P. Sexual differentiation of steroid metabolizing enzymes in the rat liver. Further studies on predetermination by testosterone at birth. *Endocrinology 91,* 374–384 (1972).

Gregory, E. H. and Pfaff, D. W. Development of olfactory-guided behavior in infant rats. *Physiol. Behav. 6,* 573–576 (1971).

Grosvenor, C. E. Evidence that exteroceptive stimuli can release prolactin from the pituitary gland of the lactating rat. *Endocrinology 76,* 340–342 (1965).

Gustafsson, B. E., Bergstrom, S., Lindstedt, S., and Norman, A. Turnover and nature of fecal bile acids in germ-free and infected rats fed cholic acid -24-^{14}C. *Proc. Soc. Exp. Biol. Med. 94,* 467–471 (1957).

Gustafsson, B. E. and Norman, A. Comparison of bile acids in intestinal contents in germ-free and conventional rats. *Proc. Soc. Exp. Biol. Med. 110,* 387–389 (1962).

Gustafsson, J. A. and Stenberg, A. Masculinization of rat liver enzyme activities following hypophysectomy. *Endocrinology 96,* 891–896 (1974).

Haslewood, G. A. D. The biological significance of chemical differences in bile salts. *Biol. Rev. 39,* 537–574 (1964).

Heaton, K. W. *Bile Salts in Health and Disease,* Churchill Livingstone, London (1972).

Holinka, C. F. and Carlson, A. D. Pup attraction to lactating Sprague-Dawley rats. *Behav. Biol. 16,* 489–505 (1976).

Kelly, P. A., Posner, B. J., Tsushima, T., and Griesen, H. G. Studies of insulin, growth hormone and prolactin binding: ontogenesis, effects of sex and pregnancy. *Endocrinology 95,* 532–539 (1974).

Kellogg, T. F. Bile acid metabolism in gnotobiotic animals, in *The Bile Acids.* Nair and Kritchevsky, eds. Plenum Press, New York (1973), pp. 283–304.

Leidahl, L. C. and Moltz, H. Emission of the maternal pheromone in the nulliparous female and failure of emission in the adult male. *Physiol. Behav. 14,* 421–424 (1975).

Leidahl, L. C. and Moltz, H. Emission of the maternal pheromone in nulliparous and lactating females. *Physiol. Behav. 18,* 399–402 (1977).

Leon, M. Maternal pheromone. *Physiol. Behav. 13,* 441–453 (1974).

Leon, M. Dietary control of maternal pheromone in the lactating rat. *Physiol. Behav. 14,* 311–319 (1975).

Leon, M. and Behse, J. H. Dissolution of the pheromonal bond: waning of approach response by weanling rats. *Physiol. Behav. 18,* 393–397 (1977).

Leon, M. and Moltz, H. Maternal pheromone: discrimination be pre-weanling albino rats. *Physiol. Behav. 7,* 265–267 (1971).

Leon, M. and Moltz, H. The development of the pheromonal bond in the albino rat. *Physiol. Behav. 8,* 683–686 (1972).

Leon, M. and Moltz, H. Endocrine control of pheromonal emission in the post-partum rat. *Physiol. Behav. 10,* 65–67 (1973).

Lindstedt, S. and Samuelsson, B. Bile acids and steroids. On the interconversion of cholic and deoxycholic acid in the rat. *J. Biol. Chem. 234,* 2026–2030 (1959).

Mekhjian, H. S. and Phillips, S. F. Perfusion of the canine colon with unconjugated bile acids. *Gastoenterology 59,* 120–129 (1970).

Moltz, H. and Leidahl, L. C. Bile, prolactin, and the maternal pheromone. *Science 196,* 81–83 (1977).

Moltz, H., Leidahl, L., and Rowland, D. Prolongation of the maternal pheromone in the albino rat. *Physiol. Behav. 12,* 409–412 (1974).

Moltz, H. and Leon, M. Stimulus control of the maternal pheromone. *Physiol. Behav. 10,* 69–71 (1973).

Moltz, H., Levin, R., and Leon, M. Prolactin in the postpartum rat: synthesis and release in the absence of suckling stimulation. *Science 163,* 1083–1084 (1969).

Nicoll, C. S. and Swearingen, K. C. Preliminary observations on prolactin and GH turnover in rat adenohypophyses *in vivo,* in *The Hypothalamus.* L. Martini, M. Motta, and F. Fraschini, eds. Academic Press, New York (1970), pp. 449–462.

Norman, A. and Sjovall, J. Microbial transformation products of cholic acid in the rat. *Biochem. Biophys. Acta 29,* 467–468 (1958a).

Norman, A. and Sjovall, J. On the transformation and enterohepatic circulation of cholic acid in the rat. *J. Biol. Chem. 233,* 872–885 (1958b).

Norman, A. and Sjovall, J. Formation of lithocholic acid from chenodeoxycholic acid in the rat. *Acta Chem. Scand. 14,* 1815–1818 (1960).

Olivecrona, T. and Sjovall, J. Bile acids in rat portal blood. *Acta Physiol. Scand. 46,* 284–290 (1959).

Porter, R. H. and Doane, H. M. Maternal pheromone in the spiny mouse (*Acomys cahirinus*). *Physiol. Behav. 16,* 75–78 (1976).

Porter, R. H. and Ruttle, K. The responses of one-day old *Acomys cahirinus* pups to naturally occurring chemical stimuli. *Z. Tierpschol. 38,* 154–162 (1975).

Posner, B. I., Kelly, P. A., and Friesen, H. G. Induction of a lactogenic receptor in rat liver: influence of estrogen and the pituitary. *Proc. Nat. Acad. Sci. 71,* 2407–2410 (1974a).

Posner, B. I., Kelly, P. A., and Friesen, H. G. Prolactin receptors in rat liver: possible induction by prolactin. *Science 188,* 57–59 (1975).

Posner, B. I., Kelly, P. A., Shiu, R. P. C., and Friesen, H. G. Studies of insulin, GH and prolactin binding: tissue distribution, species variation and characterization (monkey, rat, guinea pig, rabbit, sheep). *Endocrinology 95,* 521–531 (1974b).

Rudbach, J. A., Anacker, R. L., Haskins, W. T., Johnson, A. G., Milner, K. C., and Ribi, E. Physical aspects of reversible inactivation of endotoxin. *Ann. N.Y. Acad. Sci. 133,* 629–643 (1966).

Sar, M. and Meites, J. Effects of suckling on pituitary release of prolactin, GH, and TSH in postpartum lactating rats. *Neuroendocrinology 4,* 25–31 (1969).

Weiner, J. M. and Lack, L. Bile salt absorption; enterohepatic circulation. In *Handbook of Physiology,* Section C: Alimentary canal. Vol. III: Intestinal absorption. C. F. Code, ed. Amer. Physiol. Soc., Washington (1968), pp. 1439–1455.

Wiesner, B. P. and Sheard, N. M. *Maternal Behaviour in the Rat.* Oliver & Boyd, Edinburgh (1933).

Maternal Influences and Early Behavior

7

Maternal Behavior in the Laboratory Rat

Jay S. Rosenblatt
Harold I. Siegel

The aim of this chapter is to present research which we have carried out over the past 20 years that has led us to develop a theory of the organization of maternal behavior that is both causal and carries with it a functional explanation. Our theory proposes that the regulation of maternal behavior is divided into two main phases with a transition period joining the two and occurring around the time of parturition (Rosenblatt, 1970, 1975). In the early phase physiological processes (i.e., hormonal) predominate and give rise to the onset of maternal behavior and to the associated reproductive phenomena of parturition and lactation (Figure 1). Maternal behavior at its onset is, therefore, an extension of the reproductive physiology of the female. As Wiesner and Sheard (1933) pointed out it is essential that maternal behavior be synchronized with the birth of the young and the capacity to feed them through nursing, a basic characteristic of mammals, and this is accomplished physiologically by joining these three maternal functions to the same complex of endocrine changes which occur at the end of pregnancy.

The second phase of maternal behavior begins shortly after parturition and is based, as Schneirla (1946) and Birch (1956) foresaw early in the study of maternal behavior, upon the mother's interaction with her young. During this interaction there is an exchange of stimulation (i.e., trophallaxis) between mother and young, which, for the mother, provides the basis for the maintenance of maternal behavior during the period of lactation. This phase of maternal behavior is nonhormonal; i.e., it is not dependent upon the hormones which initiated maternal behavior at the end of pregnancy nor on any other hormones that are involved in one or another postpartum function.

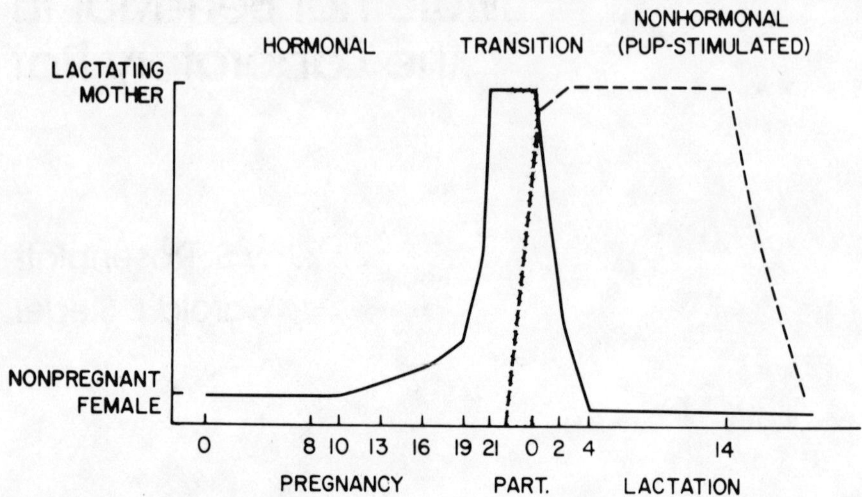

FIG. 1. Scheme of the regulation of maternal behavior during the maternal behavior cycle of the female rat. Ordinate shows levels of maternal behavior represented by lactating mother (high) and nonpregnant female (low) and abscissa shows three phases: pregnancy, parturition, and lactation.

It depends upon stimulation from the pups which the mother receives while exhibiting maternal behavior.

Maternal behavior is, therefore, self-perpetuating (i.e., enables the female to obtain pup stimulation) once it has been established until it begins to decline during the third and fourth weeks after parturition. The decline of maternal behavior is also nonhormonal, as far as the evidence indicates at the present time; the decline is in some way stimulated by pups as they grow older (Reisbick et al., 1975).

Parturition itself arises from the physiological changes which terminate pregnancy but in the course of parturition, the newly born pups appear and the female begins to interact with them, licking them, cleaning them and eating the placentas to which they are joined by the umbilical cord (Dollinger et al., 1976). The nonhormonal phase of maternal behavior is initiated at this time. Parturition is therefore transitional between the hormonal and nonhormonal phases in the regulation of maternal behavior in the female rat, and perhaps in other species of mammals as well.

This chapter is divided into four main sections in accord with the outline of the theory presented above. The first section deals with the *onset of maternal behavior* and will discuss the evidence concerning the hormonal basis of maternal behavior, the second section will deal with the *nonhormonal maintenance* of postpartum maternal behavior and will discuss as well, the phenomenon of stimulation of maternal behavior in nonpregnant females by prolonged exposure to pups (i.e., sensitization). The third section will deal with the role of parturition as a transition between the two phases of maternal behavior. Lactation and olfaction in relation to maternal behavior will be discussed in separate sections and a fourth section will propose a functional interpretation for the organization of maternal behavior as it has been already described.

THE ONSET OF MATERNAL BEHAVIOR

Descriptive Aspects

The sudden onset of maternal behavior during and after parturition has been noted by many investigators (Wiesner and Sheard, 1933; Rosenblatt and Lehrman, 1963). Most often it is initiated by body and anogenital licking of the pups and this is soon followed by lying with them, nursing, retrieving pups that have strayed from the nest and nestbuilding, which in fact often begins before parturition (Dollinger et al., 1976; Holloway et al., 1976). The female engages in placentophagia or eating of placentas at this time and although it has been suggested at times that this may contribute to the onset of maternal behavior there is little evidence to support this and strong evidence against it (Bridges, unpublished; Slotnick et al., 1973; Rosenblatt and Siegel, 1975). It is more likely that the placenta is attractive to the female because of its smell and taste and during ingestion of the placentas, the female frees the newborn from their umbilical connection, initiates breathing by the newborn (Corey, 1932), and then is attracted to the pups themselves. Sachs (1969) has shown that eating of the placenta without going on to eat the fetus can be considered an aspect of maternal behavior since it is characteristic of mothers during and shortly after parturition but not of nonpregnant or prepartum females (½ to 1½ days before parturition) who are as likely or even more likely to eat both the fetus and the placenta as the placenta alone. This behavior declines even in mothers; they are more likely to eat both the placenta and fetus than the placenta alone when tested 7–9 days postpartum.

By 24 hours after parturition nearly all females have established maternal behavior and are routinely engaging in *nestbuilding, nursing, retrieving,* and *licking of pups.* There are other components of maternal behavior in females that have recently come to light or have been studied systematically that also appear around parturition. Stern (unpublished) has shown that hoarding of food pellets which consists of carrying pellets from a distance outside the nest to nearby the nest and accumulating a store of food there starts around parturition (Herberg et al., 1972). Erskine (1978) has shown that the onset of maternal care is accompanied by the appearance of maternal aggression toward nest intruders. Still further, Korányi et al. (1976) have described the onset of responsiveness to pups calls by mothers around the time of parturition; mothers will traverse a T-maze to reach pups that are calling at the end of the maze.

Experimental Studies

It is important to know when maternal behavior begins because the hormones which are believed to stimulate its onset can be more accurately identified if the onset can be correlated with a particular period, allowing for some time for these hormones to produce their effect (i.e., latency of hormonal stimulation). Descriptive studies alone are not sufficient to provide this information since females may be ready to exhibit maternal behavior before they give birth but in the absence of pups they are unable to do so.

Several studies have shown that the onset of maternal behavior precedes parturition by at least 24 hours and even earlier. Slotnick et al. (1973) found that 25% of Wistar females exhibited retrieving and nestbuilding midday before parturition. Using a different strain of rats (Sprague-Dawley), Rosenblatt and Siegel (1975) observed nestbuilding 34 hours before parturition and retrieving of foster pups 27 hours before delivery and by the time of delivery, all the females had completed nests and 75% had already retrieved. Bridges et al. (1977) also found a prepartum onset of nestbuilding and retrieving and observed that females also crouched over young as in nursing, and licked the pups, exhibiting, therefore, all of the principal components of maternal behavior. Responses to pup calling first appear 24 hours before parturition (Korányi et al., 1976) but prepartum onset of maternal aggression has not yet been adequately tested.

These studies suggest that whatever hormones are involved in the onset of maternal behavior probably produce their effect at least 48 hours before parturition, thus allowing for an interval between the onset of hormonal stimulation and the expression of the behavior.

Blood Transfer Studies

Although it has long been believed that hormones are responsible for the onset of maternal behavior, based on the correlation of hormonal changes at the end of pregnancy and the onset of maternal behavior (Wiesner and Sheard, 1933; Beach, 1948), it was not until recently that direct evidence of blood borne factors which are capable of stimulating maternal behavior in nonpregnant females was presented. Terkel and Rosenblatt (1968) removed blood from newly maternal females, injected the plasma into nonpregnant animals, and presented them with pups to stimulate maternal behavior. These females exhibited maternal behavior in a little over 48 hours compared to control females that required more than four days after the injection of either blood from nonmaternal females or saline. Korányi et al. (1976) have confirmed these findings with latencies of 18 hours.

In a further study the blood from newly parturient mothers was cross transfused to nonpregnant females over a 6 hour period starting either 30 minutes after parturition, 24 hours after parturition, or 24 hours before parturition (Terkel and Rosenblatt, 1972). The postpartum donor females continued to exhibit maternal behavior during the cross transfusion and the recipient females were given pups to test their behavior. Those that received blood soon after parturition exhibited maternal behavior in less than two days in 88% of the cases and the average latency was 14.5 hours. Cross transfusions 24 hours before and after parturition were relatively ineffective in stimulating maternal behavior in less than two days.

These studies established that humoral factors (i.e., hormones) in the blood of new mothers are capable of stimulating maternal behavior at least in nulliparous animals and that these factors are present mainly around parturition. The problem is to identify these factors.

Hormone Administration Studies

Endocrinologists have known the general outlines of the hormonal regulation of pregnancy and parturition in the rat for some time, based upon studies of urinary secretions and biochemical and bioassays of pituitary, placental, and ovarian hormones (Zarrow 1961; Lehrman, 1961) and it was on the basis of this information that the earliest studies of hormonal stimulation of maternal behavior in rats were attempted. The principal hormones that were studied are estradiol, progesterone, and prolactin but other hormones have been tested as shown in Table 1. The early conception that prolactin was responsible for maternal behavior in the rat (Riddle et al., 1934, 1942) was not confirmed nor was estradiol or progesterone found effective in later studies by Lott (1963), Lott and Fuchs (1963) and Beach and Wilson (1963) using purified hormones and more carefully controlled procedures. Until 1970, despite the new evidence clearly indicating a humoral basis for maternal behavior (see above) no effective hormone treatment for stimulating maternal behavior was known.

Beginning in the late 1960's a large number of reports appeared (see Rosenblatt and Siegel, 1975) using radioimmunoassay procedures to measure

TABLE 1
Selected Summary of Previous Hormone Treatments in the Study of Hormonal Stimulation of Maternal Behavior in the Rat

Hormone and Other Treatments	Procedure	% Exhibit Maternal Behavior: Intact	Ovariectomized	Reference
Prolactin		71	79	1
Intermedin	Pretest days	60	77	
Luteinizing Hormone	1 to 10 (10 min)	59	60	
Desoxycorticosterone	Inject days 11 to 20	56	42	
Progesterone	Test days 21 to 23	68	66	
Testosterone		63	85	
Phenol		46	55	
Thyroxine		31	53	
Estrone withdrawal		78	50	
Progesterone	Inject days 1 to 10	21		2
Oil	Test days 11 to 13	14		
Prolactin + sensitization[5]		0		3
Prolactin + 10 min exposure to pups	Inject and test days 1 to 10	0		
Control + sensitization		33		
Control + 10 min exposure to pups		17		
Prolactin (10 mg)	Inject days 1 to 5	0		4
Prolactin (20 mg)	Test days 6 to 8	0		
Control		67[6]		
Estrogen (days 1 to 20) + Prolactin (days 21 to 30)	Test days 31 to 33	25		4
Estrogen (days 1 to 20) + water (days 21 to 30)		60		

[1]Riddle et al. (1942)
[2]Lott (1962)
[3]Lott and Fuchs (1962)
[4]Beach and Wilson (1963)
[5]Continuous exposure to pups
[6]Partial pattern of maternal behavior

the secretory rates and circulating levels of estradiol, progesterone, and prolactin during pregnancy and at parturition. Circulating levels of these hormones during pregnancy are shown in Figure 2, taken from several different sources. With this new information available renewed attempts to find the hormonal basis for the onset of maternal behavior in rats have been successful.

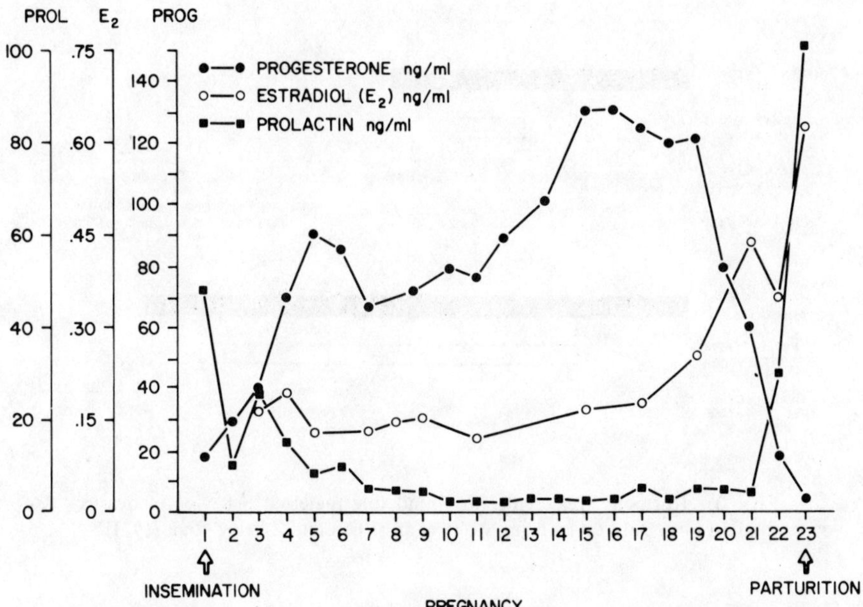

FIG. 2. Circulating levels of progesterone, estradiol and prolactin during pregnancy in the rat. Data taken from various sources: progesterone, Pepe and Rothchild (1974); estradiol, Shaikh (1971); prolactin, Morishige et al. (1973).

Moltz et al. (1970) and Zarrow et al. (1971) using basically the same combinations of hormones with slightly different schedules of injection (Figure 3) were able to stimulate short latency maternal behavior in ovariectomized females. The treatments consisted of estradiol benzoate (EB), progesterone (P), and prolactin (Prol), the latter given at the end of either 10 or 20 days of EB and P. Moltz et al. (1970) reported latencies of 35 to 40 hours following the beginning of Prol; Zarrow et al. (1971) reported immediate responding to pups in most of the females at the end of the 4th Prol injection.

Moltz et al. (1970) proposed that EB and Prol actually stimulate maternal behavior but only after P withdrawal when thresholds for EB and Prol action are lowered. Only this combination resulted in optimal responding with essentially no variability; the combination of any two of these hormones gave longer latencies and greater variability.

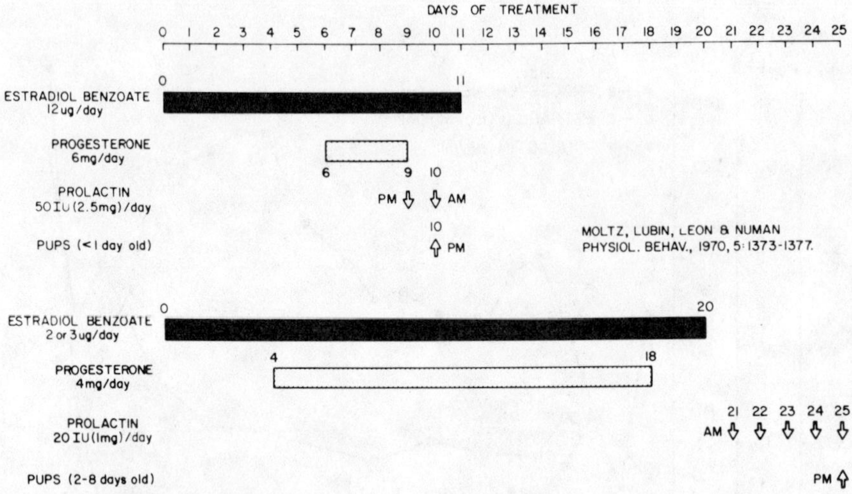

FIG. 3. Hormone treatments for stimulating maternal behavior in ovariectomized rats. Data taken from Moltz et al. (1970) and Zarrow et al. (1971).

Pregnancy Termination Studies

Maternal behavior normally arises at the termination of pregnancy. It is possible, however, to terminate pregnancy prematurely either by caesarean section (Labriola, 1953; Moltz et al., 1966) or by hysterectomizing (i.e., removing uteri with fetuses + placentas) females. The effect is to cause a premature onset of maternal behavior (Figure 4; Rosenblatt and Siegel, 1975). Since females that are not hysterectomized but are allowed to continue their pregnancies do not exhibit maternal behavior as early as those that are hysterectomized it is clear that hysterectomy provokes a change in hormone secretion from that which exists during pregnancy and that some aspect of this change is responsible for the early onset of maternal behavior. Not all of the hormonal changes which follow hysterectomy are known but there is strong evidence that once pregnancy is terminated the female initiates an estrous cycle (similar to the "postpartum estrus" of females after normal parturition).

We have taken blood samples and assayed circulating levels of P at 24 hour intervals following hysterectomy done at different times during pregnancy. In addition, we have taken vaginal smears and tested females for lordosis and then determined when ovulation takes place (Figure 5). At each of the times of

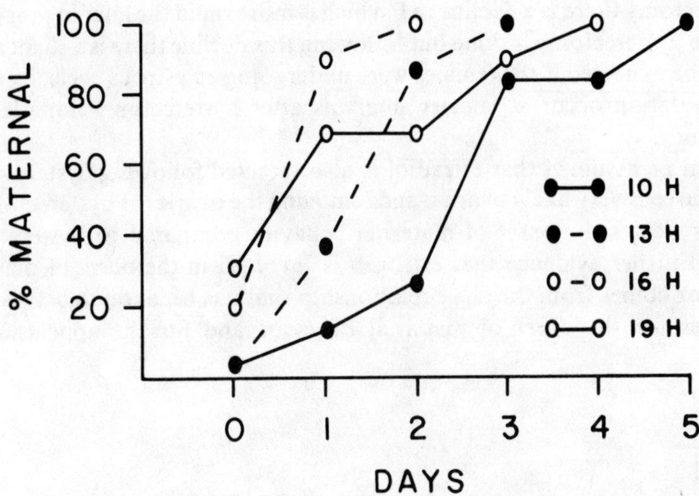

FIG. 4. Cumulative percentage of females showing Maternal behavior following hysterectomy on the 10th, 13th, 16th, and 19th days of pregnancy. First test (O) at 48 hr after surgery.

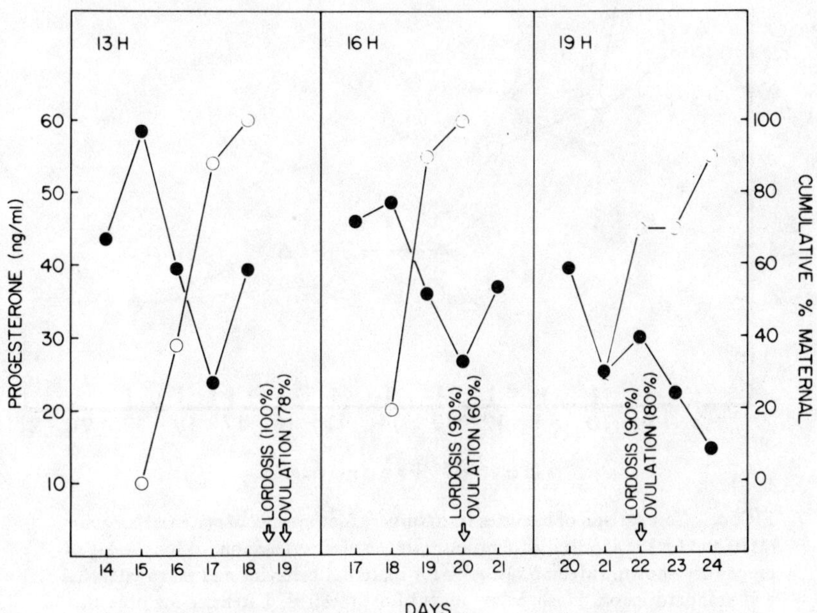

FIG. 5. Circulating levels of progesterone (filled circles) cumulative percentage of females showing maternal behavior (open circles) following hysterectomy (H) at the 13th, 16th, and 19th days of pregnancy. Time of lordosis and ovulation also shown. Maternal behavior tests started 2 days after surgery.

hysterectomy there is a decline in P which is more rapid the later in pregnancy that the hysterectomy is done but following this decline there is a slight rise as would be expected if the females were undergoing an estrous cycle. Lordosis and ovulation occur at shorter intervals after hysterectomy done later in pregnancy.

It can be assumed that estradiol is also secreted following hysterectomy. The source is very likely ovarian and removing the ovaries of hysterectomized females delays the onset of maternal behavior compared to hysterectomy alone. Further evidence that estrogen is involved in the onset of maternal behavior comes from the close relationship that has been found between the latencies for the onset of maternal behavior and for the appearance of

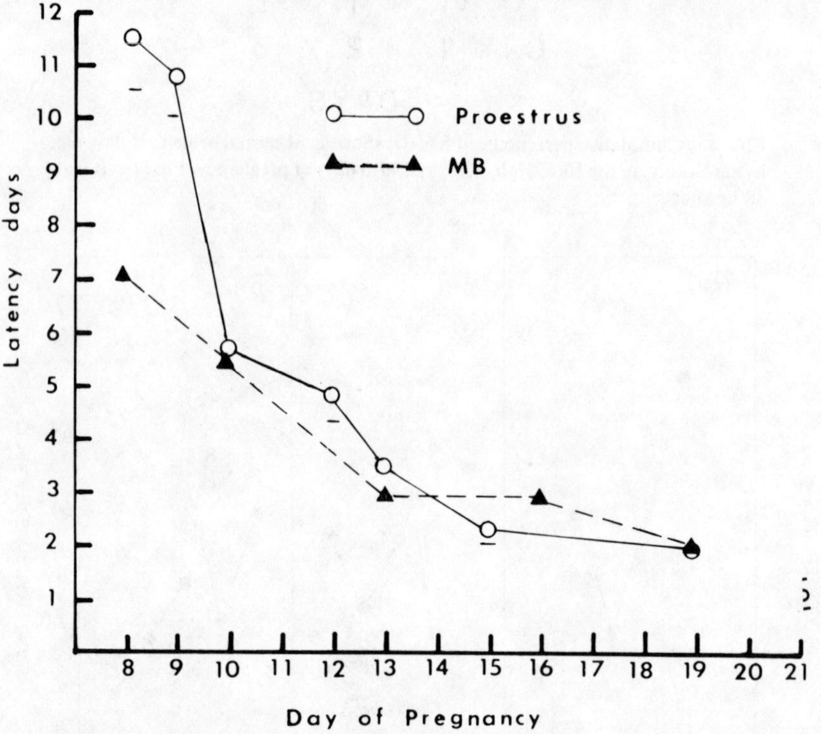

FIG. 6. Comparison of latencies from surgery for the onset of maternal behavior (MB) and for the appearance of proestrus in females hysterectomized on the day of pregnancy shown. (Median latencies for maternal behavior and mean latencies and standard errors (dash below mean) for proestrus. Latencies for proestrus taken from Morishige and Rothchild, 1974, and Johnson, 1972). (From J. S. Rosenblatt and H. I. Siegel. Hysterectomy-induced maternal behavior during pregnancy in the rat. *J. Comp. Physiol. Psychol. 89,* 685–700. Copyright 1975 by the American Psychological Association. Reprinted by permission.)

proestrus vaginal smears following hysterectomy at various times during pregnancy (Figure 6). Of course the appearance of lordosis, which requires prior estradiol stimulation, and of ovulation are additional evidence.

Females that were hysterectomized-ovariectomized (HO) on Day 16 of pregnancy, treated with EB (100 μg/kg or 20 μg/kg) at surgery and exposed to pups 48 hours postoperatively exhibited a rapid onset of maternal behavior; the latencies to maternal behavior of these animals were as short as those of females that were only hysterectomized (Figure 7; Siegel and Rosenblatt, 1975a). Although P was given initially at 44 hours after EB it was found unnecessary; in more recent research the EB dose has been reduced to 5 μg/kg (Siegel and Rosenblatt, 1977). EB implanted in the medial preoptic area of the brain of 16-day pregnant HO females resulted in equally short latencies to the onset of maternal behavior (Numan et al., 1977).

An attempt was also made to stimulate maternal behavior in nonpregnant females using the same EB treatment and employing ovariectomy to remove the endogenous source of estrogen and progesterone. Our first study using EB at 100 μg/kg was unsuccessful: females failed to respond to the treatment which had been effective in the HO pregnant females. It occurred to us that hysterectomy may have played a more important role than simply to

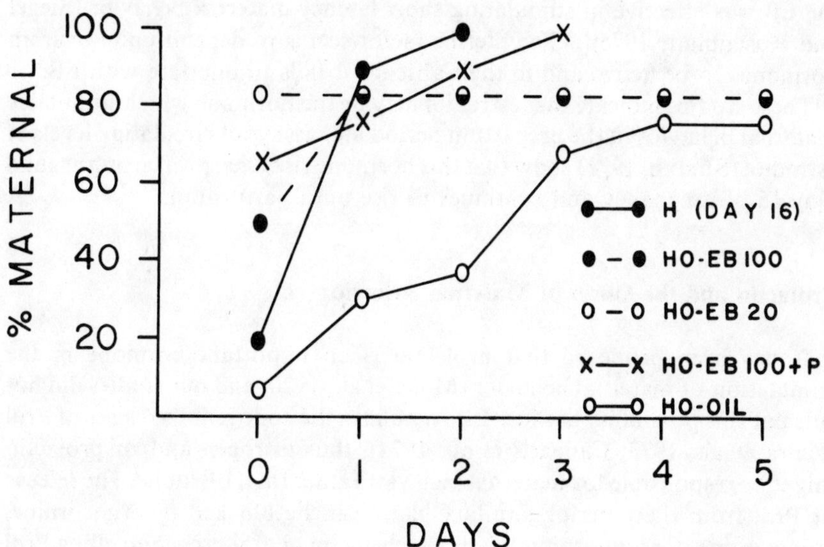

FIG. 7. Cumulative percentage of females showing maternal behavior after hysterectomy (H) or hysterectomy-ovariectomy (HO) on the 16th day of pregnancy (16) and estradiol benzoate (EB) treatments of 100 to 20 μ g/kg and progesterone (P) at 0.5 mg. Maternal behavior tests started at 48 hr after surgery and hormone treatment.

terminate the pregnancies of the pregnant females and the presence of the uteri may be interfering with the effect of EB in the nonpregnant females, a factor which we had not taken into consideration. We therefore removed the uteri and ovariectomized (HO) nonpregnant females and administered EB and found that now the EB was effective in stimulating short-latency maternal behavior (Siegel and Rosenblatt, 1975b).

This raised in our minds the question whether in the pregnant H females we were dealing with a completely artificial system as a result of removing the uteri. It was necessary to find another way to terminate pregnancy without removing the uteri to see if short-latency maternal behavior would result when pregnancy was terminated but the uteri remained. When administered on Day 16 and 19, prostaglandin $F_{2\alpha}$ ($PGF_{2\alpha}$), which has been implicated in the normal termination of pregnancy in the rat (Smalstig et al., 1974; Ford and Yoshinaga, 1975; Straus et al., 1975; Flower, 1977), induces abortion within 30 hours. These females exhibit maternal behavior as readily as hysterectomized females suggesting that the presence of the uterus at 16 or 19 days does not interfere with estrogen action (Rodriguez-Sierra and Rosenblatt, unpublished). One other study also indicates that under certain conditions the uterine factor may not be present: nonpregnant females were ovariectomized only and were treated eight weeks later with EB. At that time the EB was effective in stimulating short latency maternal behavior (Siegel and Rosenblatt, 1975b). The uterine factor seems to depend upon ovarian hormones to be active and in their absence it fails to interfere with EB.

These studies indicate that estradiol may be the hormone which stimulates maternal behavior in the prepartum period and assays of circulating levels of estradiol (Shaikh, 1971) show that this hormone rises sharply starting around Day 15 of pregnancy and continues to rise until parturition.

Prolactin and the Onset of Maternal Behavior

It has been proposed that prolactin is an important hormone in the stimulation of maternal behavior (Moltz et al., 1970) and our studies did not rule out this possibility because EB stimulates the endogenous release of Prol (Kalra et al., 1973; Caligaris et al., 1974); thus estrogen and/or prolactin might be responsible for maternal behavior rather than EB alone. The release of Prol from the anterior pituitary gland can be blocked by ergocornine, ergocryptine or apomorphine all of which act on neural sites controlling Prol secretion (Gala and Boss, 1975; Hill-Samli and MacLeod, 1975). We therefore repeated several of our studies with 16-day pregnant HO females that were given EB and one of these Prol blockers. The onset of maternal behavior after short latencies was not blocked by preventing the release of

Prol under any of these conditions (Numan et al., 1977; Rodriguez-Sierra and Rosenblatt, 1977). Zarrow et al. (1971) and more recently Stern (1977) have also reported that ergocornine or ergocryptine given to late pregnant females during the last week of pregnancy does not interfere with the onset of maternal behavior at parturition despite the failure of lactation produced by these Prol blocking agents. It should also be pointed out that the prepartum surge of circulating Prol (Figure 2) probably occurs too late to influence the onset of maternal behavior now that it is known that the onset occurs nearly a day before parturition in most females (Nagasawa and Yanai, 1972).

Progesterone Inhibition of Maternal Behavior

The decline in progesterone at the end of pregnancy (Figure 2) seems necessary for the onset of maternal behavior since several studies have shown that if progesterone levels are maintained maternal behavior fails to appear at the normal time (Moltz et al., 1969; Herrenkohl, 1971, 1974; Herrenkohl and Lisk, 1973). We were able to test this directly by giving P (0.5 mg) to EB-treated nonpregnant HO females at three different times: at the same time (0 hr) as the EB and HO, 24 hours after these two treatments or 44 hours after them (Siegel and Rosenblatt, 1975c). The results indicated that P given at 24-hour blocked EB stimulation of maternal behavior while at 44 hours it had no effect and at 0 hour it delayed the onset for a short time. This has since been duplicated with 16-day pregnant HO females given EB and P according to the same schedule (Siegel and Rosenblatt, 1977).

Progesterone Withdrawal

Does progesterone withdrawal by itself, apart from its permissive role in EB stimulation, have any direct facilitory effect on maternal behavior? This has been studied in a series of experiments by Bridges et al. (1977, 1978a,b,c). By testing 16-day pregnant HO females 24 hours following surgery after they had been given pups at the time of surgery, these investigators found that 40% were maternal compared to less than 10% of H animals. At 48 hours nearly all females of both groups were maternal. These results differed from our earlier ones in which fewer HO females were maternal at 48 hours than hysterectomized females but exposure to pups had begun at 48 hours in these earlier studies. If pups were not initially given to these HO females until 24 or 48 hours, then at 24 hours nearly 30% were still maternal but at 48 hours none were maternal, while at 48 hours nearly 60% of hysterectomized females were

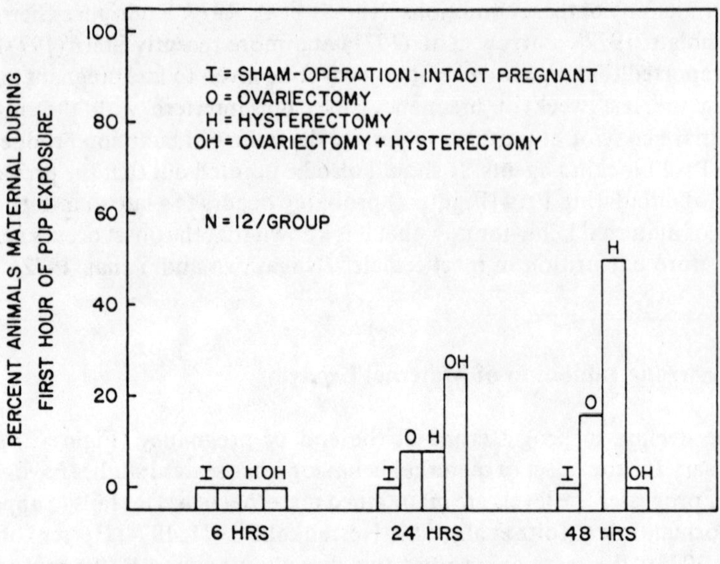

FIG. 8. Comparison of the percentage of animals that were spontaneously maternal (responded during the first hour of expsoure to foster young) after surgery at 10:00 on Day 17 of pregnancy and first presentation of pups at 6 hr, 24 hr, and 48 hr later. (From R. S. Bridges, J. S. Rosenblatt, and H. H. Feder. Stimulation of maternal responsiveness after pregnancy termination in rats: effects of time of onset of behavioral testing. *Horm. Behav. 10,* 235–245 (1978a)).

maternal upon their first exposure to pups (Figure 8). The results with HO females have been confirmed by MacKinnon and Stern (1977).

These findings indicate that the withdrawal of P may have a facilitating effect on maternal behavior for a period of 24 hours which then subsides but does not disappear since these females remain easily aroused to maternal behavior by continued exposure to pups. This effect can be blocked specifically by P implanted subcutaneously in a silastic capsule where it releases levels of P similar to those found during the latter half of pregnancy (Bridges et al., 1978c; Bridges and Feder, 1978).

The maintenance of progesterone levels, therefore, prevents the onset of maternal behavior while the subsequent withdrawal may result in short-term facilitation. However, as noted earlier, a large percentage of non-pregnant HO animals are maternal after the injection of EB alone, suggesting that prior progesterone stimulation or withdrawal are not absolutely necessary. Moreover, treating nulliparous females for two weeks with silastic capsules of progesterone followed by removal of these implants did not facilitate the display of maternal behavior (Bridges and Siegel, unpublished).

Prepartum Hormonal Onset of Maternal Behavior

Pregnancy termination effects on maternal behavior were studied because of their presumed relevance to the situation just before parturition. The same series of hormonal changes occurs following pregnancy termination by hysterectomy and $PGF_{2\alpha}$ as at the natural termination of pregnancy. Presumably, therefore, it is the prepartum rise in estradiol secretion by the ovaries which initiates maternal behavior; Prol plays no role and P withdrawal plays both a permissive and facilitating role in the onset of maternal behavior.

POSTPARTUM MAINTENANCE OF MATERNAL BEHAVIOR

Nonhormonal Maintenance of Maternal Behavior

Following parturition the female undergoes postpartum estrus around 8–13 hours after the completion of delivery (Sachs, et al., 1971; Ying and Greep, 1973; Ying et al., 1973). The pattern of anterior pituitary and ovarian hormone secretion which characterized late pregnancy undergoes rapid changes during this period and, following this single estrous cycle, the female is maintained in diestrus through suckling by the pups until 3–4 weeks after parturition. During this prolonged period, circulating levels of P and Prol are maintained at high levels while estradiol secretion is inhibited (Rothchild, 1960; Tucker et al., 1967; Gala, 1970). Females that are made pregant during postpartum estrus show a similar hormonal picture and due to the lack of estradiol the blastocysts of the new pregnancy are delayed in implanting in the wall of the uterus for as long as two weeks and delivery of the new litter may not take place until 34 days after mating (Weichert, 1940; Shelesnyak and Kraicer, 1963; Mayer, 1963).

The hormonal conditions which gave rise to the onset of maternal behavior undergo a rapid transformation immediately postpartum; it is difficult to see, therefore, how the same hormones that were present prepartum can continue to maintain maternal behavior. In support of this, there is considerable evidence that maintenance of postpartum maternal behavior does not depend upon these hormones. Hypophysectomy during the first three days does not interfere with the maintenance of maternal behavior (Bintarnihgsih et al., 1958; Rothchild, 1960; Erskine, 1978) and removal of the ovaries (Rosenblatt, unpublished) or adrenal glands (Thoman and Levine, 1970) also does not interfere wth maternal behavior postpartum. The administration of P during the first days postpartum has no effect on the maintenance of maternal behavior (Moltz et al., 1969; Herrenkohl, 1972, 1974) nor does blocking the release of Prol (Numan et al., 1972; Zarrow et al., 1971; Stern, 1978). Since none of these hormones when they are either removed from or administered to postpartum females has any effect on maintenance of maternal behavior it must be concluded either that some other hormone is involved, or, what is more likely, maternal behavior is no longer under hormonal control once it has been initiated by prepartum hormonal stimulation (Rosenblatt, 1971, 1975).

Maintenance of Maternal Behavior by Pup Stimulation

What is crucial for the maintenance of maternal behavior is that females receive stimulation from their newborn during the first few days following parturition and thereafter. When pups were removed from mothers during parturition, after the mothers had licked them clean and eaten the placentas, and the mothers were tested for maternal behavior with 5- to 10-day-old pups one week later, nearly all of the mothers failed to display maternal behavior (Rosenblatt and Lehrman, 1963). By removing pups from mothers during parturition for two or four days and testing the females on the 3rd or 5th day postpartum we were able to show that the decline in maternal responsiveness is nearly complete by the 5th day since none of the females exhibited the principal components of maternal behavior during 1-hour tests with 5- to 10-day old pups (Figure 9; Rosenblatt, 1965). Pup stimulation is required for females to establish and maintain their maternal behavior during the immediate postpartum period. However, a similar period of separation from pups after maternal behavior has been maintained for 14 days, 9 days, or as little as 3 days postpartum produces a deficit in maternal behavior in only 40 to 50% of the females and when 5- to 10-day-old young are returned to such females the pups are soon taken care of and in all cases reared to weaning (Rosenblatt and Lehrman, 1963; Rosenblatt, 1965).

Maintenance of maternal behavior involves the development of behavioral synchrony between the mother and her young in which the mother adjusts her behavior to the needs of the young by responding to stimuli from them which in the young are in some way related to these needs (Rosenblatt, 1965). The establishment of synchrony between mother and young begins at birth and progresses through the early phases of the youngs' development during which

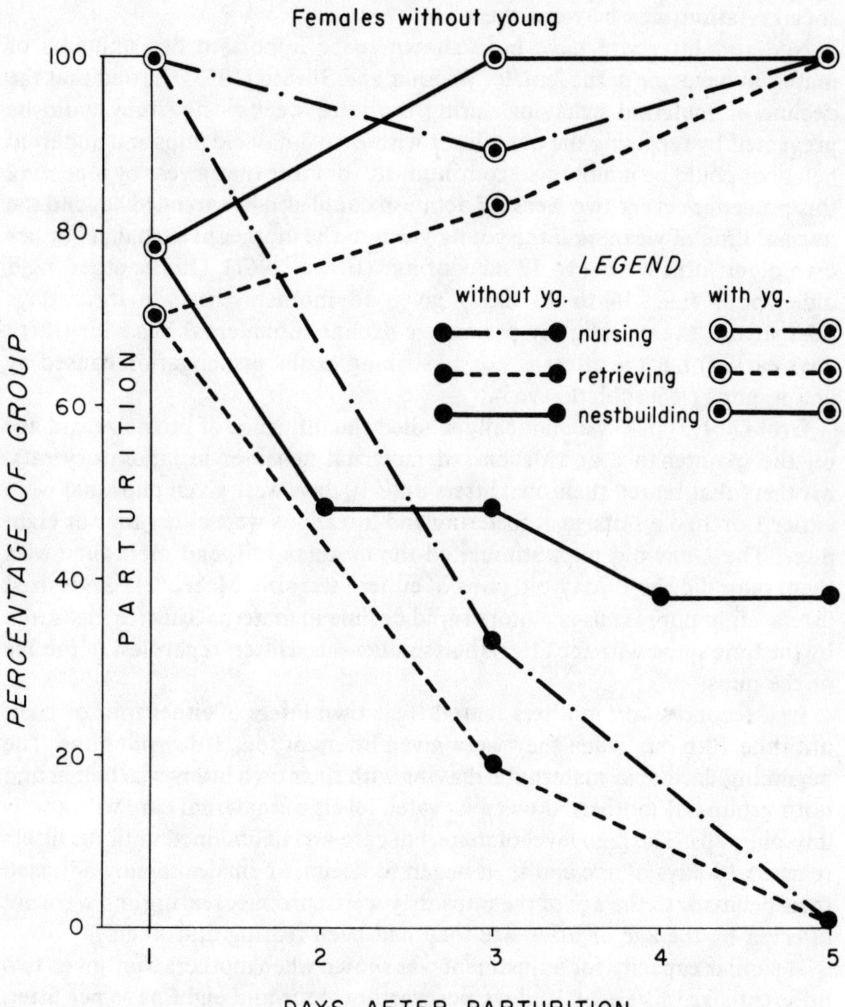

FIG. 9. Decline in maternal behavior in mothers with pups removed for 2 or 4 days and returned on the 3rd and 5th day postpartum. Comparison with mothers who kept their pups from parturition on.

the mother takes the initiative in the relationship then into later phases during which the initiative shifts to the young leading eventually to gradual weaning and dissolution of the mother-young relationship but not necessarily of all social relationships between them.

Age and litter size have been shown to be important determinants of maternal behavior in the female. Wiesner and Sheard (1933) showed that the decline of maternal behavior during the third week postpartum could be prevented by replacing the older litter with 2- to 3-day old pups and maternal behavior could be maintained continuously for more than a year by repeating this procedure every two weeks. Lactation could also be extended beyond the normal time of weaning if the young given to the mother in exchange for her own older litter were 6 to 12 days of age (Bruce, 1961). On the other hand older pups (i.e., 14 to 18 days) given to mothers that are three days postpartum cause a slightly premature decline in maternal behavior (three days earlier) but the effect is not as striking as the prolongation caused by young pups (Rosenblatt, 1965).

Grota (1973) has systematically studied the influence of litter size and age on the maintenance and decline of maternal behavior in laboratory rats. Mothers that reared their own litters until 10 days were given pups that were either 1 or 10 days of age at fostering and litter sizes were either four or eight pups. The 1-day-old pups stimulated the mothers to spend more time with them than did the 10-day-old pups of either litter size. Moreover, large-sized litters (eight pups) caused a more rapid decline in maternal care (as measured by the time spent with the litter) than smaller-sized litters regardless of the age of the pups.

In a second study mothers reared their own litters of either four or eight until the 10th day when they were given litters of four 1-day-old pups. The beginning decline in maternal behavior with their own litters was halted and both groups of mothers showed elevated levels of maternal care with the 1-day-old pups. The high level of maternal care was maintained until the litters reached 10 days of age and then began to decline. Females rapidly adjusted their behavior to the age of the pups they were currently rearing and were not affected by the age or litter size they had been rearing until then.

A similar capacity for adjustment was shown when mothers were given two different-sized litters at 10 days postpartum, four and eight pups per litter, aged 1 day at fostering. The larger-sized litter caused a more rapid decline in maternal care than the smaller litter.

What these studies show is that maintenance of maternal behavior and the eventual decline are largely determined by features of the young that are related to their age and number and that the mother has considerable flexibility in her response to her litter and to foster litters that differ from her own pups.

The age-related and litter size stimuli which mothers responded to in the above study were not determined but other studies have focussed on this problem. Most interesting is the finding that mothers may be highly responsive to certain movements made by the young and unresponsive to others. Lateral head turning in young pups is particularly pronounced in a mutant strain of Wistar rats (Gunn strain) especially the young that exhibit congenital cerebellar hypoplasia in association with jaundice (hyperbilirubinemia) (Tamaki et al., 1977). Mothers appear to be particularly solicitous of the jaundiced young, which lead Graham and Hasenstab (in press) to suspect that they were responding to this particular head movement and, in so doing, compensating for the motor disabilities which these young suffer. Graham and Hasenstab tested this idea by using wooden pegs, about the size of newborn, that could be pivoted either vertically or horizontally, simulating the head movement of the pups. Only the lateral head movement stimulated approaches by mothers, despite the fact that the amplitude of the vertical movement of the peg equalled that of the lateral movement. These findings are particularly significant in view of Tobach's (1977) observations that lateral head movement by pups is a distress response to the absence of nest odors.

The mother appears to respond to a complex of stimuli from pups which includes olfactory, auditory, visual, gustatory and thermotactile. Sensory ablation studies have been largely unsuccessful in isolating any one sensory stimulus upon which maternal behavior depends for its maintenance giving rise to the conception that the behavior is multisensory-based (Herrenkohl and Sachs, 1972). Smotherman et al. (1974) have shown, however, that odors from pups at the end of a maze that extends outward from the home cage stimulate retrieving when paired with ultrasonic vocalizations emitted by the pups (via playback). Grabon et al. (unpublished) have confirmed this but also found that odor alone could elicit a choice of the correct alley of two in a diamond-shaped runway. At close range, females appear to respond to taste and perhaps odors in their licking of pups (Charten et al., 1971). They prefer a water solution with substances wiped from the perineal region of pups (excluding urine and feces) over pure water, and they fail to respond to pups whose perineal region is covered with collodion.

While pup-emitted ultrasounds have been found to elicit search and locating pups in preparation for retrieving them to the nest (Sewell, 1970; Allin and Banks, 1971, 1972), McClinn (1978), in observing mothers and their litters daily for two 5-minute periods over the first three weeks noted only 134 instances of ultrasonic calling and 9,000 instances of sonic calls. The fact that pups were rarely out of the nest (and on these occasions did not call at all) may account for the few ultrasonic calls observed but of greater importance is the large number of sonic calls. McClinn noted that sonic calling was associated with shifts in the mother's behavior from resting, as during nursing, to movement in the nest, self-grooming, and licking the pups. When recorded sonic pups calls were played back to one-week postpartum mothers while they tended their litters, the mothers shifted on the nest and licked their pups but when either pure tones or random noise were played to the mothers the mothers only attended to the sound but did not show any particular behavior toward the pups. Mothers are therefore quite attentive to their pups' calls and alter their behavior in response to them. The calls perhaps indicate some disturbance on the part of the pups that might be caused by the mother's behavior, or in the case of ultrasonic calls, by distress resulting from separation from the mother and litter.

Mothers are also responsive to thermal stimuli from their pups as Leon et al. (1978) have shown in their study of the thermal basis of nursing and pup contact during the first 15 days postpartum. At the start of a nursing session the mother's ventral surface temperature is at its minimum within the normal range of surface temperatures and the pups' surface temperature is also at the low point of its range, having fallen during the interval from the last nursing contact with mother. During nursing the pups are warmed as is the mother's ventral surface and when both reach the high point of their normal ranges the mother leaves the pups and nursing is terminated. That the mother is responding to the pup's body temperature in determining the duration of nursing is indicated by the following: warming pups artificially and independently of the mother shortens the duration of nursing while prolonging the rise in body termperature of the pups by lowering the ambient temperature increases the duration of nursing. In both cases the ultimate determinant of nursing duration is the rate at which the mother's ventral body surface reaches its high point but in the course of monitoring this change in her own temperature the mother monitors and responds to thermal stimulation from her pups.

Stimulation of Maternal Behavior in Nonpregnant Females: Sensitization

The potency of pup stimulation is perhaps best illustrated by the phenomenon of "sensitization" which refers to the stimulation of maternal behavior in nonpregnant females by prolonged exposure to young pups. Wiesner and Sheard (1933) were the first to demonstrate this phenomenon in about 25% of their females but Cosnier and Couturier (1966) and Rosenblatt (1967) were able to show that nearly all females and males can be sensitized with average latencies of five to seven days (under specific conditions). Stern and MacKinnon (1978) have recently shown that 1- to 2-day-old pups are more effective than 3- to 12-day-old pups and above that age, pups are relatively ineffective for sensitizing females.

There is now substantial evidence that sensitization is not based upon hormones which may have been released by pup stimulation. Hypophysectomized females and females that have been ovariectomized are as readily sensitized as intact females (Rosenblatt, 1967). Moreover, females that have been sensitized do not carry in their blood any substances which when cross transfused to nonsensitized females stimulates maternal behavior as is the case in hormonally-induced newly parturient females as described earlier (Terkel and Rosenblatt, 1971, 1972).

Although latencies are not affected by high levels of circulating Prol (Baum, 1978) there is evidence that sensitization latencies may be increased by estradiol and progesterone (Leon et al., 1973, 1975). Also Marinari and Moltz (1977) have reported that during sensitization in their strain of rats (Wistar) maternal behavior is more likely to be initiated during the proestrous and estrous phases of the cycle than during other phases, a finding that differs from that reported by Rosenblatt (1967) and others (Stern and Siegel, 1978). Even if it were the case that hormones do modulate the sensitization process, it is clear that the process is not dependent upon hormones.

During sensitization the female undergoes changes that can be divided into three phases: an *early phase* during which the female investigates the pups then avoids them, a *middle phase* in which she tolerates close approach and contact by the pups and occasionally sniffs and even briefly licks them, and an *onset phase* in which the female quite abruptly begins to lick the pups, gathers them under her body, retrieves them, builds a nest and crouches over the pups as in nursing (Terkel and Rosenblatt, 1971; Fleming and Rosenblatt, 1974a). Although females vary in the rate at which they progress from one phase to another, which results in different latencies among them, they all exhibit the sequence of changes described above.

Overcoming the avoidance of pups (initial phase) appeared to us as crucial for sensitization to occur and this in turn seemed to depend upon how much contact females had with the pups (Herrenkohl and Rosenberg, 1972). To test this general hypothesis we confined females with pups in different sized cages ranging in floor area from 36 to 468 sq. inches and observed their latencies to initiate maternal behavior (Terkel and Rosenblatt, 1971). Latencies were shortest in the smallest cages (2.8 days) and were progressively longer as cage sizes increased (126 sq in = 3.5 days, 360 sq in = 4.3 days, 468 sq in = 11.6 days) and only three of five females were sensitized in the largest-sized cage which permitted females to remain at a distance of nearly 36 inches from the pups. Forced cohabitation evidently speeded the overcoming of avoidance of the pups and enabled females to exhibit maternal behavior.

Additional evidence that a reduction in the avoidance of pups is critical for sensitization to occur comes from studies on the effects of tail-pinch. Mild tail-pinch has been shown to induce anogenital licking of pups in nulliparous rats (Sherman, 1975) which does not depend upon prior experience with pups. The tail-pinch appears to "force" the females to contact the pups in this way (as it forces pellet chewing when only pellets are present) and we have shown that tail-pinch accelerates, in a dose-dependent pattern, not only pup licking but the onset of retrieving and the adoption of the nursing posture when tail-pinch is no longer administered (Szechtman et al., 1977).

The case for considering maternal behavior in sensitized females as a representation of postpartum maternal behavior, in isolation from the hormonal onset which normally precedes it during the maternal behavior cycle, would be strengthened if it could be shown that it shares the characteristics of postpartum maternal behavior. This was undertaken in two studies by Fleming and Rosenblatt (1974a) and Reisbick et al. (1975). In the first study females were sensitized and were then given pups that were the same ages, day by day, as those of lactating mothers rearing their own litters

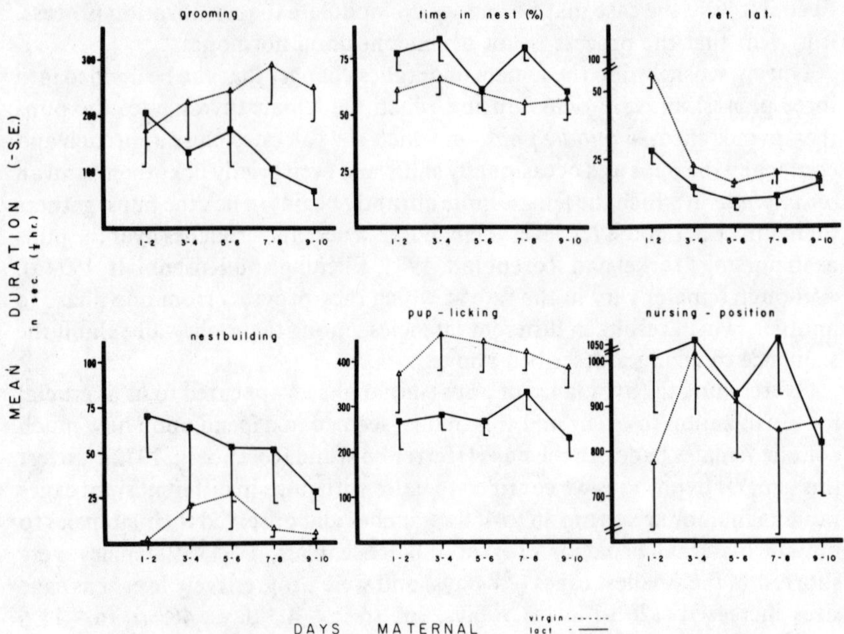

FIG. 10. Maternal behavior in the lactating and virgin female rat: mean duration (in seconds) of different maternal components as a function of days maternal. (Abbreviations: ret. lat. = retrieval latency; lact = lactating.) (From A. S. Fleming and J. S. Rosenblatt. Maternal behavior in the virgin and lactating rat. *J. Comp. Physiol. Psychol. 86*, 957–972. Copyright 1974 by the American Psychological Association. Reprinted by permission.)

from birth to the 10th day postpartum. The behavior of the sensitized "mothers" was quite similar both quantitatively and qualitatively to that of the lactating mothers with respect to time spent in the nest, retrieving latency, pup licking (both general body and anogenital licking) and nursing/crouching duration (Figure 10) and differed only in grooming and nestbuilding.

The comparison was extended to the 28th day so as to include the period of decline of maternal behavior in the second study. The similarities found during the first 10 days continued into the period of decline (Figure 11): retrieving declined at the same time in both groups but nursing/crouching declined somewhat earlier in the sensitized females and with respect to the rise of rejection and withdrawal behavior and excitable darting, hopping and shaking, only the former responses increased more rapidly in the virgins. What is most remarkable is that even without the impetus to maternal behavior given by the hormonal onset, the behavior of the sensitized females so closely resembled in overall patterns, and in most details, the maternal behavior of postpartum mothers.

There are however important differences between sensitization as the mode of establishing maternal behavior and the normal hormonal stimulation of maternal behavior. Erskine (1978) was unable to elicit maternal aggression

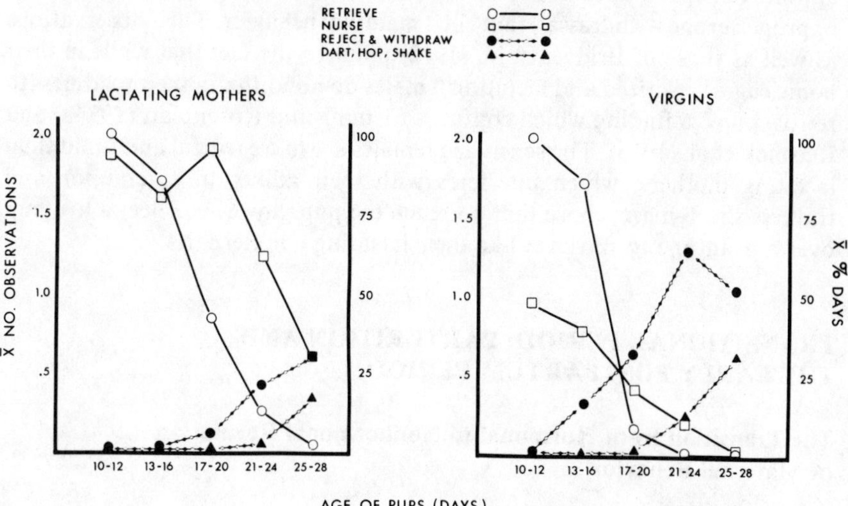

FIG. 11. Comparison of sensitized virgins and lactating mothers in the decline of maternal behavior during tests with live-in pups 10–28 days of age. (Each point represents the mean of 3- or 4-day averages for nine females.) (From S. Reisbick, J. S. Rosenblatt and A. D. Mayer. Decline of maternal behavior in the virgin and lactating rat. *J. Comp. Physiol. Psychol. 89,* 722–732. Copyright 1975 by the American Psychological Association. Reprinted by permission.)

toward introduced male intruders from sensitized females unless she extended the period of contact with pups, after the onset of maternal behavior, to 20 days or longer. Roy (1977) also was unable to elicit maternal aggression from sensitized virgins whereas EB-stimulated mothers (16-day pregnant HO females) and normal lactating mothers exhibited equally high levels of maternal aggression. This investigator also found that EB-stimulated HO virgins that were relatively poor in maternal behavior also failed to exhibit maternal aggression toward a male intruder. On the other hand, Erskine (1978) found that once maternal aggression had been established during normal delivery, hypophysectomy on Day 3 postpartum did not prevent the normal rise in maternal aggression that occurs on Day 9. This suggests that although maternal aggression is more difficult to stimulate nonhormonally during sensitization once it has been established hormonally its maintenance may be nonhormonal.

Sensitized females have also been found to differ, compared to lactating mothers, in their readiness to enter a T-maze to retrieve a pup at the other end (Bridges et al., 1972; Stern and MacKinnon, 1976; Stern, 1977; Mackinnon and Stern, 1978). The basis of this difference has been investigated by Stern and her colleague (see above) who have shown that it is not dependent upon suckling stimulation, nor even the release of prolactin during lactation, but appears to depend upon the same hormonal conditions (estradiol stimulation or progesterone withdrawal) that elicit maternal behavior. Their observations as well as those of Bridges et al. (1972) point to the fact that while in their home cages sensitized and lactating females do not differ in their readiness to retrive pups, a finding which confirms Fleming and Rosenblatt (1974a) and Reisbick et al. (1975). The sensitized females are more fearful and timid than lactating mothers, which interferes with their ability to enter upon and traverse the T-maze; those that do reach the pup, however, select a live pup over a dead one to retrieve, like their lactating counterparts.

TRANSITIONAL PERIOD: PARTURITION AND THE EARLY POSTPARTUM PERIOD

The Transition from Hormonal to Nonhormonal Regulation of Maternal Behavior

The previously described studies on separating mothers from their litters at parturition and observing the waning of maternal behavior (Rosenblatt and Lehrman, 1963; Rosenblatt, 1965) imply that the transition between hormonally-induced and pup-maintained maternal behavior occurs shortly after parturition. By allowing females 12-hour contact with pups postpartum,

Rosenblatt (unpublished observations) was able to delay waning of maternal behavior until the 8th day.

Cosnier and Couturier (1966) and Fleming and Rosenblatt (1974a) introduced another method for investigating this problem. The former investigators allowed groups of females to rear their first litters to weaning while the latter allowed females only 36-hour postpartum maternal care, and both then removed the pups and waited several weeks until the females were again undergoing estrous cycling. At that time they introduced foster pups to test whether the females' latencies for sensitization would be affected by their previous experience with their litters. Both groups of experimenters found that there was a significant reduction in latencies compared to females that were sensitized without previous experience of maternal behavior. This indicated that postpartum maternal behavior could provide the experience necessary to reduce the non-hormonally-based sensitization latency. Fleming and Rosenblatt (1974a) and Mayer and Rosenblatt (1975) then showed that prior sensitization and 36 hours of experience of maternal behavior could also provide the experience necessary to reduce sensitization latencies upon the reinduction of maternal behavior several weeks later. Postpartum maternal behavior and postsensitization maternal care, therefore, had equivalent effects upon subsequent induction of maternal behavior of nonhormonal nature. One interpretation of these findings is that the two kinds of experience, postpartum and postsensitization maternal care, are equivalent in their effects because they are both nonhormonal and as such they are easily aroused at a later time simply by exposure to pups. Support for this interpretation was provided by Cosnier and Couturier (1966) who reported that ovariectomizing the females after they had weaned their young or after removing pups from sensitized females did not alter their reduced latencies upon reinduction.

In a series of studies Bridges (1975, 1977) has employed this procedure systematically to study what he refers to as retention of maternal behavior after various kinds of earlier maternal behavior experience. Females are allowed to give birth and are given different amounts of experience with pups postpartum and during parturition followed by a 25-day separation from their litters. The results of these studies are shown in Figure 12 and they indicate that as little as 4- to 6-hour postpartum contact with pups is sufficient to enable females to reinstate maternal behavior in a little over 24 hours, 25 days later, a latency which is no longer than the latency after 21 days previous experience of rearing pups. More important, as long as females have had some contact with pups during parturition, their latencies are less than 48 hours, 25 days later, but if they are not permitted contact with pups during parturition, their latencies for sensitization 25 days later give no evidence that they have had any prior experience of maternal behavior and are equal to

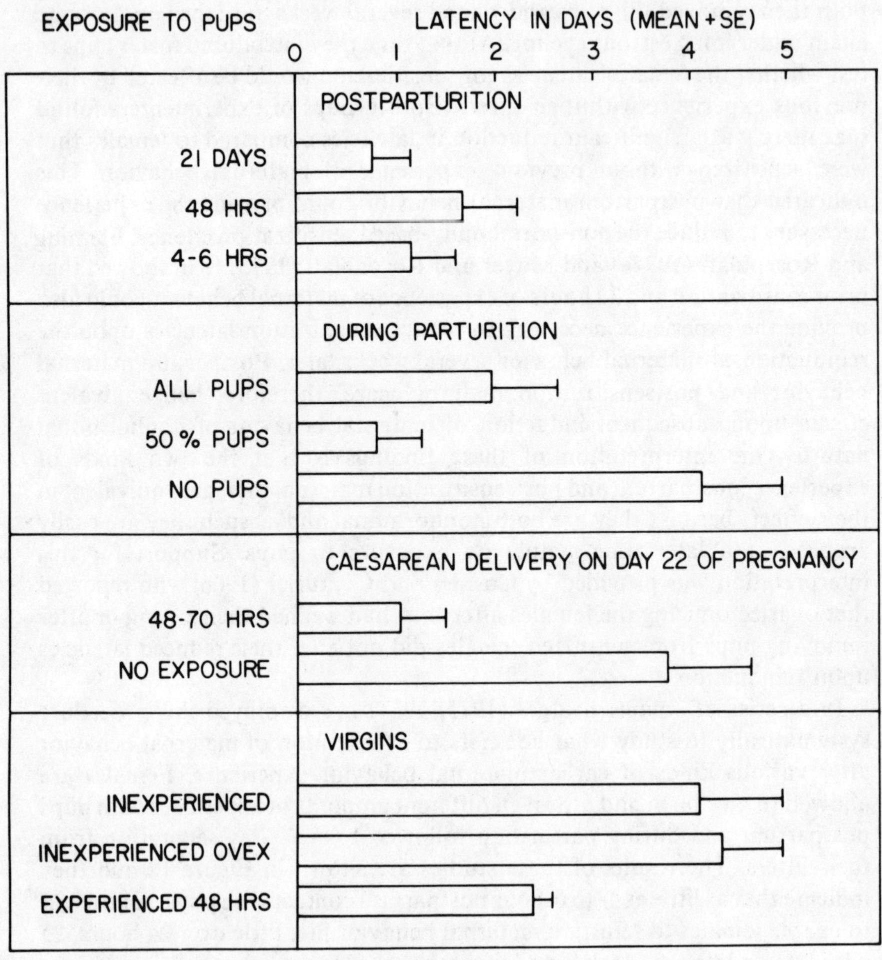

FIG. 12. Summary of the effects of parturitional and postparturitional experience with pups on maternal responsiveness after 25 days without pups. Data taken from Bridges (1975, 1977).

those of inexperienced nonpregnant females. The same results were obtained when females were delivered by Caesarean section just before parturition: if they were given pups for 48-60 hours they had short latencies at later testing but if they had no contact with pups their latencies were long like those of inexperienced nonpregnant females.

We have interpreted these findings in terms of the hypothesis of a transitional period in the establishment of nonhormonal maternal behavior during parturition. Maternal behavior is retained for 25 days only if the female has had some opportunity to establish the nonhormonal basis through contact with pups. This requires a variable period of pup contact depending upon circumstances but parturition appears to be an optimal period for beginning the transition because the female is maximally stimulated hormonally and the pups are maximally attractive and aroused by the events of parturition (Grota, 1972; Dollinger et al., 1976; Holloway et al., 1976). Even if parturition does not occur, as in cesarean-delivered females of the the studies described above, females are able to initiate maternal behavior during the first few days if provided with pups, and the transition is made at this time.

Numan (1974) and Numan et al. (1977) have provided a neural basis for the transition from hormonal and nonhormonal regulation of maternal behavior in their studies of the neural site of regulation of maternal behavior. Numan (1974) found earlier that lesions of the medial peroptic area (MPOA) of the brain eliminated maternal behavior in 5-day postpartum mothers. Using implants of EB in this region with 16-day pregnant HO females Numan et al. (1977) stimulated short latency maternal behavior (Figure 13), and effect which did not depend upon systemic effects of the hormone and was not produced by EB implants in other brain regions (i.e., ventromedial hypothalamus and mammilary bodies). In addition, when lesions were made in the MPOA in nonpregnant females before exposing them to pups for sensitization, the females failed to respond to pups by exhibiting maternal behavior. The MPOA is, therefore, one of the brain regions which mediates both hormonal and nonhormonal influences on maternal behavior. A recent study by Bridges et al. (1978c) suggests that in lactating females, lesions in the lateral neural input to the MPOA and the anterior hypothalamic area (AHA) which Numan (1974) had shown were as effective as MPOA lesions in eliminating maternal behavior, did not prevent females from exhibiting nursing/crouching over pups nor responding to suckling by releasing increased amounts of Prol.

Notwithstanding these latter findings, the MPOA provides a neural site at which hormonal and sensory stimuli may interact in mediating the transition in the regulation of maternal behavior. Once estradiol has stimulated this neural site then as the hormonal influence declines, sensory stimuli may maintain a level of neural activity required for the display of maternal

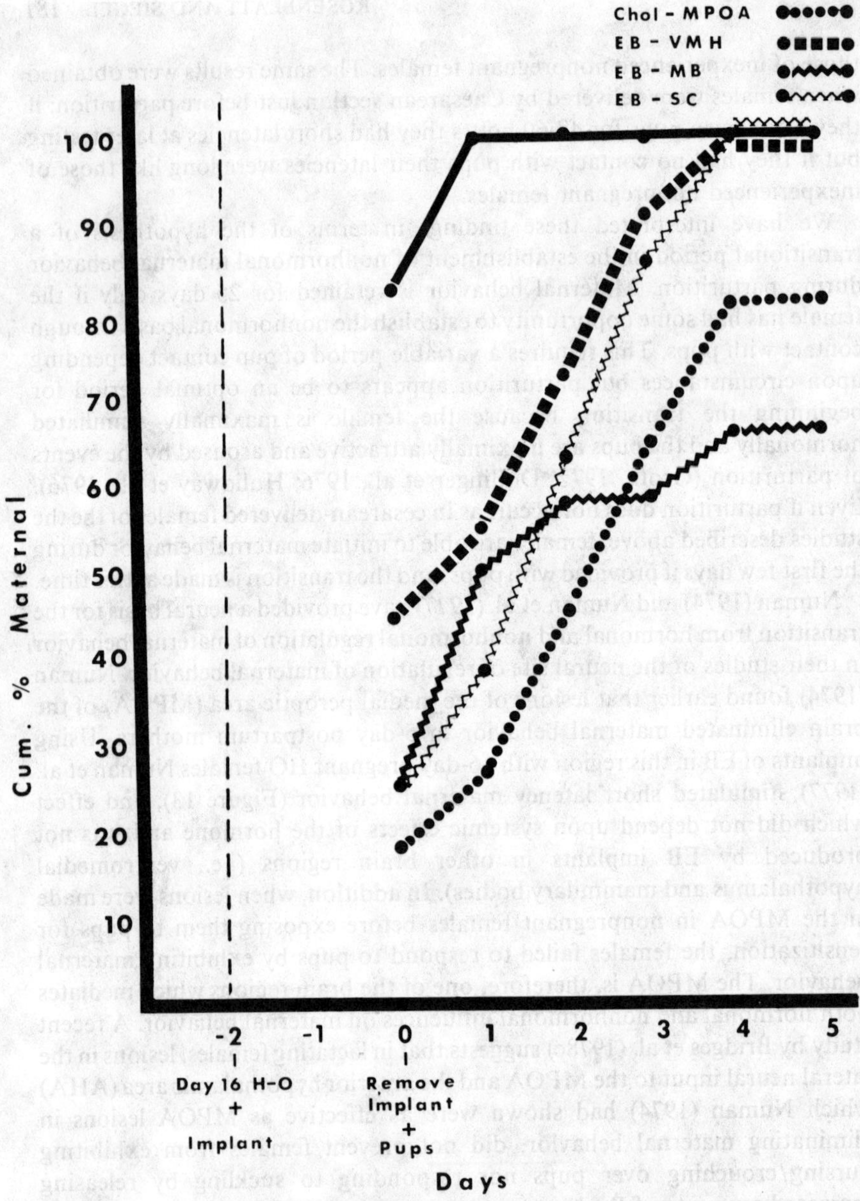

FIG. 13. Cumulative (Cum.) percentage of 16-day-pregnant, hysterectomized (H), and ovariectomized (O) female rats showing maternal behavior over the 5-day test period. (Abbreviations for identification of groups: EB = estradiol benzoate; MPOA = medial preoptic area; Chol = cholesterol; VMH = ventromedial hypothalamus; MB = mammillary bodies; SC = subcutaneously implanted control.) (From M. Numan, J. S. Rosenblatt and B. R. Komisaruk. Medial preoptic area and onset of maternal behavior in the rat. *J. Comp. Physiol. Psychol. 91,* 146–164. Copyright 1977 by the American Psychological Association. Reprinted by permission.)

behavior. A paradigm for this kind of hormone-sensory interaction can be found in the regulation of the lordosis response in the female rate and involves estradiol and various forms of genital stimulation (Komisaruk, 1974).

The timing and success of the transition between hormonal and nonhormonal regulation of maternal behavior can, therefore, be influenced by the hormonal onset as well as postparturient pup stimulation. It would be useful if we knew the duration of the hormonal stimulation of maternal behavior around parturition but this information is difficult to obtain for various reasons. Studies on 16-day pregnant HO females and on nonpregnant HO females administered EB and tested at various intervals after hormone administration provide some useful information on this problem (Siegel and Rosenblatt, 1975c, 1977; Siegel et al., 1978). In 16-day pregnant HO females the stimulating effect of EB was still evident 72 hours after administration. We could also detect an influence between 72 and 96 hours after EB treatment but this requires joint stimulation by pups. However, only females that had been treated with EB were stimulated to exhibit maternal behavior by pups they were exposed to between 72 and 96 hours. In nonpregnant HO females given 25 μg EB at surgery, 33% exhibited maternal behavior at 48 hours without prior exposure to pups but, in addition, between 48 and 72 hours, EB-treated females responded more rapidly to pup stimulation than untreated females and 33% initiated maternal behavior compared to 7% of untreated females (Siegel and Rosenblatt, 1975c).

Although following a single injection of EB there is very likely a decline in circulating hormone, nevertheless maternal behavior can be initiated 48 hours later without pup stimulation intervening and 72 and 96 hours later jointly with pup stimulation. If we consider that after estradiol secretion has risen several days earlier it normally declines just before parturition (Shaikh, 1971; Morishige and Rothchild, 1974) and circulating levels of estradiol must be low during and after parturition then prepartum estradiol may continue to exert a stimulating influence on maternal behavior for 24–36 hours postpartum and jointly with pup stimulation for another 24 hours. After that period its influence would wane and only pup stimulation would be able to maintain maternal behavior. When females are hysterectomized on Day 16 of pregnancy, about 50% initiate maternal behavior at 72 hours without prior pup stimulation and estradiol very likely is secreted only during a 2-day period before then (Rosenblatt and Siegel, 1975).

Slotnick et al. (1973) compared females that had initiated maternal behavior prepartum (i.e., hormonally) with those that did not in their ability to maintain maternal behavior with reduced stimulation from pups postpartum. Those that had initiated maternal behavior were able to maintain it when allowed only 10 minutes of pup contact each day while those that had not initiated it prepartum, failed to display it with such reduced exposure to pups. In this study inadequate development of the hormonal basis of maternal behavior before parturition in many of the females made them unable to respond to pup stimulation at such a reduced level but when the hormonal basis is well established prepartum even such brief daily exposure to pups was sufficient to maintain it.

The transition from the prepartum hormonal onset of maternal behavior to the postpartum maintenance based on pup stimulation requires an interaction between hormonal and nonhormonal stimulation. Under normal circumstances both are maximal at parturition and most females, therefore, make the transition without difficulty. Difficulties may arise if either the hormonal stimulation is inadequate or postpartum pup stimulation is absent or reduced. Where difficulties do arise they may be remedied by increasing the strength of either hormonal stimulation or pup stimulation. In the rat, at present, we are able to do either as Baum (1978) recently showed. He ovariectomized nonpregnant females and exposed them to pups for six days. A majority of females of his strain (Wistar) failed to become sensitized during that period and were then injected with 10 μg EB for two days, and presented with pups once again. Most females then exhibited maternal behavior within 18 hours after reexposure to pups.

LACTATION AND MATERNAL BEHAVIOR

At one time when peripheral theories of motivation prevailed, it was believed that maternal behavior was stimulated by intramammary pressure from filling of the mammary glands. Weisner and Sheard (1933) were the first to show that removal of the mammary glands does not prevent the onset of maternal behavior and since that time it has been shown by a number of other investigators that removal of the nipples (thelectomy) or of both the mammary glands and nipples does not interfere with maternal behavior (Moltz, et al., 1967).

An alternative theory that prolactin, the hormone of lactation that is released in large amounts during the pre- and postpartum periods, is responsible for maternal behavior has already been shown to be untrue (see Page 62). High levels of circulating prolactin are required for lactation but they do not contribute directly to the onset or maintenance of maternal behavior.

The relationship between maternal behavior and lactation is more likely the reverse of that which was originally believed: maternal behavior maintains the release of high levels of prolactin by exposing females to suckling and other nonsuckling pup stimulation. The interrelationship between maternal behavior and lactation is an interesting story that has been worked out chiefly by Grosvenor and Mena (1974).

Behavioral influences upon lactation begin before parturition during mammary glands development that occurs during pregnancy. Roth and Rosenblatt (1967) observed the licking pattern of females during pregnancy and found that as pregnancy advanced females increasingly licked more posterior body regions including the anterior and posterior nipple regions and the pelvic and genital regions. They speculated that this licking might play a role in mammary gland development since it was well known that suckling stimulation maintains mammary gland function postpartum through the release of the lactogenic complex of hormones, and mammary gland development is dependent upon the ovarian hormones and prolactin. Using a technique developed by Birch (1956) they placed wide rubber collars on pregnant females soon after mating, thereby preventing the females from licking themselves for the duration of pregnancy until the 22nd day, just before parturition, when the females were sacrificed and their mammary glands were removed and measured for the amount of secretory tissue and rated for the degree of activity of the lobulo-alveola secretory system (Roth and Rosenblatt, 1968). Females prevented from licking themselves during pregnancy had mammary glands that were retarded in development by nearly 50% and this was true at midpregnancy as well as at the end of pregnancy. This was confirmed by McMurtry and Anderson (1971) who used a biochemical measure of gland development and found a similar degree of retardation among females prevented from licking themselves during pregnancy. Herrenkohl (formerly Roth) and Campbell (1976) have restored normal gland development in collared females by applying tactile stimulation to the nipples and mammary surfaces throughout pregnancy, confirming that tactile stimulation is necessary for normal mammary gland development during pregnancy.

However, Whitworth (1972) has shown that licking of either the nipples or the pelvic and genital regions stimulates mammary gland development equally, thereby ruling out the possibility, suggested by McMurtry and Anderson (1971), that the effect is a local one at the mammary gland and, instead, suggesting that it is a systemic one based upon the release of hormones.

After parturition mammary gland growth and lactation are stimulated by suckling through the release of prolactin, adrenocorticotrophic hormone (ACTH) and growth hormone (GH)—the lactogenic complex. The release of prolactin is an immediate response to suckling, and can be measured during suckling by pups (Terkel et al., 1972; Shino et al., 1972). Grosvenor (1965) has shown that during the first two weeks of lactation, only suckling will elicit prolactic release; but after the 14th day, exteroceptive stimuli from pups are capable of eliciting the release of prolactin and the amount released during 30 minutes of nonsuckling contact with pups is equal to the amount released during actual suckling.

In seeking the exteroceptive stimulus which stimulates prolactin release, Grosvenor et al. (1970) and Mena and Grosvenor (1971, 1972) have isolated olfactory stimulation from the pups, but only pups located beneath the female are capable of eliciting the release initially. Visual stimuli may play a role when olfaction is blocked. In a recent study Terkel et al. (1978) demonstrated that ultrasonic vocalizations by pups played to mothers elicits a nine-fold increase in circulating prolactin during 30 minutes on Days 4–7 of lactation which is only slightly below that of actual suckling and is specific to pup vocalizations. Since these vocalizations cannot be heard by human experimenters without special detectors there is a good chance that they were involved in the original stuides by Grosvenor and Mena since the conditions which elicit such vocalizations from pups were present in these studies.

One implication of the exteroceptive stimulation of prolactin release is that even when suckling declines lactation may be maintained by nonsuckling stimuli. How then does the lactation decline, as it does, around the fourth week? Moreover, between 14 and 21 days pups become more effective (or females more responsive to the pups) as exteroceptive stimuli for prolactin release (Mena and Grosvenor, 1972) and females respond equally to pups that are under them as to pups that are in racks placed 3 ft in front of them. Grosvenor and Mena (1973) investigated this problem in 21-day lactating mothers by comparing the exteroceptive stimulating effect of pups located under the mother with pups located in a rack 3 ft in front of her. Pups in both situations stimulated the release of prolactin from the pituitary gland but only the females that were exposed to pups in the racks showed the expected increase in milk secretion (Grosvenor et al., 1975); females with pups under them showed no increase in milk secretion. Moreover, when pups were placed under the female either before or during exposure to pups in racks in front of the female, prolactin was released from the pituitary gland but no increase in milk secretion occurred. Grosvenor and Mena (1973, 1974) propose that 21-day-old pups beneath the female inhibit the action of prolactin on the mammary gland and they have demonstrated that this effect can be blocked by phenotoalamine, an alpha-adrenergic blocking agent, implying therefore that the inhibition may be caused by a sympathetico-adrenal secretion which either competes with prolactin for receptor sites or causes vasoconstriction of mammary gland blood vessels thus preventing prolactin from reaching the mammary glands.

The release of prolactin from the pituitary is, therefore, dependent upon the maternal state of the female and the changes in the stimuli which govern prolactin release and their effect upon the mammary glands are a function of the behavioral interactions between the mother and her young Zarrow et al. (1973). Nonpregnant females that do not lactate nevertheless exhibit exteroceptive release of prolactin after they have been sensitized by exposure to pups and have been exhibiting maternal behavior for a week or longer. Koranyi et al. (1977) first showed this by exposing 10- and 30-day sensitized females to pups for one hour after a 5-hour separation from them. Stern and Siegel (1978) have confirmed that sensitized virgin females release prolactin in response to 30-minute contact with pups after prolonged separation from them. In their study prolactin release appeared in those females that had been maternal for 8–10 days but not in animals that had been maternal for 6–7 days.

It can be said, therefore, contrary to the early belief, that it is not lactation which governs maternal behavior but rather, the maternal relationship with the young and the maternal state which govern lactation.

OLFACTION AND MATERNAL BEHAVIOR

Olfaction appears to play a special role in the onset of maternal behavior. In nonpregnant females undergoing sensitization there is occasional sniffing of pups and beyond that the female has little contact with pups until she initiates maternal behavior (Terkel and Rosenblatt, 1971; Fleming and Rosenblatt, 1974a). Even at this early state females distinguish between a pup and a plastic toy the same size as a pup and after sniffing both they lick the pup and sometimes carry it to one corner of the cage (retrieval) whereas they bite the toy and carry it from place to place in the cage (Plume et al., 1968; Rosenblatt, 1975).

Schlein et al. (1972) removed the olfactory bulbs of inexperienced nonpregnant females and found that 80% cannibalized the 2-day-old pups presented to them; none exhibited retrieving or other aspects of maternal behavior. On the other hand, Fleming and Rosenblatt (1974b) found that although 60% of their bulbectomized females cannibalized pups, an equal percentage exhibited short-latency maternal behavior, one female shifting from one to the other. The irritability produced by bulbectomy is well known (Cain, 1974) and could account for the cannibalism since bulbectomized females also kill mice when presented to them. The rapid onset of maternal behavior was unexpected, however, and required further study before it could be understood. On the assumption that the anosmia produced by bulbectomy was responsible for the short-latency maternal behavior, nonpregnant females were either treated with intranasal zinc sulfate to produce temporary anosmia or underwent lesioning of the lateral olfactory tracts (Fleming and Rosenblatt, 1974c). None of these females exhibited cannibalism when exposed to pups and nearly all exhibited maternal behavior in less than 24 hours.

These results indicated that the delay in the onset of maternal behavior during sensitization might be due to the inhibitory effect of pup odors, which may be aversive to females as well as novel. One way of testing this idea was to allow females to become maternal while anosmic due to zinc sulfate treatment then allow them to recover smell and test them again to see if the ability to smell the pups introduces an interference with maternal behavior. Mayer and Rosenblatt, (1975) compared such zinc sulfate treated females with sham treated controls with results shown in Table 2. The anosmic females showed short latency maternal behavior, both with respect to retrieving and attending pups after retrieval while the control females required the usual four days or so. However after they regained smell, the females that had already been retrieving and attending pups continued to retrieve them with short latencies but the latency for attending increased fourfold. Control females showed a reduction in latancies for both aspects of maternal behavior.

The aversive effects of pups odors, seen in nonpregnant females, is not evident in the initial responses of females during parturition (Holloway et al., 1976). This may be, as Noirot (1972) has suggested, because the pups are covered with birth fluids with which the female has become familiar through licking of her genital regions during pregnancy (Roth and Rosenblatt, 1967), a suggestion that was originally put forth by Birch (1956). Or, it may be that the hormones of pregnancy alter the female's responses to pup odors or her sensitivity to them.

TABLE 2
Retrieving Latencies (Mean days ± SD) of Zinc Sulfate-Treated and Control Females During Initial Induction and Subsequent Reinduction* of Maternal Bahavior†

	Group	
Measure	*Zinc Sulfate* (n = 14)	*Control* (n = 24)
Initial induction		
Latency to retrieve	.4 ± .7	3.6 ± 1.1
Latency to retrieve and attend	1.1 ± .8	3.8 ± 1.0
Reinduction		
Latency to retrieve	.2 ± .6	.2 ± .5
Latency to retrieve and attend	2.6 ± 2.0	2.4 ± 2.2

*Three weeks between initial induction and reinduction.
†Data taken from Mayer and Rosenblatt (1975).

FUNCTIONAL ASPECTS OF THE ORGANIZATION OF MATERNAL BEHAVIOR

The organization of maternal behavior into two phases, an initial prepartum hormonal phase during which there is the intiation of maternal behavior and a subsequent postpartum nonhormonal phase during which maintenance and decline of maternal behavior are regulated by pup stimulation arises, we believe, from functional considerations. There are adaptive advantages to the hormonal regulation at the end of pregnancy, the nonhormonal regulation thereafter, and the transition between the two around parturition.

The onset of maternal behavior must be synchronized with the termination of pregnancy and the onset of lactation (Wiesner and Sheard, 1933) all three of which are based upon different aspects of the same complex hormonal changes which occur at the end of pregnancy. The initiation of parturition, signalling the end of pregnancy, is based upon the decline in progesterone and rise in estradiol secretion (Fuchs, 1973) a process in which prostaglandin $F_{2\alpha}$ from the uterus participates (Strauss et al., 1975; Flower, 1977). The onset of lactation also is based upon these hormonal changes, but in addition, prolactin plays the principal role once the progesterone block to its activity is withdrawn (Kuhn, 1969). Synthesis and release of prolactin are dependent upon the rise in estradiol. As we have proposed, the rise in estradiol is, most likely, the stimulus for the onset of maternal behavior but this depends upon prior withdrawal of progesterone, both to remove its inhibitory effect and as a short term facilitating influence. Prolactin is not involved in the onset of maternal behavior.

Once parturition has taken place and both maternal behavior and lactation have been initiated, the reproductive processes of the female turn in two directions. The first is the maintenance of the current litter which requires maternal care and lactation and the second is the start of a second litter that will be conceived at postpartum estrus and gestated during the period of lactation (Figure 14). The reproductive strategy is an ancient one among mammals and is already present among the marsupials in which among the diprotodont marsupials mating takes place shortly after parturition and postpartum and gestation is initiated at the same time that lactation and maternal care begin (Sharman, 1963; Sharman et al., 1966).

The occurrence of estrus shortly after parturition requires a shift in the regulation of maternal behavior from its hormonal basis, which cannot be maintained except by preventing the ensuing estrus [a strategy which has evolved among certain of the marsupials in which a lengthened pregnancy prevents the establishment of a new pregnancy after parturition (Sharman, 1963)], to a nonhormonal basis, except for the continuing hormonal

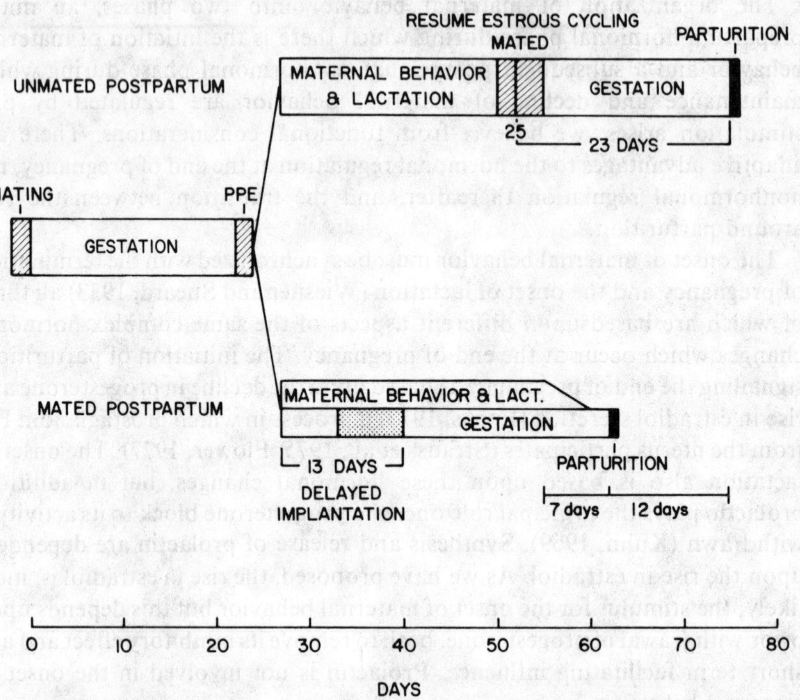

FIG. 14. Maternal behavior cycle of the rat when female is mated or remains unmated at postpartum estrus (PPE). Estrous behavior and estrous cycling (oblique lines), range of days beyond normal implantation (stipple), and parturition (black bars).

maintenance of lactation which is compatible with both the occurrence of postpartum estrus and maintenance of gestation.

There is an intervening process, however, which ensures that the new litter will not be delivered before the current litter has been fully weaned and that the female will not be drained of her metabolic resources by the simultaneous demands of lactation and gestation. This is the mechanism of "delayed implantation" which also occurs among marsupials with postpartum estrus (Sharman, 1963). The fertilized ova (blastocysts) remain in the uterus without implanting to its wall and therefore are suspended in their development. In the rat, delayed implantation may last up to 15 days and in the Red kangaroo it lasts for over 280 days. In both species implantation is under hormonal control: in the rat, there is sufficient progesterone for implantation but estradiol is lacking since there is suspension of estrous cycling during lactation and maintenance of diestrus (Shelesnyak and Kraicer, 1963; Nutting and Meyer, 1963; Dickmann et al., 1977).

Suckling by the current litter ultimately regulates when implantation of the next litter takes place and therefore determines when gestation will resume and delivery will take place. The control by the suckling pups is based upon the number of pups in the litter: with fewer than 5 pups, implantation may occur after a relatively short delay of several days but with litters consisting of more than 5 pups, and this generally means litters of 9 to 12 pups, implantation is delayed the full period of 13–15 days (Figure 14; Rothchild, 1960; Weichert, 1940). Since smaller litters gain weight more rapidly than large litters and the young develop many behavioral capacities earlier (Fleischer and Turkewitz, 1979a,b) the earlier appearance of the new litter when a small litter is suckling is not likely to interfere with its capacity to survive weaning while the same would not be true when a large litter is suckling.

Pups regulate the delay in implantation through their suckling: suckling simultaneously promotes the release of prolactin and inhibits the release of gonadotropins (follicle stimulating hormone and luteinizing hormone) thereby maintaining the ovary in a diestrus state (Gala, 1970; Ford and Yoshinaga, 1975; Tomogone et al., 1976; Mena and Grosvenor, 1968 Lu et al., 1971). As suckling declines the inhibition is lifted and the gonodotropins are secreted causing the ovary to secrete estradiol and to initiate implantation (Veomett and Daniel, 1971). One implication of this process is that should the litter be destroyed before the natural decline in suckling, implantation will be initiated almost immediately, since the inhibition of gonadotropin release will be lifted (Rothchild, 1960; Hammons et al., 1973). In this we have a hint of the adaptive significance of the entire process we have been describing: its function is to maintain a maximum rate of reproduction during the limited breeding season or reproductive life of the female.

By shifting to a nonhormonal basis for postpartum maternal behavior the female frees her reproductive processes to resume but not in such a way as to jeopardize her current litter. To ensure that this is the case, the regulation of these reproductive processes is shifted to the young both with respect to maintaining lactation for their own benefit (Kumaresan et al., 1967; Tucker et al., 1967) and to preventing gestation to their detriment (Bruce and East, 1956).

Since females who do not become pregnant during postpartum estrus only resume estrous cycling around 25 days after parturition the earliest time that they can produce a second litter is approximately 47 days after delivery of the first, assuming that they are mated at the first estrus (Figure 14). Females mated at postpartum estrus can produce second litters as early as 23 days and no later than 35 days, a saving of 12 days at the minimum and they are in a position to resume gestation immediately should their current litter fall below five pups or fail to survive for any reason. These are, apparently, sufficient advantages for this reproductive strategy to have evolved as the predominant one among the animals. This implies that the way in which maternal behavior is organized into phases in the rat may be more general among placental mammals; it even appears to characterize marsupial maternal behavior as far as the meager amount of information we now have indicates (Sharman et al., 1966; Russell and Giles, 1973).

ACKNOWLEDGMENTS

The research reported in this article and the writing were supported by USPHS Grant MH-08604 to JSR, and a Biomedical Support Grant. Institute of Animal Behavior publication number 307.

REFERENCES

Allin, J. R. and Banks, E. M. Effects of temperature on ultrasound production by infant albino rats. *Develop. Psychobiol. 4*, 149–156 (1971).

Allin, J. T. and Banks, E. M. Functional aspects of ultrasound production by infant albino rats (Rattus norvegicus). *Anim. Behav. 20*, 175–185 (1972).

Baum, M. J. Failure of pituitary transplants to facilitate the onset of maternal behavior in ovariectomized virgin rats. *Physiol. Behav. 20*, 87–89 (1978).

Beach, F. A. *Hormones and Behavior*. Paul B. Hoeber, Inc., New York (1948).

Beach, F. A. and Wilson, J. Effects of prolactin, progesterone, and estrogen on reactions of nonpregnant rats to foster young. *Psychol. Rep. 13*, 231–239 (1963).

Bintarningsih, Lyons, W. R., Johson, R. E., and Li, C. H. Hormonally-induced lactation in hypophysectomized rat. *Endocrinology 63*, 540–547 (1958).

Birch, H. G. Sources of order in the maternal behavior of animals. *Am. J. Orthopsychiat. 26*, 279–284 (1956).

Bridges, R. S. Long-term effects of pregnancy and parturition upon maternal responsiveness in the rat. *Physiol. Behav. 14*, 245–249 (1975).

Bridges, R. S. Parturition: its role in the long term retention of maternal behavior in the rat. *Physiol. Behav. 18*, 487–490 (1977).

Bridges, R., Zarrow, M. X., Gandelman, R., and Denenberg, V. H. Differences in maternal responsiveness between lactating and sensitized rats. *Develop. Psychobiol. 5*, 123–127 (1972).

Bridges, R. S., Feder, H. H., and Rosenblatt, J. S. Induction of maternal behaviors in primigravid rats by ovariectomy, hysterectomy, or ovariectomy plus hysterectomy: effect of length of gestation. *Horm. Behav. 9*, 156–169 (1977).

Bridges, R. S. and Feder, H. H. Effects of various progestins and deoxycorticosterone on rapid onset of maternal behavior induced by ovariectomy-hysterectomy during late pregnancy in rats. *Horm. Behav., 10*, 30–39 (1978).

Bridges, R. S., Feder, H. H., and Rosenblatt, J. S. Stimulation of maternal responsiveness after pregnancy termination in rats: effect of time of onset of behavioral testing. *Horm. Behav., 10,* 235–245 (1978a).

Bridges, R. S., Rosenblatt, J. S., and Feder, H. H. Serum progesterone levels and maternal behavior after pregnancy termination in rats: behavioral effects of progesterone maintenance and withdrawal. *Endocrinology, 102,* 258–267 (1978b).

Bridges, R. S., Terkel, J., and Sawyer, C. H. Maternal behavior and prolactin secretion in lactating rats after lateral deafferentation of medial preoptic and anterior hypothalamic areas. Abstract, Society for the Study of Reproduction (1978c).

Bruce, H. M. Observations on the suckling stimulus and lactation in the rat. *J. Reprod. Fertil. 2,* 17–34 (1961).

Bruce, H. M. and East, J. Number and viability of young from pregnancies concurrent with lactation in the mouse. *J. Endocrin, 14,* 19–27 (1956).

Cain, D. P. Olfactory bulbectomy: neural structures involved in irritability and aggression in the male rat. *J. Comp. Physiol. Psychol. 86,* 213–220 (1974).

Caligaris, L., Astrada, J. J., and Taleisnik, S. Oestrogen and progesterone influence on the release of prolactin in ovariectomized rats. *J. Endocrin. 60,* 205–215 (1974).

Charten, D., Adrien, J., and Cosnier, J. Déclencheurs chimiques du comportement du léchage des petits par la ratte parturiente. *Rev. Comp. Animal 5,* 89–94 (1971).

Corey, E. L. Initial inspiration in the mammalian fetus. *J. Exp. Zoöl. 61,* 1–11 (1932).

Cosnier, J. and Couturier, C. Comportement maternal provoqué chez les rattes adultes castrées. *Compte Rendu des Seances de la Société de Biologie 160,* 789–791 (1966).

Dickmann, Z., Gupta, J. S., and Dey, S. K. Does "blastocyst estrogen" initiate implantation? *Science 195,* 687–688 (1977).

Dollinger, M. J., Holloway, W. R., and Denenberg, V. H. Behavioral patterning during parturition in the rat. Paper presented at Eastern Regional Conference on Reproductive Behavior, Saratoga Springs, New York, June 13–16 (1976).

Erskine, M. S. Hormonal and experiential factors associated with the expression of aggression during lactation in the rat. Ph.D. dissertation, The University of Connecticut (1978).

Fleischer, S. F. and Turkewitz, G. Effects of neonatal stunting on the physical growth and behavioral development of rats: II. Early and late effects of large litter rearing. *Develop. Psychobiol. 12,* 137–149 (1979a).

Fleischer, S. F. and Turkewitz, G. Effects of neonatal stunting on the physical growth and behavioral devleopment of rats: III. Effects of rotation between lactating and non-lactating females. *Develop. Psychobiol.* In press (1979b).

Fleming, A. and Rosenblatt, J. S. Maternal behavior in the virgin and lactating rat. *J. Comp. Physiol. Psychol. 86,* 957–972 (1974a).

Fleming, A. and Rosenblatt, J. S. Olfactory regulation of maternal behavior in rats: I. Effects of olfactory bulb removal in experienced and inexperienced lactating and cycling females. *J. Comp. Physiol. Psychol. 86,* 221–232 (1974b).

Fleming, A. and Rosenblatt, J. S. Olfactory regulation of maternal behavior in rats: II. Effects of peripherally induces anosmia and lesions of the lateral olfactory tract in pup-induced virgins. *J. Comp. Physiol. Psychol. 86,* 233–246 (1974c).

Flower, R. J. The role of prostaglandins in parturition, with special reference to the rat, in *The Fetus and Birth.* Ciba Foundation Symposium 47 (1977), pp. 297–318.

Ford, J. J. and Yoshinaga, K. The role of prolactin in the luteotrophic process of lactating rats. *Endocrinology 96,* 335–339 (1975).

Fuchs, A.-R. Parturition in rabbits and rats, in *Endocrine Factors in Labour.* A. Klopper and J. Gardner, eds. Memoirs of the Society for Endocrinology, Cambridge University Press (1973), pp. 163–183.

Gala, R. R. Studies on maintaining the lactational diestrum after early litter weaning. *Proc. Soc, Exp. Biol. Med. 133*, 164–167 (1970).

Gala, R. R. and Boss, R. S. Serum prolactin levels of rats under continuous estrogen stimulation and 2 Br-α-ergocryptine (CB-154) injection. *Proc. Soc. Exp. Biol. Med. 149*, 330–332 (1975).

Graham, D. L. and Hasenstab, L. L. The effect of a lateral head-turning stimulus on the approach of Gunn rat dams. *Physiol. Behav.*, Submitted for publication (1978).

Grosvenor, C. E. Evidence that exteroceptive stimuli can release prolactin from the pituitary gland of the lactating rat. *Endocrinology 76*, 340–342 (1965).

Grosvenor, C. E., and Mena, F. Evidence that suckling pups, through an exteroceptive mechanism, inhibit the milk stimulatory effects of prolactin in the rat during late lactation. *Horm. Behav. 4*, 209–222 (1973).

Grosvenor, C. E. and Mena, F. Neural and hormonal control of milk secretion and milk ejection. *Lactation 1*, 227–276 (1974).

Grosvenor, C. E., Maiweg, H., and Mena, F. A study of factors involved in the development of the exteroceptive release of prolactin in the lactating rat. *Horm. Behav. 1*, 111–120 (1970).

Grosvenor, C. E., Whitworth, N., and Mena, F. Milk secretory response to the conscious lactating rat following intravenous injections of rat prolactin. *J. Dairy Sci. 58*, 1803–1807 (1975).

Grota, L. J. The effects of the placenta and fetal fluids on the acceptance of foster young. *Develop. Psychobiol. 6*, 495–502 (1972).

Grota, L. J. Effects of litter size, age of young, and parity on foster mother behaviour in *Rattus norvegicus. Anim. Behav. 21*, 78–82 (1973).

Hammons, J.-A., Valasco, M., and Rothchild, I. Effect of the suddent withdrawal or increase of suckling on serum LH levels in ovariectomized postparturient rats. *Endocrinology 92*, 206–211 (1973).

Herberg, L. J., Pye, J. G., and Blundell, J. E. Sex differences in the hypothalamic regulation of food hoarding: hormones versus calories. *Anim. Behav. 20*, 186–191 (1972).

Herrenkohl, L. R. Effects on lactation of progesterone injections administered during late pregnancy in the rat. *Proc. Soc. Exp. Biol. Med. 138*, 39–42 (1971).

Herrenkohl, L. R. Effects on lactation of progesterone injections administered after parturition in the rat. *Proc. Soc. Exp. Biol. Med. 140*, 1356–1359 (1972).

Herrenkohl, L. R. Differential effects of progesterone on lactation and nursing behavior in late pregnant and postparturient rats. *Physiol. Behav. 13*, 495–499 (1974).

Herrenkohl, L. R. and Campbell, C. Mechanical stimulation of mammary gland development in virgin and pregnant rats. *Horm. Behav. 7*, 183–198 (1976).

Herrenkohl, L. R. and Rosenberg, P. A. Exteroceptive stimulation of maternal behavior in the naive rat. *Physiol. Behav. 8*, 595–598 (1972).

Herrenkohl, L. R. and Sachs, B. D. Sensory regulation of maternal behavior in mammals. *Physiol. Behav. 9*, 689–692 (1972).

Herrenkohl, L. R. and Lisk, R. D. Effects on lactation of progesterone injections administered before and after parturition in the rat. *Proc. Soc. Exp. Biol. Med. 142*, 506–510 (1973).

Hill-Samli, M. and MacLeod, R. M. Thyrotropin-releasing hormone blockade of the ergocryptine and apomorphine inhibition of prolactin release in vitro. *Proc. Soc. Exp. Biol. Med. 149*, 511–514 (1975).

Holloway, W. R., Dollinger, M. J., and Denenberg, V. H. The parturitional environment and later growth and development of the rat. Paper presented at Eastern Regional Conference on Reproductive Behavior, Saratoga Springs, New York, June 13–16 (1976).

Johnson, N. P. Postpartum ovulation in the rat. Ph.D. dissertation, Purdue University (1972).

Kalra, P. S., Fawcett, C. P., Krulich, L., and McCann, S. M. The effects of gonadal steroids on plasma gonadotropins and prolactin in the rat. *Endocrinology 92*, 1256–1268 (1973).

Komisaruk, B. R. Neural and hormonal interactions in the control of reproductive behavior of female rats, in Sexual Behavior. W. Montagna and W. A. Sadler, eds. Proceedings of the 2nd NIH Conference, Plenum Press, New York (1974).

Korányi, L., Lissak, K., Tamasy, V., and Kamaras, L. Behavioral and electrophysiological attempts to elucidate central nervous system mechanisms responsible for maternal behavior. *Arch. Sex Behav. 5*, 503–510 (1976).

Korányi, L., Phelps, C. P., and Sawyer, C. H. Changes in serum prolactin and corticosterone in induced maternal behavior in rats. *Physiol. Behav. 18*, 287–292 (1977).

Kuhn, N. J. Progesterone withdrawal as the lactogenic trigger in the rat. *J. Endocrinol. 44*, 39–54 (1969).

Kumaresan, P., Anderson, R. R., and Turner, C. W. Effect of litter size upon milk yield and litter weight gains in rats. *Proc. Soc. Exp. Biol. Med. 126*, 41–45 (1967).

Labriola, J. Effects of caesarian delivery upon maternal behavior in rats. *Proc. Soc. Exp. Biol. Med.* 83, 556–567 (1953).

Lehrman, D. S. Hormonal regulation of parental behavior in birds and infrahuman mammals, in *Sex and Internal Secretions*, 3rd edition. W. C. Young, ed. Williams and Wilkins, Baltimore (1961), pp. 1268–1382.

Leon, M., Numan, M., and Moltz, H. Maternal behavior in the rat: facilitation through gonadectomy. *Science 179*, 1018–1019 (1973).

Leon, M., Numan, M., and Chan, A. Adrenal inhibition of maternal behavior in virgin female rats. *Horm. Behav. 6*, 165–171 (1975).

Leon, M. L., Croskerry, P. G. and Smith, G. K. Thermal control of mother-young contact in rats. *Physiol. Behav., 21*, 793–811 (1978).

Lott, D. The role of progesterone in the maternal behavior of rodents. *J. Comp. Physiol. Psychol. 55*, 610–613 (1962).

Lott, D., and Fuchs, S. Failure to induce retrieving by sensitization or the injection of prolactin. *J. Comp. Physiol. Psychol. 55*, 1111–1113 (1962).

Lu, K. H., Chen, H. T., Luang, H. H., Grandison, L., Marshall, S., and Meites, J. Relation between prolactin and gonadotrophin secretion in post-partum lactating rats. *J. Endocrin. 68*, 241–250 (1976).

MacKinnon, D. A. and Stern, J. M. Pregnancy duration and fetal number: effects on maternal behavior in rats. *Physiol. Behav. 18*, 793–797 (1977).

Marinari, K. T. and Moltz, H. Disruption of vaginal cyclicity and maternal behavor. Paper presented at Eastern Conference on Reproductive Behavior, Univeristy of Connecticut, Storrs, June 5–8 (1977)

Mayer, G. Delayed nidation in rats: a method of exploring the mechanisms of ovo-implantation, in Delayed Implantation. A. C. Enders, ed. The University of Chicago Press, Chicago (1963), pp. 213–231.

Mayer, A. D. and Rosenblatt, J. S. Olfactory basis for the delayed onset of maternal behavior in virgin female rats: Experiential effects. *J. Comp. Physiol. Psychol. 89*, 701–710 (1975).

McLinn, D. K. Rat pups' calls and rat mothers' behavior. Ph.D. dissertation, Yale University (1978).

McMurtry, J. P. and Anderson, R. R. Prevention of self-licking on mammary gland development in pregnant rats. *Proc. Soc. Exp. Biol. Med. 137*, 354–356 (1971).

Mena, F. and Grosvenor, C. E. Effects of number of pups upon suckling-induced fall in pituitary prolactin concentration and milk ejection in the rat. *Endocrinology 82*, 623–626 (1968).

Mena, F. and Grosvenor, C. E. Release of prolactin in rats by exteroceptive stimulation; sensory stimuli involved. *Horm. Behav. 2*, 107–116 (1971).

Mena, F. and Grosvenor, C. E. Effect of suckling and of exteroceptive stimulation upon prolactin release in the rat during late lactation. *J. Endocrinol. 52*, 11–22 (1972).

Moltz, H., Robbins, D., and Parks, M. Caesarean delivery and maternal behavior of primiparous and multiparous rats. *J. Comp. Physiol. Psychol. 61*, 455–460 (1966).

Moltz, H., Geller, D., and Levin, R. Maternal behavior in the totally mammectomized rat. *J. Comp. Physiol. Psychol. 64*, 225–229 (1967).

Moltz, H., Levin, R., and Leon, M. Differential effects of progesterone on the maternal behavior of primiparous and multiparous rats. *J. Comp. Physiol. Psychol. 67*, 36–40 (1969).

Moltz, H., Lubin, M., Leon, M., and Numan, M. Hormonal induction of maternal behavior in the ovariectomized nulliparous rat. *Physiol. Behav. 5*, 1373–1377 (1970a).

Morishige, W. K. and Rothchild, I. Temporal aspects of the regulation of corpus luteum function by luteinizing hormone, prolactin, and placental luteotrophin during the first half of pregnancy in the rat. *Endocrinology 95*, 260–274, (1974).

Morishige, W. K., Pepe, G. J., and Rothchild, I. Serum luteinizing hormone (LH) prolactin and progesterone levels during pregnancy in the rat. *Endocrinology 92*, 1527–1530 (1973).

Nagasawa, H. and Yanai, R. Changes in serum prolactin levels shortly before and after parturition in rats. *Endocrinol. Japon. 19*, 139–143 (1972).

Noirot, E. The onset and development of maternal behavior in rats, hamsters, and mice, in *Advances in the Study of Behavior*, Vol. 4. D. S. Lehrman, R. A. Hinde, and E. Shaw, eds. Academic Press, New York (1972).

Numan, M. Medial preoptic area and maternal behavior in the female rat. *J. Comp. Physiol. Psychol. 87*, 746–759 (1974).

Numan, M., Leon, N., and Moltz, H. Interference with prolactin release and the maternal behavior of female rats. *Horm. Behav. 3*, 29–38 (1972).

Numan, M., Rosenblatt, J. S., and Komisaruk, B. R. The medial preoptic area and the onset of maternal behavior in the rat. *J. Comp. Physiol. Psychol. 91*, 146–164 (1977).

Nutting, E. F. and Meyer, R. K. Implantation delay, nidation, and embryonal survival in rats treated with ovarian hormones, in *Delayed Implantation*. A. C. Enders, ed. The University of Chicago Press, Chicago (1963), pp. 233–252.

Plume, S., Fogarty, C., Grota, L. J., and Ader, R. Is retrieving a measure of maternal behavior in the rat? *Psychol. Rep. 23*, 627–630 (1968).

Reisbick, S., Rosenblatt, J. S., and Mayer, A. D. Decline of maternal behavior in the virgin and lactating rat. *J. Comp. Physiol. Psychol. 89*, 722–732 (1975).

Riddle, O., Lahr, E. L., and Bates, R. W. Maternal behavior induced in virgins by prolactin. *Proc. Soc. Exp. Biol. Med. 32*, 730–734 (1934).

Riddle, O., Lahr, E., and Bates, R. The role of hormones in the initiation of maternal behavior in rats. *Amer. J. Physiol. 137*, 299–317 (1942).

Rodriguez-Sierra, J. and Rosenblatt, J. S. Does prolactin play a role in estrogen-induced maternal behavior in rats: apomorphine reduction of prolactin release. *Horm. Behav. 9*, 1–7 (1977).

Rosenblatt, J. S. The basis of synchrony in the behavioural interaction between the mother and her offspring in the laboratory rat, in *Determinants of Infant Behaviour—III*. B. M. Foss, ed. Methuen, London (1965) pp. 3–41.

Rosenblatt, J. S. Nonhormonal basis of maternal behavior in the rat. *Science 156*, 1512–1514 (1967).

Rosenblatt, J. S. Views on the onset and maintenance of maternal behavior in the rat, in *Development and Evolution of Behavior: Essays in Memory of T. C. Schneirla*. L. R. Aronson, E. Tobach, D. S. Lehrman and J. S. Rosenblatt, eds. Freeman, San Francisco (1970).

Rosenblatt, J. S. Selective retrieving by maternal and nonmaternal female rats. *J. Comp. Physiol. Psychol. 88*, 678–686 (1975).

Rosenblatt, J. S. and Lehrman, D. S. Maternal behavior in the laboratory rat, in Maternal Behavior in Mammals. H. L. Rheingold, ed. John Wiley, New York (1963), pp. 8–57.

Rosenblatt, J. S. and Siegel, H. I. Hysterectomy-induced maternal behavior during pregnancy in the rat. *J. Comp. Physiol. Psychol. 89,* 685–700 (1975).

Roth, L. and Rosenblatt, J. S. Changes in self-licking during pregnancy in the rat. *J. Comp. Physiol. Psychol. 63,* 397–400 (1967).

Roth, L. and Rosenblatt, J. S. Self-licking and mammary development during pregnancy in the rat. *J. Endocrinol. 42,* 363–378 (1968).

Rothchild, I. The corpus luteum-pituitary relationship: the association between the cause of luteotrophin secretion and the cause of follicular quiescence during lactation; the basis for a tentative theory of the corpus luteum-pituitary relationship in the rat. *Endocrinology 67,* 9–41 (1960).

Roy, L. M. L. Induction of maternal behavior in the rat. Paper presented at Eastern Conference on Reproductive Behavior, University of Connecticut, Storrs, Connecticut, June 5–8 (1977).

Russell, E. M. and Giles, D. C. The effects of young in the pouch on pouch cleaning in the tammar wallaby, Macropus eugenii desmarest (marsupialia). *Behaviour 51,* 19–37 (1973).

Sachs, B. Placentaphagia and cannibalism in female rats. Abstract, Eastern Conference on Reproductive Behavior, Lansing, Michigan, June 12–14 (1969).

Sachs, B. D., Warden, A. F., and Pollak, E. Studies of postpartum estrus in rats. Paper presented at Eastern Conference on Reproductive Behavior, Haverford, Pennsylvania, June 16–19 (1971).

Sewell, G. D. Ultrasonic communication in rodents. *Nature 227,* 419 (1970).

Schlein, P. A., Zarrow, M. X., Cohen, H. A., Denenberg, V. H., and Johnson, N. P. The differential effect of anosmia on maternal behavior in the virgin and primiparous rat. *J. Repro. Fert. 30,* 39–42 (1972).

Schneirla, T. C. Problems in the biopsychology of social organization. *J. Abn. Soc. Psychol. 41,* 385–402 (1946).

Shaikh, A. A. Estrone and estradiol levels in the ovarian venous blood from rats during the estrous cycle and pregnancy. *Biol. Repro. 5,* 297–307 (1971).

Sharman, G. B. Delayed implantation in marsupials, in *Delayed Implantation.* A. C. Enders, ed. The University of Chicago Press, Chicago (1963) pp. 3–14.

Sharman, G. B., Calaby, J. H., and Poole, W. E. Patterns of reproduction in female diprotodont marsupials, in *Comparative Biology of Reproduction in Mammals.* I. W. Rowlands, ed. Academic Press, London (1966), pp. 205–232.

Shelesnyak, M. C. and Kraicer, P. F. The role of estrogen in nidation, in *Delayed Implantation.* A. C. Enders, ed. The University of Chicago Press (1963), pp. 265–279.

Sherman, K. A. Tail-pinch induces maternal behavior: evidence for the role of internal state in response selection during tail-pinch activation. Unpublished M. S. Thesis, University of Pittsburgh (1975).

Shino, M., Williams, G., and Rennels, E. G. Ultrastructural observation of pituitary release of prolactin in the rat by suckling stimulus. *Endocrinology 90,* 176–187 (1972).

Siegel, H. I. and Rosenblatt, J. S. Hormonal basis of hysterectomy-induced maternal behavior during pregnancy in the rat. *Horm. Behav. 6,* 211–222 (1975a).

Siegel, H. I. and Rosenblatt, J. S. Estrogen-induced maternal behavior in hysterectomized-ovariectomized virgin rats. *Physiol. Behav. 14,* 465–471 (1975b).

Siegel, H. I. and Rosenblatt, J. S. Progesterone inhibition of estrogen-induced maternal behavior in hysterectomized-ovariectomized virgin rats. *Horm. Behav. 6,* 223–230 (1975c).

Siegel, H. I. and Rosenblatt, J. S. Latency and duration of estrogen induction of maternal behavior in hysterectomized-ovariectomized virgin rats: effects of pup stimulation. *Physiol. Behav. 14,* 473–476 (1975d).

Siegel, H. I. and Rosenblatt, J. S. Effects of pregnancy termination on maternal behavior, lordosis, ovulation, and progesterone levels in the rat. Abstract, Eastern Conference on Reproductive Behavior, The University of Connecticut, Storrs, Connecticut, June 5–8 (1977).

Siegel, H. I., Doerr, H., and Rosenblatt, J. S. Further studies on estrogen-induced maternal behavior in hysterectomized-ovariectomized nulliparous rats. *Physiol. Behav., 21,* 99–103 (1978).

Slotnick, B. M., Carpenter, M. L., and Fusco, R. Initiation of maternal behavior in pregnant nulliparous rats. *Horm. Behav. 4,* 53–59 (1973).

Smalstig, E. B., Sawyer, B. D., and Clemens, J. A. Inhibition of rat prolactin release by apomorphine in vivo and in vitro. *Endocrinology 95,* 123–129 (1974).

Smotherman, W. P., Bell, R. W., Starzec, J., Elias, J., and Zachman, T. A. Maternal responses to infant vocalizations and olfactory cues in rats and mice. *Behav. Biol. 12,* 55–66 (1974).

Stern, J. M. Effects of ergocryptine on postpartum maternal behavior, ovarian cyclicity and food intake in rats. *Behav. Biol., 21,* 134–140 (1977).

Stern, J. M. and MacKinnon, D. A. Postpartum, hormonal, and nonhormonal induction of maternal behavior in rats: effects on t-maze retrieval of pups. *Horm. Behav. 7,* 305–316 (1976).

Stern, J. M. and MacKinnon, D. A. Sensory regulation of maternal behavior in rats: effects of pup age. *Devel. Psychobiol., 11,* 579–586 (1978).

Stern, J. M. and Siegel, H. I. Prolactin release in lactating, primiparous and multiparous thelectomized, and maternal virgin rats exposed to pup stimuli. *Biol. Reprod., 19,* 177–182 (1978).

Strauss III, J. F., Sokoloski, J., Caploe, P., Duffy, P., Mintz, G., and Stambaugh, R. L. On the role of prostaglandins in parturition in the rat. *Endocrinology 96,* 1040–1043 (1975).

Szechtman, H., Siegel, H. I., Rosenblatt, J. S., and Komisaruk, B. R. Tail-pinch facilitates onset of maternal behavior. *Physiol. Behav. 19,* 807–809 (1977).

Tamaki, Y., Semba, R., and Tooyama, S. Cerebellar hypoplasia and motor development in congenitally jaundiced Gunn rats. *Physiol. Behav. 18,* 255–259 (1977).

Terkel, J. and Rosenblatt, J. S. Maternal behavior induced by maternal blood plasma injected into virgin rats. *J. Comp. Physiol. Psychol. 65,* 479–482 (1968).

Terkel, J. and Rosenblatt, J. S. Aspects of nonhormonal maternal behavior in the rat. *Horm. Behav. 2,* 161–171 (1971).

Terkel, J. and Rosenblatt, J. S. Humoral factors underlying maternal behavior at parturition: cross transfusion between freely moving rats. *J. Comp. Physiol. Psychol. 80,* 365–371 (1972).

Terkel, J., Blake, C. A., and Sawyer, C. H. Prolactin levels in lactating rats after suckling or exposure to ether. *Endocrinology 91,* 49–53 (1972).

Terkel, J., Damassa, D. A., and Sawyer, C. H. Ultrasonic vocalizations of infant rats stimulate prolactin release in lactating females. Abstract, The Endocrine Society (1978).

Thoman, E. B. and Levine, S. Effects of adrenalectomy on maternal behavior in rats. *Develop. Psychobiol. 3,* 237–244 (1970).

Tobach, E. Developmental aspects of chemoception in the wistar (DAB) rat: tonic processes, in *Tonic Functions of Sensory Systems.* B. M. Menzel and H. P. Zeigler, eds. *Ann. N. Y. Acad. Sci. 290* (1977), pp. 226–269.

Tomogane, H., Ota, K., and Yokoyama, A. Duration of diestrous period and secretion of progestins during prolonged lactation in the rat. *Endocrinol. Japon. 23,* 137–141 (1976).

Tucker, H. A., Paape, M. J., Sinha, Y. N., Pritchard, D. E., and Thatcher, W. W. Relationship among nursing frequency, lactation, pituitary prolactin, and adrenocortocotropic hormone content in rats. *Proc. Soc. Exp. Biol. Med. 126,* 100–103 (1967).

Veomett, M. J. and Daniel, Jr., J. C. Termination of pregnancy after accelerated lactation in the rat. *J. Reprod. Fert. 26,* 415–417 (1971).

Weichert, C. K. The experimental shortening of delayed pregnancy in the albino rat. *Anta. Rec. 77,* 31–43 (1940).

Whitworth, N. Relationships between patterns of grooming, endocrine function and mammary gland development in the pregnant rat. Ph.D. dissertation, Rutgers University (1972).

Wiesner, B. P. and Sheard, N. M. *Maternal Behavior in the Rat.* Oliver and Boyd, London (1933).

Ying, S.-Y., Gove, S., Fang, V. S., and Greep, R. O. Ovulation in postpartum rats. *Endocrinology 92,* 108–116 (1973).

Zarrow, M. X. Gestation, in *Sex and Internal Secretion,* 3rd edition. W. C. Young, ed. Williams and Wilkins, Baltimore (1961) pp. 958–1031.

Zarrow, M. X., Gandelman, R., and Denenberg, V. H. Prolactin: is it an essential hormone for maternal behavior in mammals? *Horm. Behav. 2,* 343–354 (1971).

Zarrow, M. X., Johnson, N. P., Denenberg, V. H., and Bryant, L. P. Maintenance of lactational diestrum in the postpartum rat through tactile stimulation in the absence of suckling. *Neuroendocrinology 11,* 150–155 (1973).

Maternal Influences and Early Behavior

8

Maternal Mediation of Early Experience

William P. Smotherman

Robert W. Bell

Early experience studies have focused on the behavioral and physiological changes that result when young animals in their preweaning stage of development are stimulated using procedures such as handling or shock (Levine, 1969; 1975). These early experience treatments typically have prolonged and lasting effects on the animal's behavioral and physiological responses as an adult (Levine, 1962; Denenberg and Zarrow, 1971). As to how such early experience treatments exert their effects has been the source of some interest and a large literature has been generated on the topic.

EARLY EXPERIENCE HYPOTHESES

There have been several hypotheses proposed to account for the effects of handling or otherwise stimulating infant rodents (see Russell, 1971 for a review of these hypotheses). First, as suggested by the direct action hypothesis of Levine (1962), early experience outcomes result in part from the direct action of the stimulation impinging on the organism. Second, the cooling or hypothermia hypothesis (Schaefer and Weingarten, 1962) suggests that early stimulation effects result from the incidental cooling that pups receive while out of the nest during treatment. Third, Levine (1956) has suggested a stress hypothesis. In other words, all treatments employed to provide infantile stimulation are in some way noxious or stressful to the young animal and in this way serve to modify the physiological systems that mediate stress reactivity in adulthood. A fourth hypothesis focuses on the importance of changes in the maternal environment (Richards, 1966; Barnett and Burn, 1967; Meier and Schutzman, 1968). This maternal mediation hypothesis suggests that the reported effects of early stimulation result not only from the effects of the stimulation on the pups per se but are also in part mediated by changes in the nature of the mother–infant interaction. These changes occur subsequent to the stimulation and return of the stimulated pups to the nest. This hypothesis has been redefined and more precisely stated as of late in the work of Bell et al. (1974) and Smotherman et al. (1977b).

Typical early stimulation procedures are administered to the pups directly. However these procedures have the additional effect of altering ongoing mother–infant interactions. Any developmental outcomes produced by early stimulation could represent the indirect effects of altered mother–infant interactions rather than the direct effects of stimulation on the pups. This explanation is based on the premise that changes in mother–infant interactions have the capacity to influence the ontogeny of behavior in the pup. Villescas et al. (1977) have shown that prohibiting interaction between mother and pups after handling the pups significantly alters the developmental outcomes typically produced by this treatment. Levine and Weiner (1977), Hennessy et al. (1978) and Villescas (1978) have summarized how any interpretation of the literature on malnutrition has become complicated by the recognition that other factors, non-nutritional in nature (i.e., maternal environment) affect developmental outcomes. It would seem important, if not necessary to assess the role of changes in maternal caretaking activities in programs of investigation which entail direct or indirect manipulation of the maternal environment.

Ressler (1962, 1963) showed that mother–infant interactions in rodents were dyadic and reciprocal in nature. Rodent offspring provide cues which initiate (Herrenkohl and Sachs, 1972), and direct mother–infant interactions early in lactation (Smotherman et al., 1975) and coordinate the decline of maternal behaviors as lactation proceeds (Reisbick et al., 1975). Smotherman et al. (1978) have further suggested that the sensory/stimulus control of mother–infant behavior sequences changes as the 4-week lactation period proceeds. Early (during weeks 1–2) the pups provide cues—odors, vocalizations, etc. to which the mother responds both behaviorally and physiologically. As lactation proceeds, pup-produced cues diminish and the mother's physiological state proceeds to a condition where she begins to secrete a pheromone to which the pups are attracted. This is brought about in part by the changing pattern of stimulation provided by the pups (Moltz and Kilpatrick, 1978). Attraction to the mother by the pups ceases at the end of the fourth week thereby coordinating the weaning process. This cessation is most likely due to the young establishing their own odor environment (Leon, 1975).

The stimulus qualities of the pups e.g., their size, vocalizations, odors, body hair, mobility all show ontogenetic changes. There is data showing that these stimulus attributes of pups interact with one another (Smotherman et al., 1974) and with other nest cues—maternal or conspecific odors (Oswalt and Meier, 1974; Conely and Bell, 1978) to coordinate mother and infant behaviors. Further evidence suggests that treatments such as those typically employed in early stimulation experiments alter these pup stimulus characteristics. The clearest evidence of this shows that early stimulation among other things produce changes in the rate of ultrasound production (Bell et al., 1971). Bell et al. (1971) speculated that changes in maternal behavior elicited by these pup ultrasounds may mediate early experience outcomes. This was the first report suggesting a direct link between changing pup cues elicited by early stimulation, maternal behavioral responsiveness and developmental outcomes. Bell et al. (1974) went a step further to demonstrate convincingly that maternal behavior and ultrasonic vocalizations varied systematically as a function of the intensity of stimulation the pups had received. In this study groups of litters were exposed to 3 minutes of handling (H), 2 minutes of 5–6° c cooling (2C) or 5 minutes of 5–6° c cooling (5C) for the first five days postpartum. The authors measured ultrasounds and maternal behaviors simultaneously. They reported parallels between the rate and persistance of vocalizations and the effectiveness of mothering the pups received. Specifically, pups in the H group vocalized infrequently and elicited little maternal attention. In the 2C condition pups initially vocalized at high rates which triggered effective mothering. The rate of vocalizations in this group declined steadily across the recording session. In the 5C condition pups vocalized somewhat less initially but the vocalizations persisted across the recording period. Pups in this condition also received ineffective mothering. Smotherman et al. (1977a) also reported maternal behavior changes that corresponded to pup treatment. Litters were assigned to handled (H) or shocked (S) conditions and mother–infant interactions were observed following these treatments on Days 2, 9, and 16 of lactation. On Days 2 and 9 mothers that interacted with pups in the S condition showed more pup-directed activity than mothers interacting with pups after the pups experienced the H treatment.

ROLE OF MATERNAL BEHAVIOR

Bell et al. (1974) have suggested that a maternal factor enters into the curvilinear relationship between the intensity of early stimulation and adult behavior (Denenberg, 1964). Pups in the H and 2C litters would receive effective mothering as a result of their stimulation and would both differ from non-stimulated control and 5C litters both of which would receive ineffective mothering—pups exposed to the latter two treatments would not differ from one another. Mothers detect and respond to the telereceptive cues from pups as reflected by both behavioral (Bell et al., 1974; Smotherman et al., 1976) and physiological (Smotherman et al., 1976; Mendoza et al., 1978) indices of maternal responsiveness.

While most studies have examined maternal behavior changes that take place during the interval immediately after the pups are returned to the nest there also exists evidence showing that changes in the maternal environment i.e., changes in mother–infant interactions, are long lasting (Lee and Williams, 1974) and are present during periods of time not specifically associated with a disturbance of the mother–infant dyad (Lee and Williams, 1975). In the same context it has been shown that prior litter experience may affect the way mothers respond to pups of subsequent litters. Wright et al. (1977) have shown that parity interacts with the degree of stimulation (stress) litters have received to alter mother–infant interactions. These data suggest that compared to primiparae, multiparae are initially more responsive to pups and further that over the 20 day pup treatment period they employed the multiparous mothers did not change their behavior due to the stress their pups had received. This latter finding suggests a stability in the maternal behavior of multiparous mothers which was not as contingent upon pup cues as was the primiparous mothering. Villecas et al. (1977) have also demonstrated parity effects. In this case they found parity effects on the developmental outcomes elicited by early handling. When the treatment (the pups were handled or left non-handled) imposed upon multiparous pups was factorially combined with the treatment that had been imposed upon the primiparous pups (again handled or left non-handled) the emotionality (e.g., open field behavior) of the second litter offspring varied as a function of the treatment of their mother's initial litter, not as a function of their having been handled or not. These data show that there exists a change in mothering style which results from the differential treatment of her primiparous litter. This change influences her behavior with subsequent litters. As was stated above, the importance of changes in caretaking behaviors for affecting developmental outcomes needs to be specified. According to Wright et al. (1977) it is evident that to fully understand the consequences of early experience phenomena it will be necessary to explore them within a larger ecological context including manipulations of maternal characteristics, stress-induced changes in mothering and other features of the pups early life situation.

MATERNAL MEDIATION HYPOTHESIS

Figure 1 summarizes some of the major points of the previous discussion. Early experience treatments are generally applied to the litter directly and no

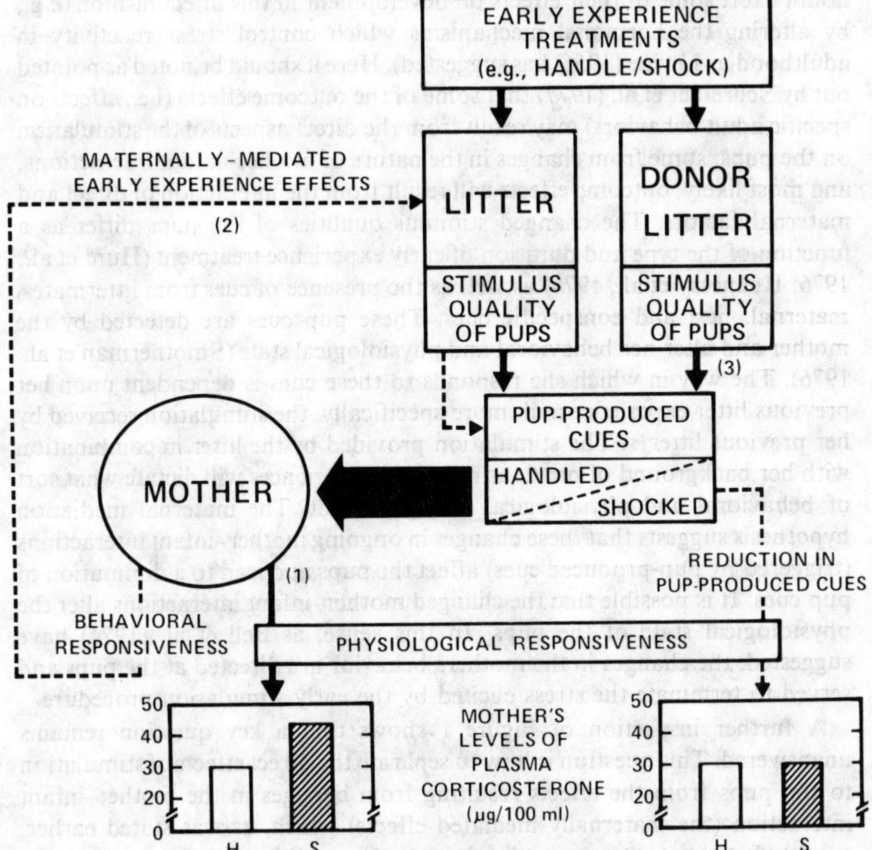

FIG. 1. A schematic representation of events triggered by early experience treatment (e.g., handling, shock) to a litter. Early experience treatments cause a change in the stimulus quality of the litter. The pups emit cues (e.g., odors, ultrasounds) which differ as a function of the intensity of the early experience treatment. These telereceptive cues are detected by the mother. These cues trigger physiological changes even in situations where mother and pups are prevented from contact interaction (1). Behavioral changes by the mother occur which vary systematically as a function of the pup treatment. Alterations in maternal caretaking activities effect the litter resulting in both a reduction in pup produced cues and maternal (and perhaps pup) physiological responsiveness (2). It is further illustrated that similar treatments to a donor litter (3) would also be expected to trigger similar physiological and behavioral responses in mother. This chain of events leading to alterations in mother–infant interactions has been implicated as a contributing factor in typical early experience outcomes. This process is collectively referred to as the maternal mediation of early experience effects.

doubt exert some of their effects on development in this direct fashion (e.g., by altering the hormonal mechanisms which control stress reactivity in adulthood as Levine (1956) has suggested). Here it should be noted as pointed out by Schreiber et al. (1977) that some of the outcome effects (i.e., effects on specific adult behaviors) may result from the direct aspects of the stimulation on the pups, some from changes in the nature of mother–infant interactions, and most likely, outcome effects will result from the interaction of direct and maternal factors. The changed stimulus qualities of the pups differ as a function of the type and duration of early experience treatment (Hunt et al., 1976; Hennessy et al., 1978) as well as the presence of cues from littermates, maternal, nest and conspecific cues. These pup cues are detected by the mother and alter her behavioral and physiological state (Smotherman et al., 1976). The way in which she responds to these cues is dependent upon her previous litter experience and, more specifically, the stimulation received by her previous litter/s. The stimulation provided by the litter in combination with her background of previous maternal experiences will dictate what sort of behavioral and physiological changes result. The maternal mediation hypothesis suggests that these changes in ongoing mother–infant interactions (triggered by pup-produced cues) affect the pups and lead to a diminution of pup cues. It is possible that the changed mother–infant interactions alter the physiological state of the pups. In this sense, as Bell et al. (1974) have suggested, the changes in the mothers behavior are directed at the pups and served to terminate the stress elicited by the early stimulation procedure.

A further inspection of Figure 1 shows that a key question remains unanswered. This question is how to separate the direct effects of stimulation to the pups from the effects resulting from changes in the mother–infant interaction (the maternally mediated effects) which, as was stated earlier, persist after the pup treatment has been terminated. Looking at the right side of the diagram (Fig. 1) an alternate pathway has been drawn. The experimenter can apply early experience treatments to a donor litter. These treatments would change the stimulus properties of the pups in the donor litter resulting in pup-produced cues (telereceptive). Test mothers nursing their own undisturbed litters (undisturbed in that they do not receive any added stimulation from the experimenter) could be exposed to these telereceptive cues emanating from the stimulated donor litter. Such a procedure has been used effectively by at least two investigators to alter ongoing maternal behaviors, i.e., to increase pup directed activities. Brown et al. (1977) first showed that such a procedure was effective in increasing pup-directed activities engaged in by the mother—whose litter had not received any direct stimulation. Noirot (1974) using a similar procedure found that virgin mice exposed to cues from donor litters increased their nestbuilding activity in response to such cues. In neither of these studies however were the litters of pups receiving this extra maternally-mediated stimulation tested as adults for early experience outcomes.

Test mothers in this situation did exhibit an increase in pup-related behaviors which they directed toward their own undisturbed litters. The important question for the matter of the present discussion is whether or not this added maternal stimulation, in the absence of any direct, i.e., experimenter stimulation would effect a "typical early experience outcome" (Smotherman, 1975). Such a question and experimental arrangement are presented in Figure 2.

Schreiber (1978) has used such a donor litter preparation effectively in a

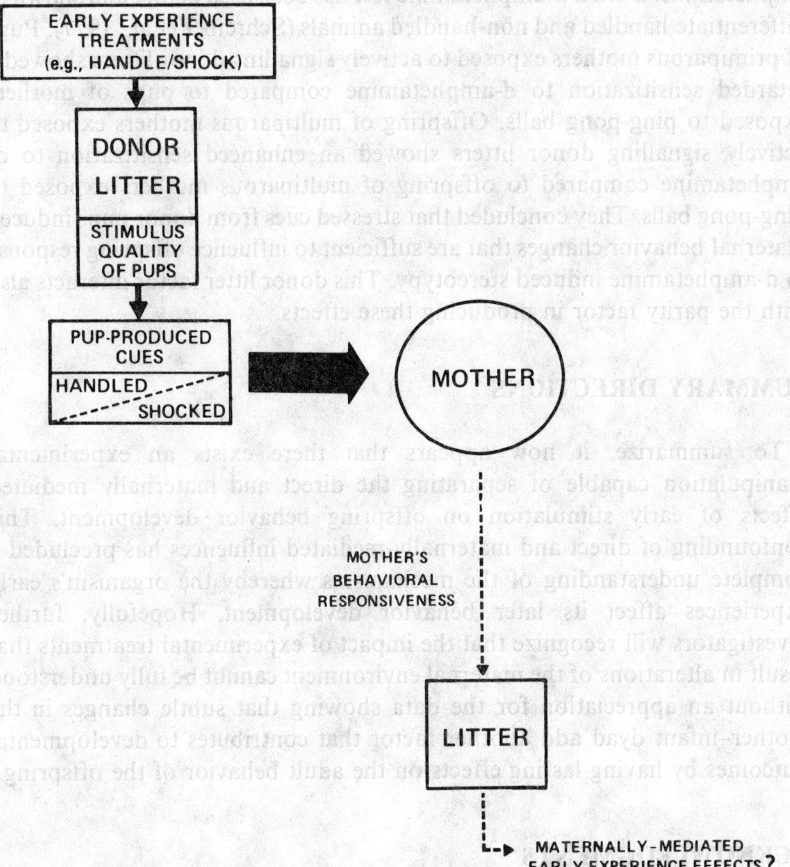

FIG. 2. A schematic representation of how donor litters could be used to test out assumptions about maternal factors as they influence developmental outcomes.

paradigm designed to look at developmental outcomes following daily exposure of mothers/litters to cues from donor litters. Experimental groups of primiparous and multiparous mothers were exposed to baskets (donor litters) of actively signalling cold-stressed pups, baskets of anesthesized non-signalling pups or baskets of ping-pong balls daily for the first week of lactation while their own pups were undisturbed. Maternal behaviors were measured during and after the exposures to the baskets and pups were tested as adults for developmental outcomes. The results suggested that both primiparous and multiparous mothers responded to the actively signalling and anesthesized pups with increased maternal care of their own pups.

Following weaning the offspring were tested for their reaction to d-amphetamine. Such a d-amphetamine test has been used before and shown to differentiate handled and non-handled animals (Schreiber et al., 1977). Pups of primiparous mothers exposed to actively signalling donor litters showed a retarded sensitization to d-amphetamine compared to pups of mothers exposed to ping-pong balls. Offspring of multiparous mothers exposed to actively signalling donor litters showed an enhanced sensitization to d-amphetamine compared to offspring of multiparous mothers exposed to ping-pong balls. They concluded that stressed cues from donor pups induced maternal behavior changes that are sufficient to influence offspring response to d-amphetamine induced stereotypy. This donor litter factor interacts also with the parity factor in producing these effects.

SUMMARY DIRECTIONS

To summarize, it now appears that there exists an experimental manipulation capable of separating the direct and maternally mediated effects of early stimulation on offspring behavior development. This confounding of direct and maternally-mediated influences has precluded a complete understanding of the mechanisms whereby the organism's early experiences affect its later behavior development. Hopefully, further investigators will recognize that the impact of experimental treatments that result in alterations of the maternal environment cannot be fully understood without an appreciation for the data showing that subtle changes in the mother–infant dyad add another factor that contributes to developmental outcomes by having lasting effects on the adult behavior of the offspring.

ACKNOWLEDGMENTS

William P. Smotherman is supported by Oregon State University College of Liberal Arts Research Grant (30-050-5302).

REFERENCES

Barnett, S. A. and Burn, J. Early stimulation and maternal behavior. *Nature* (London) *213,* 150–152 (1967).

Bell, R. W., Nitschke, W., Bell, N. J., and Zachman, T. Early experience, ultrasonic vocalizations, and maternal responsiveness in rats. *Dev. Psychobiol. 7,* 235–242 (1974).

Bell, R. W., Nitschke, W., Gorry, T. H., and Zachman, T. Infantile stimulation and ultrasonic signalling: A possible mediator of early handling phenomena. *Dev. Psychobiol. 4,* 181–191 (1971).

Brown, C. P., Smotherman, W. P., and Levine, S. Interaction-induced reduction in differential maternal responsiveness: An effect of cue reduction or behavior? *Dev. Psychobiol. 10,* 273–280 (1977).

Conely, L. and Bell, R. W. Neonatal ultrasounds elicited by odor cues. *Dev. Psychobiol. 11,* 193–197 (1978).

Denenberg, V. H. Critical periods, stimulus input and emotional reactivity: A theory of infantile stimulation. *Psych. Rev. 71,* 335–351 (1964).

Denenberg, V. H. and Zarrow, M. X. Effects of handling in infancy upon behavior and adrenocortical activity: Suggestions for a neuroendocrine mechanism. In *Early Childhood: The Development of Self-Regulatory Mechanisms,* D. N. Walcher and D. L. Peters, eds. Academic Press, New York (1971), pp. 40–74.

Hennessy, M. B., Laughlin, N. K., Weiner, S. G., and Levine, S. Malnutrition and maternal behavior in the rat. In *Maternal Influences and Early Behavior,* R. W. Bell and W. P. Smotherman, eds. Spectrum Publications, New York (1979) pp. 211–234.

Hennessy, M. B., Smotherman, W. P., Kolp, L., Hunt, L., and Levine, S. Stimuli from pups of adrenalectomized and malnourished mother rats. *Physiol. and Behav. 20,* 509–513 (1978).

Herrenkohl, L. R. and Sachs, B. D. Sensory regulation of maternal behavior in mammals. *Physiol. and Behav. 9,* 689–692 (1972).

Hunt, L. E., Smotherman, W. P., Wiener, S. P., and Levine, S. Nutritional variables and their effect on the development of ultrasonic vocalizations in rat pups. *Physiol. and Behav. 17,* 1037–1039 (1976).

Lee, M. H. S. and Williams, D. I. Changes in licking behavior of rat mother following handling of young. *Anim. Behav. 22,* 679–681 (1974).

Lee, M. H. S. and Williams, D. I. Long term changes in nest condition and pup grouping following handling of rat litters. *Dev. Psychobiol. 8,* 91–95 (1975).

Leon, M. Dietary control of maternal pheromone in the lactating rat. *Physiol. and Behav. 14,* 311–319 (1975).

Levine, S. A further study of infantile handling and adult avoidance learning. *J. Personal. 25,* 70–80 (1956).

Levine, S. The psychophysiological effects of infantile stimulation. In *Roots of Behavior,* E. Bliss, ed. Paul Hoeber and Co. New York (1962) pp. 246–253.

Levine, S. An endocrine theory of infantile stimulation. In *Stimulation in Early Infancy,* A. Ambrose, ed. Academic Press, London (1969) pp. 45–63.

Levine, S. The potential influence of infantile stimulation on emotional disorders. In *Society, Stress and Disease.* Vol. 2. *Childhood and Adolescence,* L. Levi, ed. Oxford Univ. Press, London (1975) pp. 411–415.

Levine, S. and Weiner. Malnutrition and early environmental experience: Possible interactive effects on later behavior. In *Environments as Therapy for Brain Dysfunction,* R. N. Walsh and W. T. Greenough, eds. Plenum Publishing Corp. New York (1976) pp. 51–70.

Meier, G. W. and Schutzman, L. H. Mother–infant interactions and experimental manipulation: Confounding or misidentification? *Dev. Psychobiol. 1,* 141–145 (1968).

Mendoza, S. P., Coe, C. L., Smotherman, W. P., and Levine, S. Functional consequences of attachment: A comparison of two species. In *Maternal Influences and Early Behavior.* R. W. Bell and W. P. Smotherman eds. Spectrum Publications, New York (1979) pp. 235–251.

Moltz, H. and Kilpatrick, S. J. Pheromonal control of maternal behavior. In *Maternal Influences and Early Behavior,* R. W. Bell and W. P. Smotherman, eds. Spectrum Publications, New York (1979) pp. 135–154.

Noirot, E. Nestbuilding by the virgin female mouse exposed to ultrasounds from inaccessible pups. *Anim. Behav. 22,* 410–420 (1974).

Oswalt, G. L. and Meier, G. W. Olfactory, thermal and tactual influences on infantile ultrasonic vocalizations in rats. *Dev. Psychobiol. 8,* 129–135 (1975).

Reisbick, S., Rosenblatt, J. S., and Mayer, A. D. Decline of maternal behavior in the virgin and lactating rat. *J. Comp. Physiol. Psych. 89,* 722–732 (1975).

Ressler, R. H. Parental handling in two strains of mice reared by foster parents. *Science 137,* 129–130 (1962).

Ressler, R. H. Genotype-correlated parental infuences in two strains of mice. *J. Comp. Physiol. Psych. 56,* 882–886 (1963).

Richards, M. P. M. Infantile handling in rodents: A reassessment in light of recent studies of maternal behavior. *Anim. Behav. 14,* 582 (1966).

Russell, P. A. "Infantile stimulation" in rodents: A consideration of possible mechanisms. *Psych. Bull. 75,* 192–202 (1971).

Schaefer, T. and Weingarten, F. S. Temperature change: The basic variable in the early handling phenomenon. *Science 135,* 41–42 (1962).

Schreiber, H. L. Maternal behavior and offspring amphetamine response. Unpublished Doctoral Dissertation. Texas Tech University (1977).

Schreiber, H. L., Bell, R. W., Kufner, M., and Villescas, R. Maternal behavior: A determinant of amphetamine toxicity in rats. *Psychopharm. 52,* 173–176 (1977).

Smotherman, W. P., Bell, R. W., Starzec, J., Elias, J., and Zachman, T. Maternal responses to infant vocalizations and olfactory cues in rats and mice. *Behav. Biol. 12,* 55–66 (1974).

Smotherman, W. P. The maternal mediation of early experience. Paper presented at the Southwestern Psychological Assoc. Meeting, April, Albuquerque (1975).

Smotherman, W. P., Wiener, S. G., Mendoza, S. P., and Levine, S. Maternal pituitary-adrenal responsiveness to noxious and pup-produced stimuli. In *Ciba Foundation Symposium on Breastfeeding and the Mother,* K. Elliot and D. W. Fitzsimons, eds. Elsevier, Amsterdam (1976) pp. 5–25.

Smotherman, W. P., Brown, C. P., and Levine, S. Maternal responsiveness following differential pup treatment and mother-pup interactions. *Horm. Behav. 8,* 242–253 (1977a).

Smotherman, W. P., Mendoza, S. P., and Levine, S. Ontogenetic changes in pup-elicited maternal pituitary-adrenal activity: Pup age and stage of lactation effects. *Dev. Psychobiol. 10,* 365–371 (1977b).

Smotherman, W. P., Bell, R. W., Hershberger, W., and Coover, G. D. Orientation to rat pup cues: Effects of maternal experiential history. *Anim. Behav. 26,* 265–273 (1978).

Villescas, R. The effects of maternal protein-restriction during gestation on the maternal behavior of the lactating rat and on the physical and behavioral development of the neonatal rat. Unpublished Doctoral Dissertation, Texas Tech University (1978).

Villescas, R., Bell, R. W., and Kufner, M. Interactive effects of parity and early handling. Paper presented at the International Society of Developmental Psychobiology Meeting, November, Toronto (1976).

Villescas, R., Bell, R. W., Wright, L., and Kufner, M. Effects of handling on maternal behavior following return of the pups to the nest. *Dev. Psychobiol. 10,* 323–329 (1977).

Wright, L., Bell, R. W., Schreiber, H. L., Villescas, R., and Conely, L. Interactive effects of parity and pup stress in maternal behavior. *Dev. Psychobiol. 10,* 331–337 (1977).

Maternal Influences and Early Behavior

9

Malnutrition and Maternal Behavior in the Rat

Michael B. Hennessy
Nellie K. Laughlin
Sandra G. Wiener
Seymour Levine

Maternal nutrition, particularly during the periods of gestation and lactation, can have important consequences for the developing young. Nutritional deprivation of the mother has been reported to produce alterations in the behavior and physiological functioning of the offspring which may persist beyond the brief, early period of deprivation. These abnormalities have been hypothesized to arise from inadequate nourishment during the time of most rapid development of the young organism (Smart and Dobbing, 1971a,b; Winick and Noble, 1966; Zamenhof et al., 1968).

Recently, increasing attention has been paid to the impact of dietary manipulations on the quality of maternal care provided for the offspring (Levine and Wiener, 1976; Plaut, 1970). If dietary restriction influences the mother's treatment of her young, then any long-term effect of maternal malnutrition on the young may result from these modifications in maternal care, rather than from malnutrition per se. Alterations in the young organism's maternal environment are known to produce various long-term behavioral and physiological consequences (Denenberg et al., 1968; Harlow et al., 1971; Levine and Thoman, 1969; Thoman and Levine, 1969). In fact, it has been suggested that the many lasting effects of early handling and other forms of stimulation in young rodents may, at least partially, result from changes in maternal behavior following the return of the pups to the nest (Bell et al., 1971; Richards, 1966; Russell, 1971). Clearly then, the quality of maternal care represents a potentially critical and contaminating variable in studies of early malnutrition effects.

Unfortunately, assessment of the effects of malnutrition on maternal behavior is in itself difficult, for the various procedures used to produce malnutrition may also disrupt maternal behavior to some degree. That is, observed differences in the maternal behavior of malnourished animals may result not only from poor nutrition of the mother or young per se, but also from some additional disturbance (e.g., handling, social isolation) inherent in the implementation of the malnutrition regimen. Moreover, some of the presently used techniques produce malnutrition in the offspring, but not in the mother. These techniques may be useful to specifically examine the capacity of malnourished pups to elicit maternal behavior, but they shed no light on the effects of the mother's own nutritional state on her behavior. A more comprehensive understanding of the results of malnutrition on maternal behavior might best be achieved by examining the composite of effects seen with various procedures, while recognizing the limitations of each individual technique. In the next section we will examine the techniques used to produce malnutrition in rats, and discuss the applicability of these various methods for maternal behavior studies.

CRITIQUE OF TECHNIQUES FOR IMPOSING MALNUTRITION IN RATS

One method used to produce malnutrition is to separate the mother from the pups for several hours each day (Eayrs and Horn, 1955). This technique is one which selectively malnourishes the pups, not the mother, and thereby permits no examination of any direct effect of malnutrition on the mother's behavior. Further, since handling of pups is known to alter maternal behavior (Lee and Williams, 1975; Smotherman et al., 1977), any disturbance to the litter while separating it from the mother may affect her behavior. This technique not only deprives the young of mother's milk, but also of all forms of maternal stimulation during the daily period of separation. The potential effect of this deprivation on mother–pup interactions following reunion needs to be controlled. These effects might be ameliorated to some degree by replacing the mother with a virgin female which has been induced to act maternally through previous exposure to pups (Slob et al., 1973) or with a nipple-ligated (nonlactating) female (Lynch, 1976), or by incubating the pups (Salas et al., 1974), which at least provides warmth during the period of separation.

A second procedure used to produce malnutrition is to increase the litter size to 15–20 pups (Kennedy, 1957). This technique limits each pup's access to a nipple and thereby malnourishes the pups without affecting the nutritional condition of the mother. In general this procedure suffers from an inability to equally malnourish all members of the litter. Galler and Turkewitz (1975) found the coefficient of variability of pup weights ($\bar{X}$ standard deviation/$\bar{X}$ pup weight) to be about twice as great in litters of 16 as compared to litters of eight. Another problem with this procedure is that the size of the litter becomes a contaminating variable. Different-sized litters undoubtedly afford the mother different amounts of pup-associated stimuli, which could alter maternal behavior patterns. Possible empirical support for this notion is provided by studies in which mothers of larger litters were found to score lower on a composite index of maternal behavior (Seitz, 1954, 1958) and to spend less time with their litters (Grota and Ader, 1969) than were mothers of smaller litters. In both of these cases, the effect would appear to be more likely due to the altered litter size than to pup nutrition. Seitz (1958) found that mothers caring for three pups differed from mothers with litters as small as nine, a litter size which would not seem to be too large to restrict normal intake of milk. (Pup body weights were not reported in this study.) Similarly the finding that large litters receive diminished maternal contact (Grota and Ader, 1969) would also appear to be due to litter size rather than nutrition, since pups malnourished with other procedures have consistently been found to receive increased maternal contact relative to controls. (These results will be discussed at greater length in a later section of this chapter.) The fact that neither of these effects of large litters on maternal behavior can be unequivocally attributed to either litter size or pup nutrition points up the hazards of using this technique in maternal behavior studies.

A third method used to produce malnutrition is to substitute gastric infusion or intubation of a limited quantity of food or an unbalanced diet as the pups' sole source of nutrition (Hall, 1975; Hofer, 1973; Messer et al., 1969; Miller and Dymsza, 1963). The mother's nutrition is, of course, unaffected by this technique, but if the mother is to remain with the pups at all, she must be rendered unable to provide milk. Any potential effect of this sort of intervention (e.g., removal of all nipples) on maternal behavior must then also be taken into account. In addition, these artificial feeding procedures require handling of pups, which may alter maternal behavior (Lee and Williams, 1975; Smotherman et al., 1977).

A fourth technique for producing malnutrition is to adrenalectomize the mother (Wiener et al., 1977). Since adrenal corticoids are necessary for normal lactation (Cowie, 1961; Cowie and Folley, 1947), removal of the adrenals reduces the amount of milk available to the young. Adrenalectomy thus selectively malnourishes the litter, not the mother. However, with this technique, any effect of the absence of adrenal hormones on the mother's behavior becomes a confounding variable and needs to be considered.

A fifth technique used to produce malnutrition is to limit the mother rat's daily intake of a good diet to some percentage of normal (Chow and Lee,

1964). This technique results in malnutrition of both mother and pups, and unlike the above-mentioned procedures can be applied prenatally as well as after birth. One problem with this technique is that maternal behavior may be disrupted not by malnutrition, but by the mother's increased food-seeking behaviors which may be performed to the exclusion of other (maternal) behavior patterns (Simonson et al., 1969). Also, feeding mothers during only the lights-on period can cause a shifting of the normal circadian rhythm of maternal behavior (Stern and Levin, 1976), thereby producing a further disruption of mother–infant activities.

A final procedure, which results in malnutrition of both mother and young, is to allow the mother unlimited access to a low-protein diet (Barnes et al., 1968). This technique reduces the quantity of milk produced by the mother without altering its protein content (Mueller and Cox, 1946; Venkatachalam and Ramanathan, 1964) and can be used both pre- and postnatally. This procedure seems to be the most suitable for maternal behavior studies since disturbance of the mother and litter is minimized. However, factors such as the amount of protein provided by the low-protein diet need to be considered. Protein levels which have been employed to produce malnutrition range from about 5–12% of the diet (normal laboratory diets contain approximately 24% protein), so that mothers and pups in some studies may be more-severely malnourished than mothers and pups in others. More generally, with this technique as with the others, small differences in experimental protocol can make comparisons of findings difficult. Since, as noted above, handling of pups can alter maternal behavior, differences in the frequency with which pups are weighed to obtain a growth curve can lead to spurious differences among laboratories in the results of maternal behavior studies. Similarly, such variables as the length and timing of the deprivation period, the size and age of the experimental subjects, as well as the host of more usual experimental concerns (e.g., time and conditions of testing, strain of rat) need to be taken into account when comparing experimental outcomes.

We will next describe the findings available at this time on the effects of malnutrition on: (a) maternal retrieval, (b) other pup-directed activities, (c) non-pup-directed activities, and (d) pup-associated stimuli. At the present state of investigation, much of the information is fragmentary or inconclusive, and discrepancies among findings exist. Possible explanations or integrative hypotheses will be presented when available.

MATERNAL RETRIEVAL

The efficiency with which the mother retrieves scattered pups to the nest is probably the most often employed measure of rodent maternal behavior.

While one early study (Cowley and Griesel, 1964) found no differences in the retrieval behavior of malnourished and well-nourished mothers, several more-recent reports have noted retrieval deficiencies in poorly nourished mothers. Fraňková (1971) compared the retrieval of mothers which were either maintained on a control diet, or switched at parturition to a low (10%) protein diet which contained large quantities of either fat or carbohydrate. In retrieval tests conducted on Days 6, 8 and 10 postpartum, mothers fed either low protein diet took longer to begin retrieving pups to the nest and retrieved a smaller percentage of the litter during the 3-minute testing period than did controls. Similar results have been obtained with intake-restricted mothers. Smart and Preece (1973) fed experimental animals approximately half as much of a good quality diet as consumed by control animals. The dietary regimens began at conception and retrieval tests were conducted on Days 4, 6, 8 and 10 postpartum. Underfed mothers took significantly longer to initiate retrieval on Days 8 and 10 than did controls. The undernourished mothers also retrieved fewer pups on Day 10 and showed less retrieval of the entire litter on Days 8 and 10. Thus retrieval performance was impaired only during the second week of lactation.

In analyses of retrieval as well as other aspects of mammalian maternal behavior, it has become almost axiomatic to regard the mother–infant bond as reciprocal in nature. Not only do different patterns of mothering have different consequences for the development of the offspring (e.g., Denenberg et al., 1968; Ressler, 1963), but various characteristics of the offspring also influence the behavior of the mother (e.g., Beach and Jaynes, 1956; Nicoll and Meites, 1959; Young, 1965). Thus the retrieval deficits observed in malnourished mothers might result from a direct effect of the mother's own nutritional condition on her behavior, or alternatively, the malnourished condition of the pups might make them less effective elicitors of retrieval. A third possibility is that a poorly nourished mother and poorly nourished offspring are both necessary conditions for the observed deficits. In the previously-mentioned studies it is not possible to distinguish between these alternatives because inadequately nourished mothers were always tested with their own malnourished offspring. However, several studies have attempted to parcel out the separate influences of the mother and the pups in producing the retrieval impairment. In one such study (Smart, 1976), well-fed and underfed (permitted approximately half of normal intake of good diet beginning at conception) mothers were tested for retrieval with either well-nourished or undernourished pups on Days 5, 7, 9 and 11 postpartum. Regardless of the nutritional condition of the young, control mothers showed a shorter latency to retrieve the first pup on Days 7, 9 and 11 and retrieved more young to the nest on Days 9 and 11, than did their underfed counterparts. Thus, this study suggests that the previously found retrieval deficits of underfed mothers (Smart and Preece, 1973) are a function of the mother's nutritional condition, rather than that of her pups. Similar findings have been reported by Crnic (1976). Mothers were either well nourished or fed approximately 40% of normal intake of a good diet beginning on about the 20th day of gestation. The mothers were tested for retrieval with either well-nourished or poorly nourished young on the 8th day after birth. The nutritional condition of the mother was again found to be the critical variable. Well-fed mothers retrieved the entire litter in a shorter time than did underfed mothers, regardless of the pup's nutritional condition.

The relative importance of the nutritional condition of the mother and the pups has also been examined in animals fed low-protein diets. Wiener et al. (1977) fed experimental animals an 8% protein diet beginning on Day 14 of gestation, and tested for retrieval on Days 2–12 postpartum. In a first experiment, low-protein mothers tested with their own pups retrieved a smaller percentage of their litters on Days 9–12 than did well-nourished control mothers tested with their own pups. A second experiment attempted to examine the relative importance of the nutritional states of the mother and young in producing these retrieval deficits. In addition to the low-protein and control groups, this experiment also included a group of adrenalectomized mothers and their young. Since maternal adrenalectomy malnourishes only the litter, and not the mother, a similar pattern of retrieval deficits in low-protein fed and adrenalectomized mothers would suggest that the impaired retrieval was primarily due to the altered stimulus qualities of the malnourished pups, rather than to the nutritional condition of the mother. The low-protein and adrenalectomy preparations produced similar degrees of malnutrition in the pups during the first eight days of life as determined by pup body weights. However, the patterns of retrieval in these two groups were markedly different (see Fig. 1). The low-protein mothers again showed a progressive deterioration of retrieval across days, retrieving significantly fewer pups than did controls on Days 6–12. The adrenalectomized mothers showed no such deterioration. Although the adrenalectomized females retrieved a somewhat smaller percentage of pups than did the controls on each of the testing days, on no day was the difference between the two groups significant. Thus, the different patterns of retrieval observed in malnourished and adrenalectomized mothers favor an interpretation of the retrieval deficits of low-protein fed mothers as being due to the nutritional condition of the mother, rather than that of the young. In a later study, Hennessy et al. (1977) found that adrenalectomized mothers would evidence retrieval deficits (smaller percentage of litter retrieved; longer latency to retrieve first pup) in a similar test paradigm. However, these findings do not appear to alter the interpretation of the Wiener et al. (1977) study. The percentage of pups retrieved by adrenalectomized mothers in the two studies was similar.

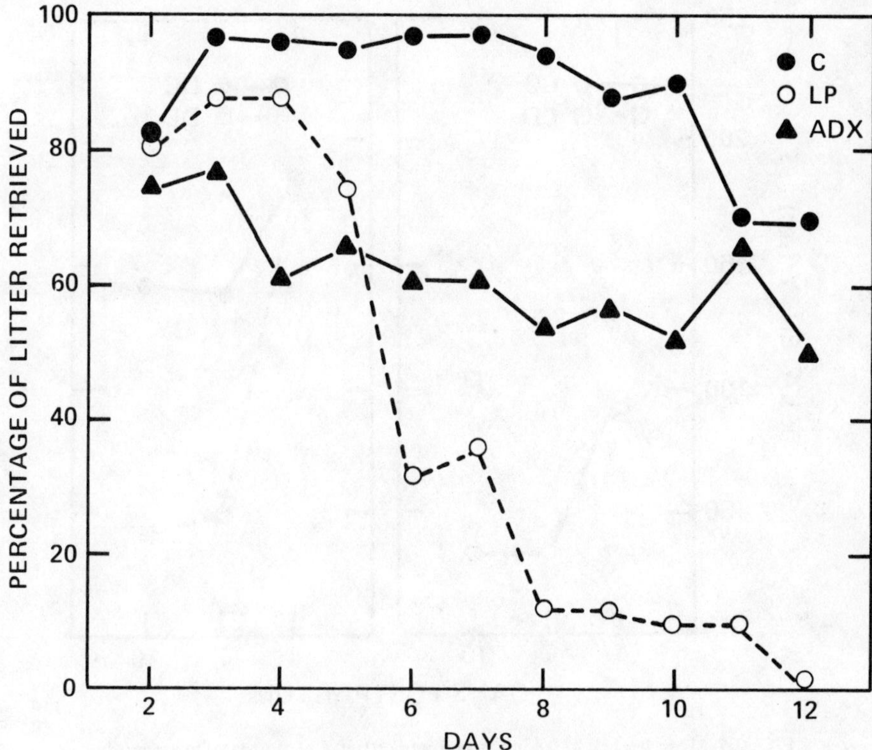

FIG. 1. Daily percentage of litter retrieved by control (C), low-protein (LP), and adrenalectomized (ADX) mothers during a 10-min retrieval test on Days 2–12 postpartum (C > LP on Days 6–12; ADX > LP on Days 8–12; from Wiener et al., 1977).

Moreover, testing in the Hennessy et al. (1977) study was terminated on Day 4, before the patterns of retrieval of low-protein fed and adrenalectomized mothers were found to differ by Wiener et al. (1977).

The retrieval behavior of low-protein fed mothers was also examined by Laughlin et al. (1976). Mothers were either well nourished or maintained from the 14th day of gestation on an 8% protein diet. At birth, mothers in each group were fostered either pups of well-nourished mothers or pups of low-protein fed mothers. Thus pups experienced either: (a) a malnourished mother both pre- and postnatally; (b) a malnourished mother prenatally and a well-nourished mother postnatally; (c) a well-nourished mother prenatally and a malnourished mother postnatally; or (d) a well-nourished mother both pre- and postnatally. Each foster mother was tested for retrieval of her litter on Days 4, 7, 10, and 13. The results indicated that latency to begin retrieval

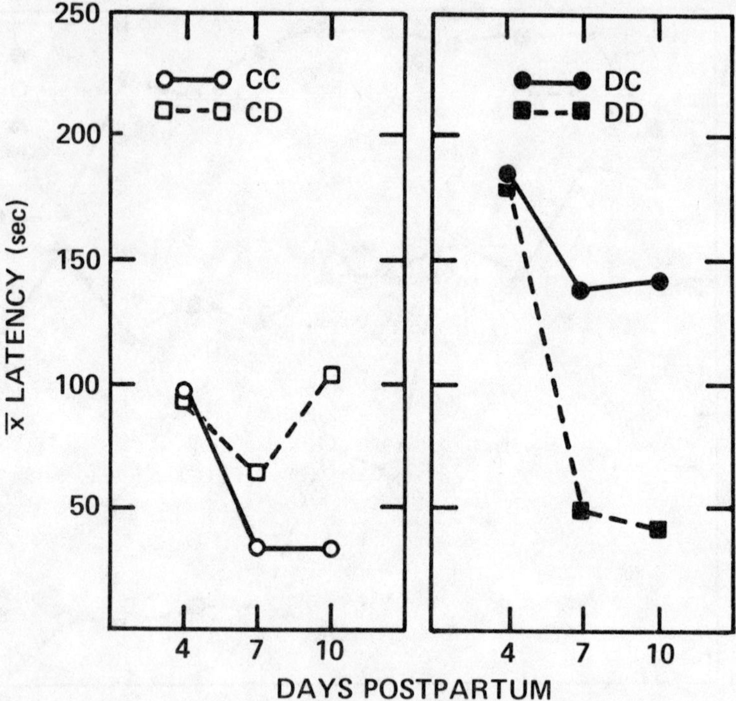

FIG. 2. Mean latency in seconds to initiate retrieval by postnatal foster mother on Days 4, 7 and 10 postpartum. For each group, the first letter indicates the nutritional condition of the pup's prenatal mother; the second letter indicates the nutritional condition of the pup's postnatal foster mother. C = well nourished, D = protein deprived (from Laughlin et al., 1976).

was affected by an interaction of prenatal and postnatal nutritional conditions (Fig. 2). Mothers which were fostered pups of the same nutritional condition (well-fed mothers fostered pups of well-fed mothers; low-protein fed mothers fostered pups of low-protein fed mothers) showed more-efficient retrieval than did mothers which were fostered pups of a different nutritional condition (well-fed mothers fostered pups of low-protein fed mothers; low-protein fed mothers fostered pups of well-fed mothers). Mothers fostered pups of the same nutritional condition displayed a moderately long latency on Day 4, and marked improvement on Days 7 and 10. Mothers fostered pups of a different nutritional condition showed a similar prolonged latency on Day 4 but no noticeable improvement on Days 7 and 10. By Day 13, a large number of pups in each group were crawling back to the nest, so that retrieval scores were not analyzed. The percentage of the litter retrieved did not differ among the four groups.

The results of this study indicate a different pattern of retrieval deficits in low-protein mothers than described by Wiener et al. (1977). This discrepancy might be accounted for in terms of the severity of malnutrition imposed. While both Laughlin et al. (1976) and Wiener et al. (1977) employed similar experimental regimens (8% protein diet from Day 14 of gestation, litters culled to eight), there are indications that Laughlin et al.'s animals were less severely malnourished. The weight loss of malnourished pups in the Wiener et al. (1977) and Laughlin et al. (1976) studies differed markedly, although similar weights for control animals were obtained in both studies. Wiener et al.'s well-nourished pups weighed approximately 21 g at 10 days of age, and 47 g when weaned at 21 days. The corresponding figures for Laughlin et al.'s controls were 20 and 43 g. In contrast, pups malnourished during both gestation and lactation weighed approximately 10 and 17 g in Wiener et al.'s study, and 14 and 33 g in Laughlin et al.'s study at 10 and 21 days of age, respectively. While malnourished pups in both studies showed a significant weight loss as compared to controls, a more drastic weight loss and growth retardation was observed in the Wiener et al. study. A procedural difference between the two studies which might, at least partially, account for the differential weight gain of pups is the age at which the adult females were malnourished. Wiener et al.'s animals were approximately 3 months old when dietary restriction began, while Laughlin et al.'s females were about 5 months of age. There is some evidence that lactating females of the age used by Laughlin et al. require less nutrients than do those of the age employed by Wiener et al. Altman et al. (1971a) found that, during lactation, 5–8-month-old multiparous females consumed less of a well-balanced diet than did 3–4-month-old primiparous females. Thus, the same malnutrition regimen might constitute a less severe deprivation for older animals (as in Laughlin et al.) than for younger animals (as in Wiener et al.).

Overall, it would appear that malnutrition of mother and young, whether produced by underfeeding or by administration of a low-protein diet, produces retrieval deficits. Retrieval efficiency deteriorates across days, usually becoming significantly impaired at about the beginning of the second week of lactation. Moreover, the deficits appear to be due primarily to the nutritional condition of the mother, rather than to that of the pups. Under other conditions (less severe protein malnutrition), these deficits may not appear, but the effects of less obvious factors are manifested. Retrieval appears normal as long as the nutritional condition of the mother matches that of the pup. When the gestational nutrition of the mother and pup do not match, retrieval is initiated more slowly. Whether this deficit is due to some desynchronization in the speed of progression through various phases of interaction by the mother and pup, some cue specific to the gestational nutrition of the pup, or some other factor is not clear.

OTHER PUP-DIRECTED MATERNAL ACTIVITIES

Poorly and well-nourished mothers have also been found to differ in terms of other pup-directed activities. Wiener and Levine (unpublished) found that low-protein mothers (8% protein from Day 14 of gestation) licked their pups less than did well-fed mothers during unobtrusive observations on Days 2–21. Likewise, Smart and Preece (1973) reported that underfed mothers showed less licking of their young than did well-fed mothers during retrieval tests on Days 4, 8 and 10. In a subsequent study, Smart (1976) showed that the difference in licking was apparently due primarily to the nutritional condition of the pup, rather than to that of the mother. Control and underfed mothers spent more time licking pups when presented with well-nourished young than they did when presented with malnourished offspring.

Differences between inadequately- and well-nourished mothers have also been found in the amount of time spent in contact with the young. Smart and Preece (1973) observed that well-fed mothers were found more often in their nests at 0900 hr on Days 1–20 postpartum than were underfed mothers. At 1300 hr, the control mothers were still found in their nests more frequently than were the underfed mothers, though the difference was less pronounced. By 1700 hr the pattern had reversed with the underfed mothers more often in their nests than were the controls. However, the underfed mothers were given their daily rations at 0930 hr, and it is not possible to determine if the altered pattern of nest occupation and absence was due to the actual nutritional state of mother and/or young, or to a shifting of circadian activity patterns in response to the time of feeding. Massaro et al. (1974) used time-lapse photograpy to observe mothers which were either maintained on a control diet or switched at parturition to a low-protein diet (12% casein; casein is approximately 87% protein). The photographs, taken during the dark phase of the light-dark cycle, revealed that low-protein mothers spent more time in the nesting area with the litter on Days 12, 17, 22 and 28 than did the control mothers. No differences were observed on Days 1 and 6.

Lynch (1976) rotated lactating and nonlactating (nipple-ligated) mothers between litters every 12 hr so that the pups were provided with a lactating mother during only half of the preweaning period. Control mothers were either rotated with other control mothers, or left undisturbed. Mothers and litters were observed in the home cage six times daily until weaning. In general, mothers (both nipple-ligated and lactating) exposed to malnourished pups spent more time in contact with the young than did mothers (both rotated and undisturbed controls) exposed to well-nourished offspring. Of particular interest, at each of the six times of day, lactating mothers rotated between malnourished pups spent more time in contact with pups than did lactating mothers rotated between well-nourished pups. This finding suggests that the increased contact time observed by Massaro et al. (1974) in malnourished mothers and litters is primarily a function of the pup's, rather than the mother's nutritional state. Wiener et al. (1977) found that mothers maintained on a low-protein diet from Day 14 of gestation were more often in contact with their young during unobtrusive observation periods in both the lights-on and lights-off phases of the light-dark cycle. These differences became apparent at about Day 3–4 and were maintained until observations were terminated at Day 12. Adrenalectomized mothers were found to show levels of contact with their malnourished young which were virtually identical to those of the low-protein group. These findings support the conclusion of Lynch that more contact is elicited by malnourished than by well-nourished pups.

This conclusion was further corroborated in a study (Robinson, unpublished) which employed both the litter-rotation and protein restriction techniques. Pups were malnourished by either administering the mother a low-protein diet (12% casein) beginning on Day 14 of gestation or by rotating the pups between well-fed lactating and nonlactating (nipple thelectomized) mothers. Control pups were either suckled by their own well-fed mother, or rotated between well-fed lactating females. Overall, mothers of malnourished pups spent more time in the nest area, more time nursing, and less time lying away from the pups during unobtrusive observations on Days 3–18 than did mothers nursing well-fed pups.

There is also evidence that time spent with the young may be influenced by the prenatal nutritional history of the pups. Massaro et al. (1977) fed mothers throughout gestation with either control or low-protein (7% casein) diets. At birth, all pups were fostered to well-fed mothers. Time-lapse photographs were taken of all litters during the dark phase of the light-dark cycle on every fourth postnatal day. The amount of time spent in the nest by the foster mothers of the two groups did not differ until Days 25 and 29, when more time was spent with the gestationally deprived, than with the gestationally nondeprived pups. The previously deprived young were also found to differ from control offspring in showing lower levels of climbing, rearing, and litter fragmentation during the later stages of lactation. The authors suggest that the differences in the mothers' behaviors may reflect a retarded development, in the gestationally deprived pups, of behaviors which facilitate weaning.

Laughlin et al. (1976) also found that the pups' prenatal nutritional history influenced the amount of time that the mother spent crouching over the young. During retrieval tests, prenatally malnourished pups elicited a different pattern of crouching from both well- and low-protein fed mothers than did well-fed pups. Overall, gestational malnutrition appeared to retard the developmental course of this behavior. Mothers of gestationally-well-nourished pups showed a peak of crouching at Day 7 and an appreciable decline by Day 10. The mothers of the gestationally-malnourished young showed their highest levels of crouching at Day 10 and a decline at Day 13. Thus, while many of the particulars of the Laughlin et al. (1976) and Massaro et al. (1977) studies differ, they agree in the finding that gestational malnutrition of the young affects the postnatal behavior of the mother in ways which tend to delay the waning of mother–infant contact.

The above studies show that pre- and postnatal malnutrition influence measures reflecting the amount of time the mother spends with the young. Wiener and Levine (unpublished) have found that the various activities that the mother engages in while with the young may be differentially affected by malnutrition, and further, that these activities may be differentially sensitive to other aspects of the early postnatal environment. These authors found the characteristic increase in time spent with the young in low-protein fed, as compared to control, mothers during both lights-on and lights-off observation periods. In addition, examination of active and passive nursing behaviors during the time spent with the young showed that low-protein mothers spent more time crouched over the litter in an active nursing posture than did well-nourished mothers during both lights-on and lights-off. Daily handling (4 hr prior to the lights-on observation period) altered the pattern of active nursing behavior similarly for both types of mothers. Handling decreased active nursing during lights-on and increased the amount of this activity during lights-off. However, a different pattern was observed for passive nursing. Unhandled control animals were found to display more passive nursing than unhandled low-protein mothers during the lights-on phase and no difference was observed during lights-off. In contrast, handling increased the amount of passive nursing received by low-protein, but not control young, during both observation periods. The increase in active nursing observed in malnourished litters appears to be a consequence primarily of the nutritional state of the young, since Thoman and Levine (1970) found adrenalectomized mothers to show a similar increase in the active, but not passive, nursing of their own malnourished pups. The results of Wiener and Levine show how easily small differences in experimental protocol might lead to conflicting conclusions in various laboratories. In labs where pups are handled daily (as they would be during daily weighing sessions) malnutrition may be found to produce quite different effects on maternal behavior than would be the case in labs where daily handling is not performed. Moreover, the effects of handling may also depend on the time at which the behavioral observations occur.

One general conclusion from the findings reviewed in this section thus far is that malnourished pups tend to elicit more maternal contact than do well-nourished pups, regardless of whether the malnutrition is imposed during gestation (Laughlin et al., 1976; Massaro et al., 1977), lactation (Lynch, 1976; Massaro et al., 1974; Robinson, unpublished), or both periods (Smart and Preece, 1973; Wiener et al., 1977; Robinson, unpublished; Wiener and

Levine, unpublished). One exception to this conclusion is reported by Fraňková (1974). She fed mothers a 5% protein diet beginning at birth and examined behaviors toward pups in a maze situation on Days 6 and 7 and in an open field on Days 21 and 28. On Days 6 and 7 low-protein mothers showed a lower frequency and shorter duration of contacts with their young than did controls. Malnourished mothers also approached their young less often on Day 21 and made fewer contacts with the pups on Days 21 and 28 than did controls. Further, negative responses toward pups (e.g., pushing pup away, attempting to escape) were more common in the malnourished group on both of the latter two test days. This study differed from others reported here not only in the direction of the effects of malnutrition, but also in testing conditions. Fraňková tested her animals in a novel apparatus, rather than in the home cage. Thus the discrepancy between her results and others reported in the literature might reflect differences between inadequately and well-nourished mothers in responsiveness to novel environments.

In summary, inadequately and well-nourished mothers have been found to differ in a number of pup-directed behaviors other than retrieval. Nutritionally-deprived mothers have been reported to lick their young less than do control mothers, and there is evidence that this deficit is due to a failure of the malnourished offspring to elicit maternal licking. However, on other measures, malnourished pups appear to be more potent elicitors of maternal care. In general, mothers of malnourished pups tend to spend more time in contact with their young than do mothers of well-fed pups. When nutritional deprivation is imposed during the prenatal period, the deprived pups tend to elicit high levels of maternal contact over a longer postnatal period than do nondeprived controls. The effects of malnutrition on the mother's behavior also appear to be modulated to some degree by other environmental factors such as whether the infants have been handled, the time at which observations occur, and perhaps the novelty of the testing situation.

NON-PUP-DIRECTED ACTIVITIES

Malnutrition has been found to affect a number of maternal behaviors which do not involve direct mother–pup interaction. Some of these behaviors (e.g. immobility in a novel testing apparatus, rearing, ambulation) may not, at first glance, appear relevant to a discussion of mother–infant relationships. But these behaviors may reflect changes in motivation (e.g., exploratory tendencies) or other internal states (e.g., emotional reactivity) which, in turn, may affect the quality of care the mother administers the litter.

One of the non-pup-directed behaviors which is affected by malnutrition, nest building, is obviously related to the care provided for the pups. Protein-deficient mothers have been found to build heavier nests than controls (Cowley and Griesel, 1964). Further, Wiener et al. (1977) found that perinatal malnutrition affected the speed of nest building. Following retrieval tests on Days 2–12, the old nest was removed and new nesting material presented to the mother. One hour later more control animals had built nests than had low-protein mothers. By 5 hours, the number of nests of low-protein and control mothers did not differ. This slower nest building by the malnourished mothers appears to be attributable to the nutritional condition of the mother rather than to that of the pup, since adrenalectomized mothers built nests as rapidly as did well-nourished controls.

Various authors have reported that inadequately-nourished mothers rear more than do controls. While not all investigators report this effect (Fraňková, 1974), increased rearing has been found in mothers which have been either underfed (Crnic, 1976; Smart, 1976; Smart and Preece, 1973) or protein malnourished (Massaro et al., 1974; Wiener and Levine, unpublished), in females deprived during either lactation (Massaro et al., 1974) or both gestation and lactation (Crnic, 1976; Smart, 1976; Smart and Preece, 1973; Wiener and Levine, unpublished), and in animals observed either unobtrusively in the home cage (Massaro et al., 1974; Wiener and Levine, unpublished), during retrieval tests in the home cage (Crnic, 1976; Smart and Preece, 1973), or in a separate test in a novel environment (Smart, 1976). Deprived mothers have been found to rear more than controls regardless of the nutritional condition of the pups with which they are tested (Crnic, 1976) and in the absence of pups (Smart, 1976), indicating that the effect is not due to differences in pup stimuli which elicit rearing, but rather to some more direct effect of poor nutrition on the mother's behavior.

The increased rearing probably reflects a tendency of malnourished animals to explore more than controls. Fraňková (1971) found low-protein mothers to score higher than their well-nourished counterparts on an overall exploratory measure which included rearing as one component. In another study, rearing was also found to correlate highly with sniffing, another exploratory measure (Crnic, 1976). Increased sniffing by deprived mothers has also been reported by Fraňková (1974). One explanation for these exploration effects would be that a poor diet increases the animal's food-seeking behaviors, and general exploration is one such behavior. A second, and not necessarily mutually exclusive, hypothesis would be that poor nutrition increases the animal's distractibility so that normally insignificant features of the environment begin to elicit active investigation. Poorly nourished mothers have also been found to differ from controls in ways which reflect increased emotional reactivity to the environment. Malnourished mothers have been reported to take longer to return to the nest from an elevated platform (Cowley and Griesel, 1964), to be more active in an open field on the first day of testing (high ambulation has been reported to indicate high emotionality on the first day of testing; Whimbey and Denenberg, 1967) and to freeze more during the second day of testing in a maze situation (Fraňková, 1974) than do controls.

The effect of malnutrition on self-grooming is less clear. Low-protein mothers have been found to spend more time self-grooming during the dark phase of the light-dark cycle (Massaro et al., 1974; Wiener and Levine, unpublished) than well-fed mothers. However, Wiener and Levine (unpublished) found that low-protein fed mothers self-groomed less than controls during the light phase of the light-dark cycle, suggesting that a low-protein diet alters the circadian pattern, rather than overall frequency of self-grooming. In contrast, Smart (1976) found underfed mothers to spend less time grooming than controls during tests in the dark phase of the cycle. Whether this finding is due to differential effects of underfeeding and protein deprivation on self-grooming, or to some other difference between the Smart (1976) and other investigations (Massaro et al., 1974; Wiener and Levine, unpublished) of self-grooming effects is unclear.

Feeding behaviors can also be affected by malnutrition. Massaro et al. (1974) observed that during the lights-off period low-protein mothers were fed more often than controls. No differences in drinking were found. In contrast, Wiener and Levine (unpublished) found that low-protein mothers ate as well as drank less often than controls during both lights-off and lights-on. Reasons for this discrepancy are not readily apparent. Laughlin et al. (1976) weighed the food containers of well-nourished and low-protein mothers to determine total amount of food eaten. The two preparations did not differ in food intake throughout gestation, even during the last week, when the dietary restriction was imposed (Fig. 3). During lactation, low-protein mothers ate less than controls, particularly during the final week, supporting the results of Wiener et al. (1977). In addition, it was found that mothers which were fostered gestationally malnourished pups ate less during lactation than did mothers which were fostered gestationally well-nourished pups, regardless of the mother's own nutritional condition. Thus, postpartum maternal food intake was influenced by the prenatal nutritional condition of the foster pup.

Overall, the findings reported in this section indicate that malnutrition affects many non-pup-directed behaviors. Malnourished mothers build heavier nests and are slower to rebuild the nest following a disturbance than are controls. Malnutrition has also been found to increase rearing and other apparent exploratory behaviors. Other behaviors which are affected suggest that malnourished mothers are more emotional than well-nourished controls.

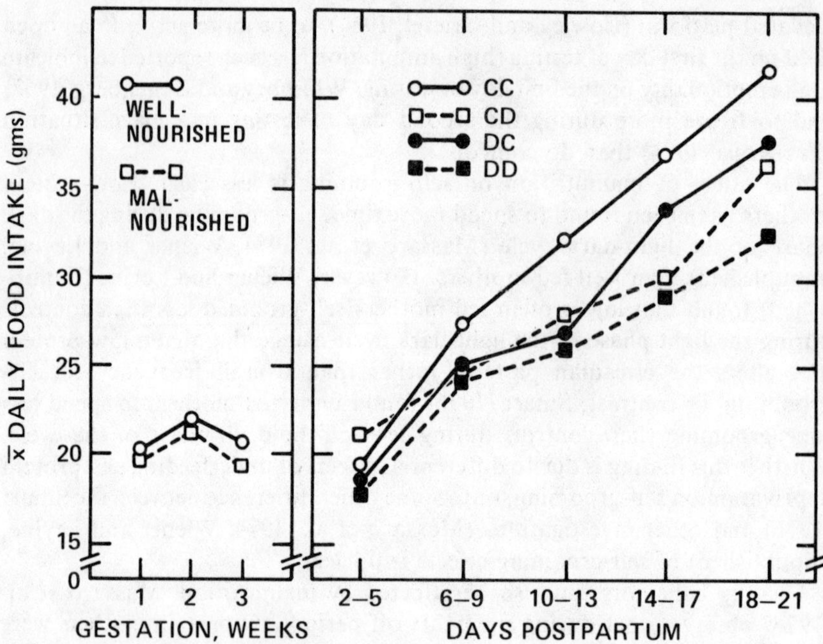

FIG. 3. Mean daily maternal food intake in grams. Left: amount eaten during gestation by well-nourished and malnourished females. Right: amount eaten during lactation. For each group, the first litter indicates the prenatal nutritional condition of the mother's foster pups; the second letter indicates the mother's own nutritional condition. C = well nourished, D = protein deprived (from Laughlin et al., 1976).

Changes in self-grooming and measures of eating and drinking have also been noted. The available evidence suggests that at least two of the behavioral changes, speed of nest building and amount of rearing, are primarily a result of the mother's own altered nutritional state, while postnatal maternal food intake can be influenced by the prenatal nutrition of the young.

Many of these findings might be parsimoniously accounted for by assuming that malnutrition increases the distractibility of the mother. Thus, normally insignificant aspects of the environment become more salient and elicit exploration. Substantial changes in the environment [e.g., placing the animal on an elevated platform (Cowley and Griesel, 1964); testing in a novel testing apparatus (Fraňková, 1974; Smart, 1976)] are likely to elicit emotional responses in malnourished animals. Following a somewhat milder disturbance (retrieval testing and nest removal), the distracted malnourished mother takes longer to build a new nest.

PUP-ASSOCIATED STIMULI

As reported above, several of the behavioral differences found between inadequately and well-nourished lactating rats appear to be a consequence primarily of the nutritional state of the pups rather than that of the mother. Malnourished pups have been found to elicit different amounts of licking (Smart, 1976), contact (Laughlin et al., 1976; Massaro et al., 1974; Wiener et al., 1977) and food intake (Laughlin et al., 1976) by the mother than do well-fed pups. Poorly and well-nourished pups clearly appear to differentially elicit various maternal activities. The stimulus properties of the pups which are responsible for these differences have not been delineated. However, there are a number of documented differences between well- and malnourished pups which could potentially elicit differential maternal behavior patterns. The two types of pups are different sizes and therefore afford different amounts of visual and tactual stimulation. In addition, the malnourished pup shows delayed development of other characteristics of physical growth (e.g., eye opening, incisor eruption and hair growth; Sykes and Cheyne, 1976), social development (Fraňková, 1973), reflex emergence (e.g., startle and righting reflexes; Sykes and Cheyne, 1976), and various locomotor activities (e.g., head lifting, rearing, climbing, grooming, and ambulation in the open field; Altman et al., 1971b; Massaro et al., 1974; Sykes and Cheyne, 1976). Thus same-aged well- and malnourished pups provide different stimulus constellations for the mother.

Nutritional deprivation might also alter the infant's odor or ultrasonic vocalizations, two cues known to influence maternal behavior in this species (Allin and Banks, 1972; Fleming and Rosenblatt, 1974a,b; Smotherman et al., 1974). Two studies of the effects of malnutrition on infantile ultrasounds are available. Hennessy et al. (1978) compared the rate of ultrasonic vocalizations of handled and shocked pups of normal, low protein-fed (8%) and adrenalectomized mothers. Pup malnutrition, whether imposed by maternal protein restriction or adrenalectomy, resulted in a retardation of normal vocalization development. Although the shape of the developmental curves was similar for all three preparations (Fig. 4), normal pups showed a peak rate of vocalizing on the 4th postpartum day, while malnourished pups did not reach their peak until Day 11. Thus malnutrition retarded this aspect of development by an entire week, or approximately one-fourth of the normal preweaning period.

In a second, similar study Hunt et al. (1976) found virtually no vocalizations in pups of low protein-fed (8%) mothers following either handling, shock, or cooling during the first two weeks postpartum. The discrepancy between the two studies is probably due to one of two procedural differences: an altered cage temperature during recording sessions, or the use

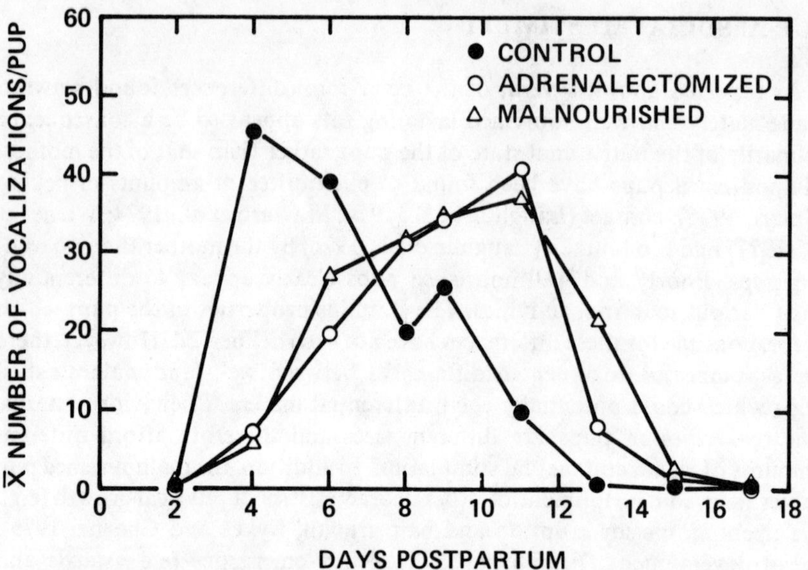

FIG. 4. Mean frequency of ultrasonic signals per pup following disturbance (handling or shock) during first 17 days postpartum. The pups' mothers had been either fed a control diet, adrenalectomized or malnourished. (Control > Adrenalectomized and Malnourished on Day 4; Adrenalectomized and Malnourished > Control on Day 11; from Hennessy et al., 1978).

of different recording equipment. The colder cage temperature employed by Hennessy et al. may have facilitated vocalizing in the malnourished group. Alternatively, since the equipment used by Hennessy et al. seemed to record signals of lower amplitude than that used by Hunt et al., the discrepant results might indicate that the growth-stunted malnourished animals signal less intensely than do well-fed pups.

Another approach taken in the study of the effects of malnutrition on pup stimuli has been to examine the capacity of pup cues to elicit a state of arousal or excitation in the mother, as measured by pituitary-adrenal activity. Wiener et al. (1976) tested mothers which either were fed an 8% protein diet from the 14th day of gestation or were well nourished. On postpartum Days 2, 9 and 16, mothers had their litters removed from the nest and were presented with a stimulus litter which was either well nourished or malnourished and which had been either handled or shocked. Litters were presented in wire baskets which prevented direct interaction between mother and pups. (See Mendoza et al. in this volume for a more complete description of methods and review of related literature.) Control pups were found to elicit a greater elevation of plasma levels of corticosterone than were malnourished pups from both control (Days 2, 9 and 16) and malnourished (Days 9 and 16) mothers.

Further, shocked control pups elicited a greater pituitary-adrenal response from both types of mothers than did handled control pups, while shocked and handled malnourished pups evoked equivalent corticoid elevations. Thus, as measured by pituitary-adrenal responsiveness, stimuli from pups whose mothers had been fed a low-protein diet were less arousing than were those from control pups. Following the more severe intervention (shocking), stimuli from the control pups were more arousing to the mother than were stimuli from controls receiving the less severe intervention (handling). In malnourished animals, stimuli following either type of intervention had equivalent effects on the mother.

In a second study (Hennessy et al., 1978), the stimulating properties of pups malnourished by maternal adrenalectomy were compared with those of controls. Shocked control pups were found to elicit a greater pituitary-adrenal response in control mothers than did handled control pups on Day 9, but not on Day 2. The opposite pattern was seen for adrenalectomized pups. In these animals, shocking produced greater plasma corticoid elevations in normal mothers than did handling on Day 2, but not on Day 9. Thus pup malnutrition, whether imposed by feeding the mother a low-protein diet or by removing her adrenals, alters the arousal-eliciting properties of pup stimuli, although the effects seen in the two malnutrition preparations also differ from each other.

In summary, the stimulating properties of malnourished and well-fed pups are known to differ in several respects. Compared to well-nourished controls malnourished pups are smaller, and show retardation of various physiological and anatomical features and aspects of psychomotor development, including ultrasonic signalling. The ultrasonic signals of well- and malnourished pups also probably differ in other ways (e.g., amplitude, responsiveness to cold). Undoubtedly additional parameters of the vocalizations as well as other modalities of stimulation, most notably olfaction, need to be examined before any comprehensive description of the effects of malnutrition on pup cues can be attained. However, the importance of pup cues in explaining malnutrition outcomes is evidenced by the different patterns of maternal pituitary-adrenal responsiveness and behavior, which are elicited by well- and malnourished pups.

CONCLUSIONS

As documented by the studies reviewed in this paper, the interactions between inadequately nourished mother rats and their litters differ in a number of respects from those occurring between well-nourished mothers and young. Several aspects of the malnourished mother's behavior appear to be deficient. These females are less efficient retrievers, lick their young less, are slower to rebuild the maternal nest following a disturbance, and in general seem to be more distractible and easily influenced by environmental perturbations, than are normal healthy mother rats. However, it would be inaccurate to characterize malnutrition effects as reflecting an overall impairment or suppression of maternal behavior. Rather, in some ways the poorly nourished mother appears superior to her well-nourished counterpart. Malnourished mothers typically spend more time in contact with their young and have been observed to actively nurse their litters more than do controls. Of course it would be premature to unequivocally label any change in maternal behavior as an impairment or improvement until the consequences, both short and long range, of that behavioral change have been thoroughly examined. At present it would seem best to bear in mind that maternal behavior is not a unitary concept, but is comprised of many diverse components. The end result of malnutrition on maternal behavior is to alter a number of these components in various ways.

Given that nutritional deficiencies can alter particular features of mother–young interactions, the question then becomes: How does malnutrition exert its effects? A first step toward an adequate answer might be to identify those behavioral differences which appear to be primarily the result of the mother's nutritional condition and those resulting primarily from the nutritional state of the young. As this review indicates, a number of researchers have successfully focused their attention on this problem. It would be an oversimplification, however, to stop the search for causative factors at this stage. At every point in lactation the mother's present condition is affected, to some degree, by her past experiences with her pups; and likewise, at every point beyond conception, the pup's present condition is influenced by its past experiences with its mother. To say that an effect is a "mother effect" is not to say that the pup contributes nothing to that effect. The pup may exert no direct influence at the time of investigation, but the importance of the pup's past interactions with its mother in shaping her present condition or behavior cannot be overlooked.

Another approach to identifying the causal agents in the effects of malnutrition on maternal behavior is to examine the developmental processes which are retarded by malnutrition. The mother–pup dyad has evolved to work in harmony. As the pup grows, its changing needs must be responded to appropriately by the mother. That is, there is a dynamic synchronous quality to mother–infant interactions throughout the preweaning period. The studies reviewed above indicate that malnutrition disrupts this synchrony by delaying or retarding various aspects of the pup's development. The malnourished infant grows more slowly than the healthy pup. The development of various physical features, reflexes, aspects of locomotion, and social behaviors, including ultrasonic vocalizations, are similarly delayed. We feel that this desynchronization of the normal mother-pup relationship may contribute substantially to the altered patterns of interactions observed in malnourished mothers and young.

ACKNOWLEDGMENTS

This study was supported by Research Grant NICH&HD-02881 from the National Institutes of Health to Seymour Levine who is supported by USPHS Research Scientist Award K5-MH-19936 from the National Institute of Mental Health. Michael Hennessy was supported by a postdoctoral training grant (MH-15147) from the National Institute of Mental Health. Nellie Laughlin was supported in part by the Palo Alto Veterans Administration Hospital.

REFERENCES

Allin, J. T. and Banks, E. M. Functional aspects of ultrasound production by infant albino rats, *Rattus norvegicus*. *Anim. Behav. 20,* 175–185 (1972).

Altman, J., Das, G. D., Sudarshan, K., and Anderson, W. J. The influence of nutrition on neural and behavioral development. II. Growth of body and brain in infant rats using different techniques of undernutrition. *Dev. Psychobiol. 4,* 55–70 (1971a).

Altman, J., Sudarshan, K., Das, G. D., McCormick, N., and Barnes, D. The influence of nutrition on neural and behavioral development. III. Development of some motor, particularly locomotor, patterns during infancy. *Dev. Psychobiol. 4,* 97–114 (1971b).

Barnes, R. H., Neely, C. S., Kwong, E., Labadan, B. A., and Fraňková, S. Postnatal nutritional deprivations as determinants of adult rat behavior toward food, its consumption and utilization. *J. Nutr. 96,* 467–476 (1968).

Beach, F. A. and Jaynes, J. Studies of maternal behavior in rats. III. Sensory cues involved in the lactating female's response to her young. *Behaviour 10,* 104–125 (1956).

Bell, R. W., Nitschke, W., Gorry, T. H., and Zachman, T. A. Infantile stimulation and ultrasonic signaling: A possible mediator of early handling phenomena. *Dev. Psychobiol. 4,* 181–191 (1971).

Chow, B. F. and Lee, C. J. Effect of dietary restriction of pregnant rats on body weight gain of the offspring. *J. Nutr. 82,* 10–18 (1964).

Cowie, A. T. The hormonal control of milk secretion. In *Milk: The Mammary Gland and its Secretions,* Vol. I, S. K. Kon and A. T. Cowie, eds. Academic Press, New York (1961), pp. 163–203.

Cowie, A. T. and Folley, S. J. Adrenalectomy and replacement therapy in lactating rats. 2. Effects of deoxycorticosterone acetate on lactation in adrenalectomized rats. *J. Endocrinology 5,* 14–23 (1947).

Cowley, J. J. and Griesel, R. D. Low protein diet and emotionality in the albino rat. *J. Gen. Psychol. 104,* 89–98 (1964).

Crnic, L. S. Maternal behavior in the undernourished rat (*Rattus norvegicus*). *Physiol. Behav. 16,* 677–680 (1976).

Denenberg, V. H., Rosenberg, K. M., Paschke, R., Hess, J. L., Zarrow, M. X., and Levine, S. Plasma corticosterone levels as a function of cross-species fostering and species differences. *Endocrinology 83,* 900–902 (1968).

Eayrs, J. T. and Horn, G. The development of cerebral cortex in hypothyroid and starved rats. *Anat. Rec. 121,* 53–61 (1955).

Fleming, A. S. and Rosenblatt, J. S. Olfactory regulation of maternal behavior in rats. I. Effects of olfactory bulb removal in experienced and inexperienced lactating and cycling females. *J. Comp. Physiol. Psychol. 86,* 221–232 (1974a).

Fleming, A. S. and Rosenblatt, J. S. Olfactory regulation of maternal behavior in rats. II. Effects of peripherally induced anosmia and lesions of the lateral olfactory tract in pup-induced virgins. *J. Comp. Physiol. Psychol. 86,* 233–246 (1974b).

Fraňková, S. Relationship between nutrition during lactation and maternal behaviour of rats. *Activ. Nerv. Sup. 13,* 1–18 (1971).

Fraňková, S. Effect of protein-caloric malnutrition on the development of social behavior in rats. *Dev. Psychobiol. 6,* 33–43 (1973).

Fraňková, S. Effects of protein deficiency in early life and during lactation on maternal behaviour. *Baroda J. Nutr. 1,* 21–28 (1974).

Galler, J. R. and Turkewitz, G. Variability of the effects of rearing in a large litter on the development of the rat. *Dev. Psychobiol. 8,* 325–331 (1975).

Grota, L. J. and Ader, R. Continuous recording of maternal behaviour in *Rattus norvegicus. Anim. Behav. 17,* 722–729 (1969).

Hall, W. G. Weaning and growth of artificially reared rats. *Science 190,* 1313–1315 (1975).

Harlow, H. F., Harlow, M. K., and Suomi, S. J. From thought to therapy. Lessons from a primate laboratory. *Amer. Sci. 59,* 538–549 (1971).

Hennessy, M. B., Harney, K. S., Smotherman, W. P., Coyle, S., and Levine, S. Adrenalectomy-induced deficits in maternal retrieval in the rat. *Horm. Behav. 9,* 222–227 (1977).

Hennessy, M. B., Smotherman, W. P., Kolp, L., Hunt, L., and Levine, S. Stimuli from pups of adrenalectomized and malnourished female rats. *Physiol. Behav. 20,* 509–513 (1978).

Hofer, M. A. The role of nutrition in the physiological and behavioral effects of early maternal separation on infant rats. *Psychosom. Med. 35,* 350–359 (1973).

Hunt, L. E., Smotherman, W. P., Wiener, S. G., and Levine, S. Nutritional variables and their effect on the development of ultrasonic vocalizations in rat pups. *Physiol. Behav. 17,* 1037–1039 (1976).

Kennedy, G. C. The development with age of hypothalamic restraint upon the appetite of the rat. *J. Endocrinology 16,* 9–17 (1957).

Laughlin, N. K., Favor, M. A., and Lints, C. E. Effects of perinatal malnutrition on maternal responsiveness in the rat. Paper presented at Annual Meeting of the Animal Behavior Society, Boulder, Colorado, June 20–25 (1976).

Lee, M. H. S. and Williams, D. I. Long-term changes in nest condition and pup grouping following handling of rat litters. *Dev. Psychobiol. 8,* 91–95 (1975).

Levine, S. and Thoman, E. B. Physiological and behavioral consequences of postnatal maternal stress in rats. *Physiol. Behav. 4,* 139–142 (1969).

Levine, S. and Wiener, S. Malnutrition and early environmental experience: possible interactive effects on later behavior. In *Environments as Therapy for Brain Dysfunction,* R. N. Walsh and W. T. Greenough, eds. Plenum Publishing Corp., New York (1976), pp. 51–70.

Lynch, A. Postnatal undernutrition: an alternative method. *Dev. Psychobiol. 9,* 39–48 (1976).

Massaro, T. F., Levitsky, D. A., and Barnes, R. H. Protein malnutrition in the rat: Its effects on maternal behavior and pup development. *Dev. Psychobiol. 7,* 551–561 (1974).

Massaro, T. F., Levitsky, D. A., and Barnes, R. H. Early protein malnutrition in the rat: Behavioral changes during rehabilitation. *Dev. Psychobiol. 10,* 105–111 (1977).

Messer, M., Thoman, E. B., Terrasa, A. G., and Dallman, P. R. Artificial feeding of infant rats by continuous gastric infusion. *J. Nutr. 98,* 404–410 (1969).

Miller, S. A. and Dymsza, H. A. Artificial feeding of neonatal rats. *Science 141,* 517–518 (1963).

Mueller, A. J. and Cox, W. M., Jr. The effect of changes in diet on the volume and composition of rat milk. *J. Nutr. 31,* 249–259 (1946).

Nicoll, C. S. and Meites, J. Prolongation of lactation in the rat by litter replacement. *Proc. Soc. Exp. Biol. Med. 101,* 81–82 (1959).

Plaut, S. M. Studies of undernutrition in the rat: Methodological considerations. *Dev. Psychobiol. 3,* 157–167 (1970).

Ressler, R. Genotype-correlated parental influences in two strains of mice. *J. Comp. Physiol. Psychol. 56,* 882–886 (1963).

Richards, M. P. M. Infantile handling in rodents: a reassessment in the light of recent studies of maternal behaviour. *Anim. Behav. 14,* 582 (1966).

Robinson, W. M. Effects of malnutrition and maternal responses on pup vocalizations, behavior, and brain development of malnourished and nutritionally rehabilitated rats. *Unpublished manuscript.*

Russell, P. A. "Infantile stimulation" in rodents: A consideration of possible mechanisms. *Psychol. Bull. 75,* 192–202 (1978).

Salas, M., Diaz, S., and Nieto, B. Effects of neonatal food deprivation on cortical spines and dendritic development of the rat. *Brain Res. 73,* 139–144 (1974).

Seitz, P. F. D. The effects of infantile experiences upon adult behavior in animal subjects: I. Effects of litter size during infancy upon adult behavior in the rat. *Am. J. Psychiat. 110,* 916–927 (1954).

Seitz, P. F. D. The maternal instinct in animal subjects: I. *Psychosom. Med. 20,* 215–226 (1958).

Simonson, M., Sherwin, R. W., Anilane, J. K., Yu, W. Y., and Chow, B. F. Neuromotor development in progeny of underfed mother rats. *J. Nutr. 98,* 18–24 (1969).

Slob, A. K., Snow, C. E., and de Natris-Mathot, E. Absence of behavioral deficits following neonatal undernutrition in the rat. *Dev. Psychobiol. 6,* 177–186 (1973).

Smart, J. L. Maternal behaviour of undernourished mother rats towards well fed and underfed young. *Physiol. Behav. 16,* 147–149 (1976).

Smart, J. L., and Dobbing, J. Vulnerability of developing brain. II. Effects of early nutritional deprivation on reflex ontogeny and development of behaviour in the rat. *Brain Res. 28,* 85–95 (1971a).

Smart, J. L. and Dobbing, J. Vulnerability of developing brain. VI. Relative effects of foetal and early postnatal undernutrition on reflex ontogeny and development of behaviour in the rat. *Brain Res. 33,* 303–314 (1971b).

Smart, J. L. and Preece, J. Maternal behaviour of undernourished mother rats. *Anim. Behav. 21,* 613–619 (1973).

Smotherman, W. P., Bell, R. W., Starzec, J., Elias, J., and Zachman, T. Maternal responses to infant vocalizations and olfactory cues in rats and mice. *Behav. Biol. 12,* 55–66 (1974).

Smotherman, W. P., Brown, C. P., and Levine, S. Maternal responsiveness following differential pup treatment and mother–pup interactions. *Horm. Behav. 8,* 242–253 (1977).

Stern, J. M. and Levin, R. Food availability as a determinant of the rat's circadian rhythm in maternal behavior. *Dev. Psychobiol. 9,* 137–148 (1976).

Sykes, S. E. and Cheyne, J. A. The effects of prenatal and postnatal protein malnutrition on physical and motor development in the rat. *Dev. Psychobiol. 9,* 285–296 (1976).

Thoman, E. B. and Levine, S. Role of maternal disturbance and temperature change in early experience studies. *Physiol. Behav. 4,* 143–145 (1969).

Thoman, E. B. and Levine, S. Hormonal and behavioral changes in the rat mother as a function of early experience treatments of the offspring. *Physiol. Behav. 5,* 1417–1421 (1970).

Venkatachalam, P. S. and Ramanathan, K. S. Effect of protein deficiency during gestation and lactation on body weight and composition of offspring. *J. Nutr. 84,* 38–42 (1964).

Whimbey, A. E. and Denenberg, V. H. Two independent behavioral dimensions in open-field performance. *J. Comp. Physiol. Psychol. 63,* 500–504 (1967).

Wiener, S. G., and Levine, S. Influences of early handling of rat pups on the maternal behavior of mothers receiving a low protein diet.Unpublished manuscript.

Wiener, S. G., Smotherman, W. P., and Levine, S. Influence of maternal malnutrition on pituitary-adrenal responsiveness to offspring. *Physiol. Behav. 17,* 897–901 (1976).

Wiener, S. G., Fitzpatrick, K. M., Levin, R., Smotherman, W. P., and Levine, S. Alterations in the maternal behavior of malnourished rats. *Dev. Psychobiol. 10,* 243–254 (1977).

Winick, M. and Noble, A. Cellular response in rats during malnutrition at various ages. *J. Nutr. 89,* 300–306 (1966).

Young, R. D. Influence of neonatal treatment on maternal behavior: a confounding variable. *Psychonom. Sci. 3,* 295–296 (1965).

Zamenhof, S., van Marthens, E., and Margolis, F. L. DNA (cell number) and protein in neonatal brain: alteration by maternal dietary protein restriction. *Science 160,* 322–323 (1968).

Maternal Influences and Early Behavior

10

Functional Consequences of Attachment: A Comparison of Two Species

Sally P. Mendoza
Christopher L. Coe
William P. Smotherman
Joel Kaplan
Seymour Levine

In mammals nurturance of young by the mother is a requisite for survival of the offspring. Mothers must therefore have the capacity to selectively respond to stimuli from the infant. However, responsiveness to infant-produced stimuli is not equivalent to attachment. Attachment presumes at least three additional criteria: (1) ability to recognize the object of attachment, (2) preference for the attachment figure, (3) response to removal of the object of attachment (Ainsworth, 1972). In order to understand the attachment process and perhaps the functions of attachment more clearly, a comparison will be made between a species in which attachment occurs (the squirrel monkey) and a species in which there is little evidence of attachment as we understand it (the rat).

Since mother–infant interactions are species-specific, it is often difficult to compare the behaviors between two species in a meaningful way. However, it is possible to contrast the nature of the mother–infant relationship in the rat with that of the squirrel monkey by assessing an equivalent physiological response following similar experimental manipulations. As previous work has suggested, the pituitary–adrenal system in both rats (Levine et al., 1972) and squirrel monkeys (Brown et al., 1970; Coe et al., 1978a) can be a sensitive indication of the organism's state of arousal. Therefore, emphasis in this paper will be placed on those studies which have utilized changes in corticoid levels to assess the response to manipulations of the mother–infant relationship.

RECOGNITION

Squirrel monkey infants have been shown to be capable of recognizing their mothers when given a choice between the mother and a familiar (Rosenblum, 1968) or unfamiliar (Kaplan and Schusterman, 1972) adult female. Squirrel monkey mothers also show a preference for their own infants over infants of a comparable stage of development (Rosenblum, 1968). As early as 4 weeks of age surrogate-reared infants have been shown to be capable of discriminating their own surrogate from a perceptually identical clean surrogate (Kaplan and Russell, 1974). Both squirrel monkey mothers and infants, then, are capable of recognizing their respective attachment figure, illustrated by the active preference shown when presented with a choice.

The evidence suggests that neither recognition nor preference plays a primary role in maternal behavior in the rat. Rat mothers indiscriminately retrieve and show maternal behavior to pups of any litter (Moltz, 1971). In addition, maternal behavior in rats can be indefinitely extended by continuously replacing older pups with pups from another litter but of a younger age (Rosenblatt, 1965). There are reports which indicate specificity of response of a given rat mother to her young in wild populations (Beach and Jaynes, 1956; King, 1939). However, if the maternal diet is held constant the specificity of response of mother to young as well as young to mother is no longer apparent (Leon, 1975). Thus it appears that rat mothers respond discriminately to their own odors rather than to other specific characteristics of their young.

RAT SEPARATION AND MATERNAL RESPONSIVENESS

Since mother rats do not specifically discriminate their own offspring, it was of interest to determine whether or not mother rats respond to separation from their infants. In the following experiment changes in the plasma levels of adrenal corticosteroids were used to evaluate the response of lactating rats to removal of their infants (Smotherman et al., 1977c). Mothers on Days 7 and 14 of lactation were removed from their home cages for a 2-minute period. During this time pups were either removed prior to the return of the mother (R Condition, the mother was returned to an empty cage) or the pups were left undisturbed and the mother was simply returned to her cage (C Condition), thus serving as a control for the disturbance of handling. The blood of the mothers was then sampled 15, 30, 60 or 180 minutes later.

Both mothers that were returned to an empty cage and those that were returned to their pups showed an initial elevation in steroids. However, the fact that there was no difference between groups R and C suggests that this elevation was due to the disturbance caused by removing the lactating female from her home cage. Separation from young did not result in an additional increment in plasma corticosteroid levels (see Fig. 1).

Infant rats do respond to brief periods of separation from the mother. However, if the infant is provided with compensatory stimuli (e.g. warmth and contact) normally provided by the mother, the separation response is eliminated (Hofer, 1975). When the infant is not provided compensation for maternal characteristics the infant shows an increased rate of ultrasonic vocalizations. Further increases in vocalization have been reported when the infant rat is handled, shocked or exposed to cold during separation. The more intense the stimuli that the infant is exposed to the more vigorous the vocalizations appear to be (Bell et al., 1974).

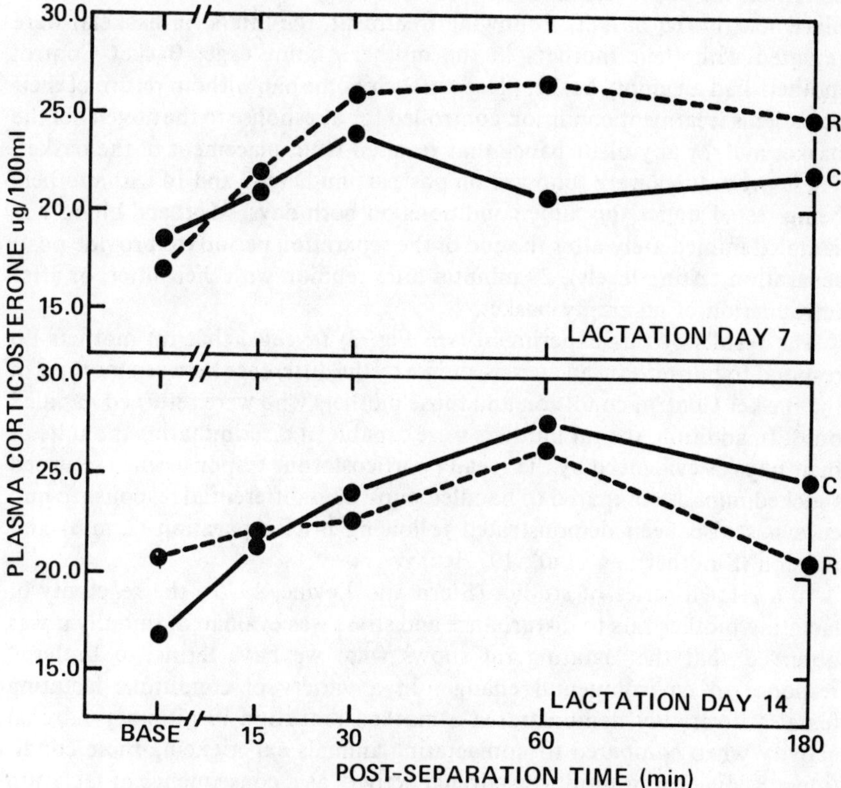

FIG. 1. Rat mothers' plasma corticosterone response to separation from her pups. Data are plotted separately for Litter Removal (R) and Disturbance Control (C) groups. Mothers were sampled after treatment on Days 7 and 14 of lactation.

In an extension of the separation experiment described above, differentially treated litters were returned to their mothers following a 3-hour separation. Prior to return pups were either shocked or handled. The pups were returned to their mother in a wire mesh basket in order to prevent direct mother–infant interaction, thus allowing a determination of whether or not rat mothers are capable of discriminating the stimulus quality of their pups. Mothers were assigned to one of three experimental groups, depending on treatment prior to blood sampling: return of Handled Pups, Shocked Pups or an empty basket (Basket Control). The blood of an additional group of mothers was sampled to determine corticosterone levels after the 3-hour period of separation.

In the Handled Pups condition the pups were removed from their home cage and placed into a circular wire mesh basket. In the Shocked Pups condition the pups were given 90 seconds of scrambled shock (.4 mA) before placement in the basket. Following treatment, the litters (in baskets) were reunited with their mothers in the mother's home cage. Basket Control mothers had an empty basket placed in their home pan without return of their litter. This treatment condition controlled for a response to the novelty of the basket and/or any disturbance that resulted from placement of the basket. These procedures were followed on postpartum Days 7 and 14 with mothers being tested under the same conditions on both days. Mothers' blood was sampled immediately after the end of the separation period (to provide post-separation resting levels), 20 minutes after reunion with their litter, or after introduction of an empty basket.

The results of this experiment (see Fig. 2) revealed that rat mothers do respond to pup-produced cues as shown by the difference between mothers in the Basket Control condition and those mothers who were returned handled pups. In addition, the rat mothers were capable of discriminating the state of their pups as evidenced by the greater corticosterone response when returned shocked pups as compared to handled pups. This differential response to pup cues has also been demonstrated following brief separation (2 min) and reunion (Smotherman et al., 1977b,c).

In a related series of studies (Stern and Levine, 1975), the reactivity of lactating mother rats to disturbance and stress was evaluated. Initially it was observed that the lactating rat shows what we have termed a buffered response to environmental change. In a variety of conditions lactating females invariably demonstrated a marked reduction in pituitary–adrenal activity when compared to nonlactating animals experiencing these conditions. Reduction in pituitary–adrenal activity as a consequence of lactation minimizes the physiological response to stress. Nonlactating females without previous experience with pups, however, do not respond to pup cues regardless of pup treatment (Smotherman et al., 1976). Thus, we have

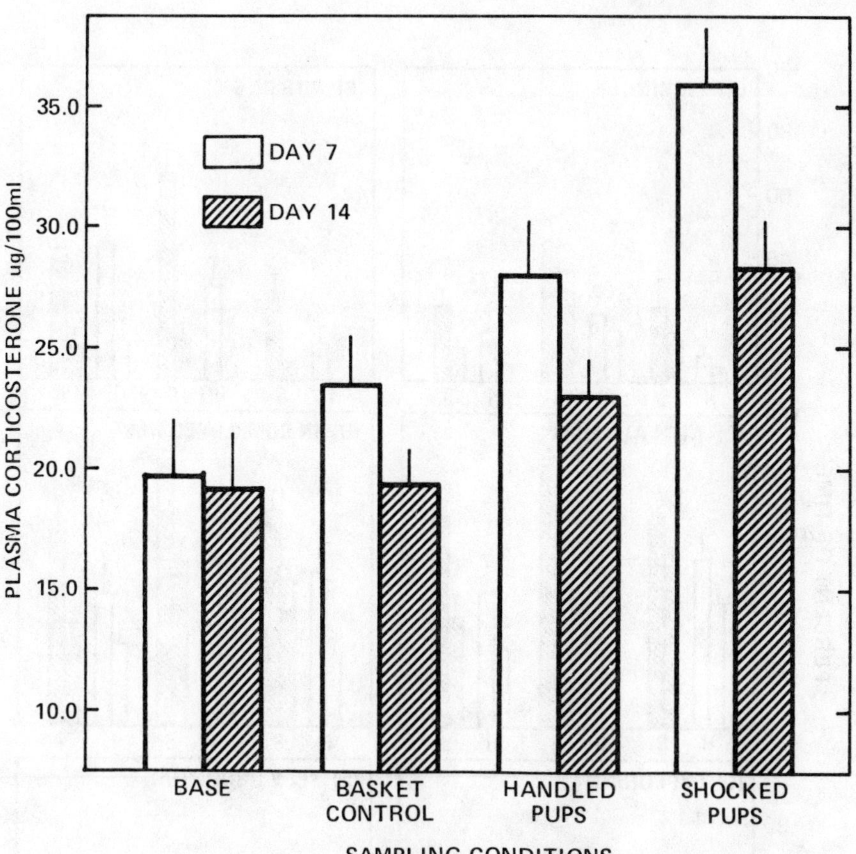

FIG. 2. Rat mothers' plasma levels of corticosterone after reunion with handled or shocked pups or an empty basket. Pups were returned after 3 hr of separation and mothers were sampled 20 min after the reunion. Entries are means (±S.E.M.).

demonstrated that the lactating rat, although hyposensitive to many aspects of her environment, is highly responsive to stimuli emitted by her pups.

When mothers and pups are permitted to interact directly following brief separation (2 min) and pup manipulation, the intensity of maternal behaviors is much greater when mothers are reunited with shocked pups than when reunited with handled pups (Smotherman et al., 1977a) (see Fig. 3). With direct interaction, however, the rat mother no longer shows a differential corticoid response to handled and shocked pups when her blood is sampled 20 minutes following reunion with her litter. The response to shocked pups is diminished when the mother is allowed to interact directly with her pups. However, the pituitary–adrenal response to handled pups does not change as

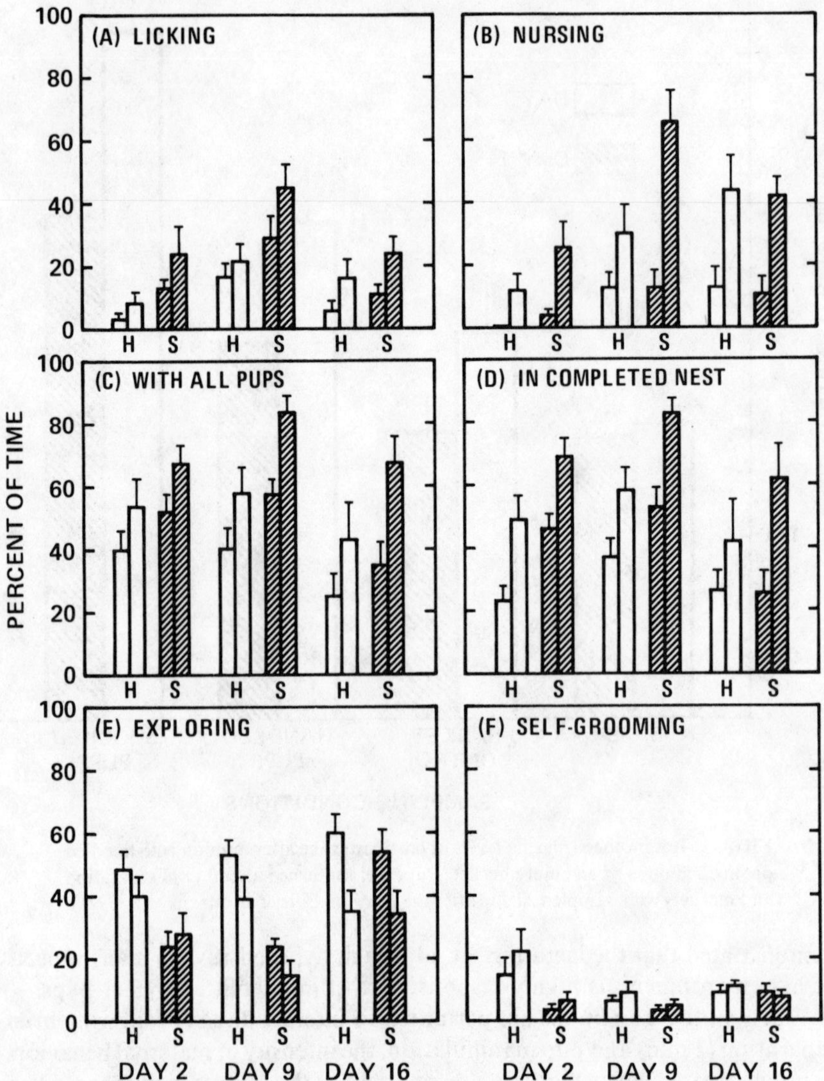

FIG. 3. Incidence of six maternal activities in the rat within the first and second 10-min observation periods following pup manipulation, plotted separately and sequentially, in handled (H) and shocked (S) pups. Standard errors are shown by vertical bars. Activities A, B, C and D indicate time spent attending to pups. Activities E and F indicate time spent in activities not directed to pups.

a function of mother–pup interaction. These data were interpreted as indicating that the buffering of the stress response noted earlier provides a condition whereby the mother filters out irrelevant stimuli which would normally be arousing. This permits her sensitivity to specific stimuli related to the pups. These stimuli now become more arousing and cause the mother to give greater attention to the offspring, particularly in a condition where the offspring are in distress.

SQUIRREL MONKEY SEPARATION AND RESPONSIVENESS

Although data comparable to those just presented on the rat are not available for the primates, there are sufficient behavioral data to indicate that squirrel monkeys do respond to stimuli from their infants. Although squirrel monkeys of all age/sex classes respond to separated infants as evidenced by approach and investigatory behaviors, it is only females, particularly preparturition females, who will actually retrieve separated infants (Rosenblum, 1972). Thus, just prior to giving birth squirrel monkeys show an accentuated sensitivity to infant stimuli. Rosenblum (1971) has reported that the response of late-term females can actually lead to the failure of infants to survive, as these females will "aunt" infants of other mothers and then prevent their return to the mother for feeding. It was particularly interesting in this study that females with infants of their own did not retrieve separated infants. Following parturition responsiveness narrows to the mother's own infant, and as previously mentioned, mother and infant squirrel monkeys can selectively recognize one another.

Following involuntary separation from its mother the infant squirrel monkey shows increased locomotion and vocalization as well as a reduction in object manipulation, activity play and social play (Jones and Clark, 1973). The squirrel monkey mother has also been shown to display increased vocalization and locomotion when separated from her infant (Kaplan, 1970). In order to make the data on separation and reunion in the squirrel monkey comparable with those of the rat, emphasis will be placed on studies of the pituitary–adrenal response in the monkey. The squirrel monkey has been shown to have extraordinarily high circulating levels of plasma corticoids (Brown et al., 1970). Preliminary studies in our laboratory have revealed, however, that the response characteristics of the adrenal are similar to other species although considerably magnified in terms of response capacity (Coe et al., 1978a).

In the following experiment (Mendoza et al., 1978) pituitary–adrenal response in mother and infant squirrel monkeys after brief separation was assessed. Each mother–infant pair was subjected to each of three experimental conditions: (1) Base sampling—mother and infant were removed from their home cage, separated, immediately anesthetized, and blood sampled; (2) Separation—mother and infant were removed from their cage, the mother returned to her cage, and the infant placed in an identical holding cage in a different room until 30 minutes following separation when mother and infant were anesthetized and their blood was sampled; (3) Separation-Reunion—mother and infant were removed, separated, immediately reunited and returned to their home cage; 30 minutes following this regimen the pair was again removed, anesthetized and blood samples were obtained. A similar paradigm was used to assess the response to separation and reunion in surrogate-reared infants. The mothers in this study were all wild-born squirrel monkeys imported from Columbia and Peru. The infants were 3 months of age at the beginning of the study. The infants raised on inanimate surrogates were placed with the surrogates at 1 week of age (Kaplan and Russell, 1973).

The results indicate that mothers, infants, and surrogate-reared infants respond to 30-minute separation with a substantial increase in plasma cortisol (see Fig. 4). The values obtained in the Separation-Reunion condition did not differ significantly from Basal values in any of the three groups, suggesting that the effect of separation on the pituitary–adrenal system is not due to the disturbance involved in the separation procedure. Furthermore, the adrenal responses of surrogate-reared infants following separation from their surrogates demonstrated that these infants develop attachments to the surrogate which are similar to those between normal infants and their own mothers.

In addition, this experiment indicated that the disturbance involved in removal, separation, and reunion is either not stressful or that contact between mother and infant as well as between infant and surrogate buffers the adrenal response to this disturbance. A second experiment (Mendoza et al., 1978) was designed to distinguish between these alternative hypotheses.

Seven nonlactating females were tested under each of two conditions: (1) Basal sample—subjects were removed from their cage, immediately anesthetized, and blood sampled; (2) Handling—subjects were removed briefly from their home cage and returned; 30 minutes later the females were again removed, anesthetized, and their blood was sampled.

The nonlactating females, unlike lactating females and infants, did show a significant elevation in plasma cortisol concentrations in response to the handling procedure (see Fig. 5). Thus, it appears that the resumption of contact between mother and infant ameliorates the response to the stress of capture and brief separation.

The mothers and infants in the previous study were housed as mother–infant pairs or infants housed individually with their surrogates. In a

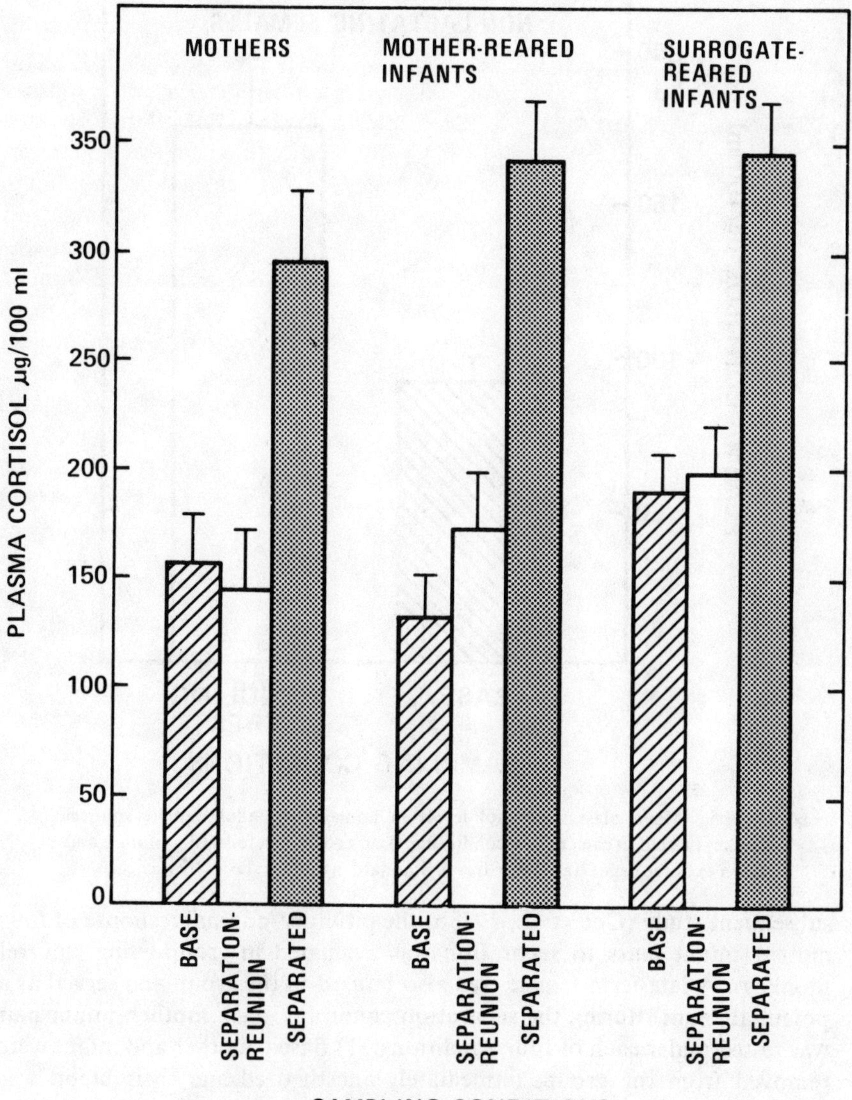

FIG. 4. Mean plasma cortisol levels in squirrel monkey mothers, mother-reared infants and surrogate-reared infants, in each of three conditions: Base; 30 min following brief separation and immediate reunion (Separation-Reunion); and 30 min following Separation. Standard errors are shown by vertical bars.

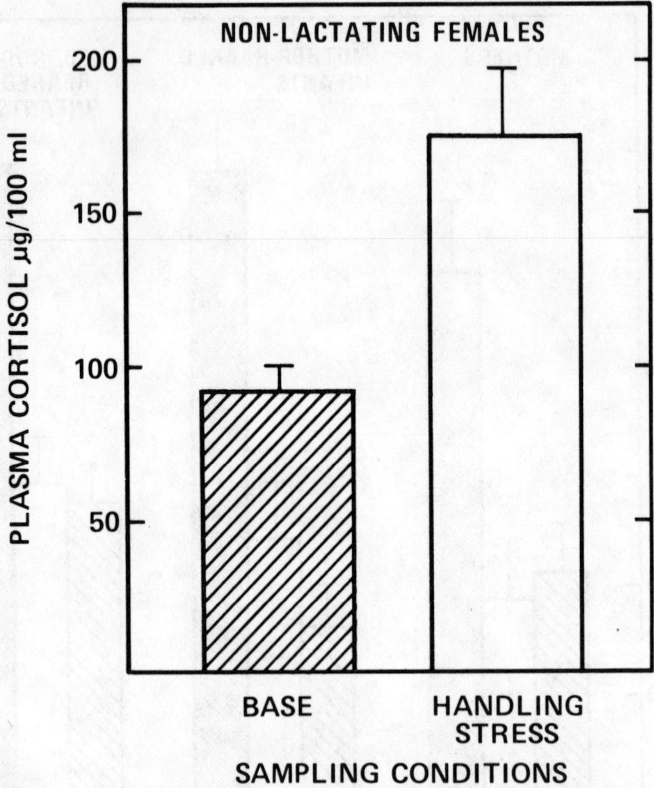

FIG. 5. Mean plasma cortisol levels in nonlactating adult female squirrel monkeys tested in each of two conditions: Base and 30 min following capture and return to home cage (Handling Stress). Standard errors are shown by vertical bars.

subsequent study (Coe et al., 1978b) the pituitary–adrenal response of four mother–infant pairs to separation was evaluated in group-living squirrel monkeys. A late-term female was also housed in the group and served as a potential "aunt" during the separation condition. Each mother–infant pair was tested under each of four conditions: (1) Base—mother and infant were removed from the group, immediately anesthetized and their blood was sampled; (2) Separation-Reunion—mother and infant were removed from the group, briefly separated, immediately reunited and then returned to the group. Thirty minutes following this procedure the pair was again removed from the group, anesthetized and blood samples obtained from each; (3) Infant-Removal—the mother–infant pair was caught, separated, and the mother returned to the group. The infant was housed individually in a holding cage. Thirty minutes later both mother and infant were caught, anesthetized and their blood was sampled; (4) Mother-Removal—same as condition #3 except the infant was returned to the group and the mother placed in a holding cage. The infants were approximately 10 weeks of age at the beginning of the study. The adults were wild-born squirrel monkeys of the Guyanese variety. In this experiment it was possible to evaluate the effects of the social group on both the mother and infant during separation. In addition, the effect of non-mother contact was evaluated since three of the four infants were "aunted" by the pregnant female (i.e., retrieved and carried on the back), consistent with the prior findings by Rosenblum (1972).

The results indicated that the levels of plasma cortisol were significantly elevated in both mothers and infants following separation and the response was not reduced by the presence of familiar animals. Again, separation followed by immediate reunion did not result in elevated values (see Fig. 6). These data indicate that a specific attachment relationship develops between mother and infant, and that the arousal induced by separation is reduced only by reunion with the object of attachment.

In the infant squirrel monkey we have demonstrated that, although the infant may be aunted during separation, the infant still remains highly aroused. In fact, the infant's adrenal response when in the group and aunted was indistinguishable from its response when removed from the group altogether. These data alter the interpretation by Rosenblum that aunting eliminates the effects of separation. Although aunting does tend to reduce the behavioral agitation which is observed in the separated infant, a state of high arousal as indicated by the activity of the pituitary–adrenal system is still apparent.

In another study we have evaluated further the effects of reunion with the attachment figure (Levine et al., 1978). The aim of the following experiment was to examine the manner in which reunion of mothers and infants influenced the high plasma cortisol levels already occurring after sustained separation. Seven mother–infant pairs, which were individually housed, were used in this experiment. The mothers were wild-born and the infants were approximately 3 months of age. The blood of each dyad was sampled at weekly intervals in each of three conditions: (1) Basal—immediately sampled after removal from their home cage, (2) Separation—both mother and infant were sampled after a 30-minute separation, and (3) Reunion—the dyads were sampled 30 minutes after reunion in their home cage following a 30-minute separation.

As can be seen in Figure 7, the 30-minute separation resulted in similar elevations in the levels of plasma cortisol in both mothers and infants. However, the responses of the mothers and infants differed significantly following reunion. The mothers' plasma cortisol levels rapidly returned to basal levels whereas the infants continued to show vigorous pituitary–adrenal

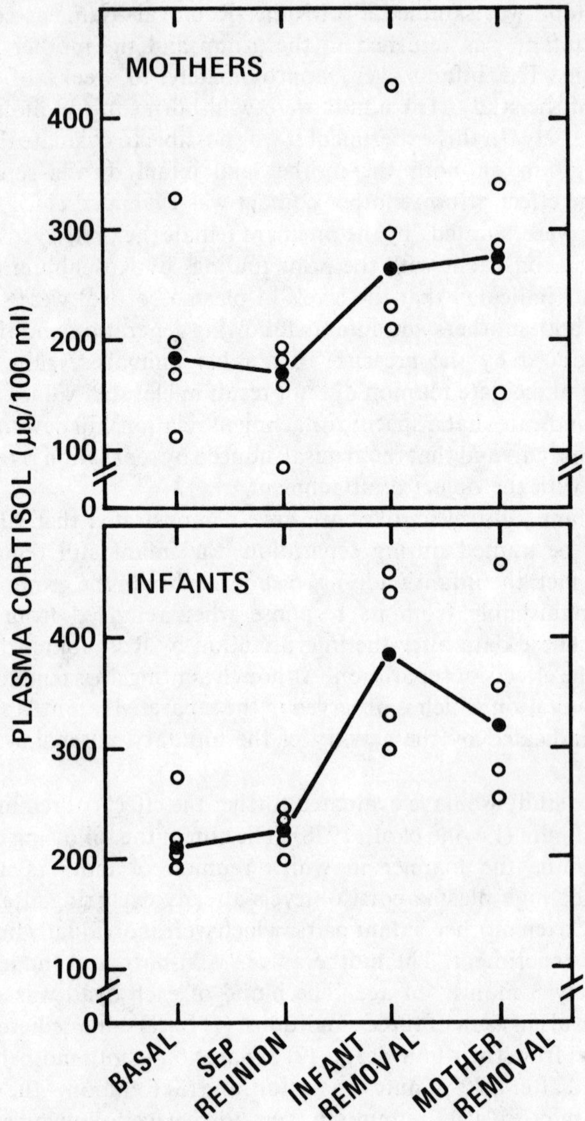

FIG. 6. Median (closed circles) and individual (open circles) levels of plasma cortisol for mother and infant squirrel monkeys sampled in each of four conditions: Basal; 30 min following brief separation and immediate reunion (Separation-Reunion); and 30-min following either Mother-Removal or Infant-Removal from the group.

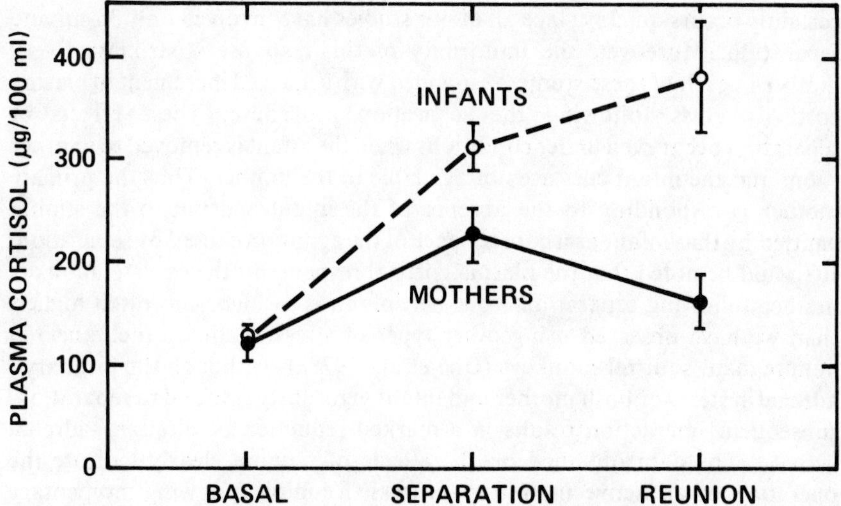

FIG. 7. Mean plasma cortisol levels in mother (closed circles) and infant (open circles) squirrel monkeys in each of three conditions: Basal; 30 min after mother-infant separation; and 30 min following Reunion after a brief (30 min) separation. Vertical bars represent standard errors.

activation. These latter data are open to several possible interpretations at this point. It is possible that the infant pituitary–adrenal system differs from that of the adult, in that the return to basal levels may take longer in the infant. In the rat, at least, the development of negative feedback requires a certain period of maturation (Goldman et al., 1973). However, an alternative hypothesis is more likely which may indicate an important aspect of mother–infant interaction. Resumption of contact between mother and infant may reduce arousal more rapidly in the mother since the mother's ability to provide adequate care could be impaired if she were to remain disturbed, while sustained arousal in the infant may serve to increase mother–infant interactions upon reunion.

CONCLUSIONS

Utilizing the data from these studies as a whole we can characterize the nature of mother–infant attachment in the squirrel monkey. The squirrel monkey mother shows a striking elevation in plasma cortisol following separation from her infant. This response occurs whether the mother is permitted to remain in her own cage, permitted to remain with her group, or removed from the group. Although a time course of when plasma cortisol elevates following infant removal has not been looked at, the response certainly occurs quickly since all of our studies have involved only 30-minute separation. Moreover, the uniformity of this response is striking. Every mother in each of these studies responded with a marked increment in plasma cortisol values following the separation procedure. These effects of separation occur even under conditions when the infant is removed to another room and the infant cues are not available to the mother. Thus the primate mother is responding to the absence of the infant and not to the stimuli emitted by that infant as a consequence of the agitation caused by separation. It should be noted that the plasma cortisol response of the squirrel monkey mother following separation from her infant, is as high, and often higher, than we have observed using other types of stressful stimuli (i.e. ether) in nonpregnant squirrel monkeys (Coe et al., 1978a). Although the pituitary–adrenal systems of both mother and infant vigorously respond to separation, subsequent interaction results in a marked reduction of pituitary–adrenal activity. The data obtained on the effects of reunion clearly indicate the operation of an active inhibitory process. Reunion following momentary separation inhibited the activation of the pituitary–adrenal systems in both mother and infant and reunion after a sustained separation was initially more effective in reducing the mother's elevated cortisol levels.

In the rat, however, separation from the pups did not cause a more significant elevation in plasma corticosteroids than has been observed when the mother was simply disturbed. Thus, there appears to be a striking difference between the squirrel monkey and the rat mother in that the primate mother clearly responds to the absence of her infant whereas the rat mother responds only when infants emit specific stimuli. The rat mother's response to pup-produced cues, however, is not specific to her own litter (Smotherman et al., 1977b). In the squirrel monkey, on the other hand, only nonlactating females appear to show a nondiscriminant response to infant cues (Rosenblum, 1972). The squirrel monkey mother's response is restricted to her own infant. Thus, the capacity to respond to separation on the part of the primate mother may be related to her ability to recognize her own infant.

Recognition of the object of attachment appears to be equally important in the infant's response to separation. The response to separation is not attenuated by familiar surroundings or the presence of an "aunt" for the infant squirrel monkey. Separation of surrogate-reared infants from their cloth "surrogate mother" also led to a similar response of the pituitary–adrenal system. We would expect that if one were to examine the physiological response of the infant when placed on a surrogate mother that was different from the one that it had become attached to, that this infant should also exhibit a plasma cortisol response.

Infant rats when separated from their mothers do show a response to separation as measured by increased ultrasonic vocalizations. This response appears to be a consequence of the physical events that occur with separation (e.g., reduction in body temperature, response to handling) rather than a response to removal of the mother per se. Thus in the rodent there does not appear to be a specific attachment process and the mother–infant interactions are based primarily on certain generalized cues emitted by the pup and the physiological state of the mother. In contrast, attachment is a very active process in the squirrel monkey and disruption of this attachment bond causes an active behavioral and physiological distress which is ameliorated only by the presence of the specific object of attachment. The results of these experiments indicate further that, in addition to the many roles attachment plays in the development of the primate offspring, yet another function can be ascribed to the attachment process. The availability of the mother–infant interaction appears to suppress or even eliminate the normally occurring hormonal response to environmental disturbances in both the mother and the infant.

Although the rat mother does not manifest a specific attachment to her offspring, she can respond differentially to distress stimuli emitted by the pups. The effect of mother–pup interaction was to eliminate the differential pituitary–adrenal responsiveness as a result of a reduction in the corticoid response to shocked pups. The response to handled pups remained the same, whether or not direct interaction was permitted. Thus, although the opportunity for interaction with pups does have some effect in reducing the rat mother's pituitary–adrenal response to shocked infants, it does not eliminate the response to either handled or shocked pups. This is in clear contrast to the data obtained with squirrel monkeys which indicated amelioration of the response to disturbance when mother and infant were immediately reunited. Similar findings have been reported in other primates. In surrogate-reared infant rhesus macaques the pituitary–adrenal response to novelty is markedly reduced when the infant's surrogate is present (Hill et al., 1973). Furthermore, in chimpanzee infants the response to electric shock as measured by the infant's vocalization is reduced when the infant is being held by the "caregiver" (Mason and Berkson, 1962).

Differences in the pituitary–adrenal responses of the rat and the squirrel monkey reflect distinctive aspects of the mother–infant interactions in each species. The rat mother did not respond specifically to the absence of her own litter but did react to the disturbance of her litter. Her pituitary–adrenal responses also indicated that she reacted differentially to distress signals from the pups. These data are in keeping with the fact that the rat is a nesting animal and must at times be away from its litter. In addition, the relatively asocial rat may not normally need to discriminate its young from other offspring. With regard to each of the stated criteria defining attachment, it appears as though the rat does not manifest attachment. However, the rat mother is clearly sensitive to the status of the pups and is able to show appropriate behaviors necessary for their maintenance. Our data support, therefore, the growing emphasis on the influence of infants on the regulation of maternal behavior. The distress signals emitted by the rat pups in our studies had a marked effect on the mother's plasma corticosteroid levels and appear to induce maternal behavior which in turn serves to reduce the pups' arousal.

The initial interactions between the primate mother and neonate are continuous and the infant plays an active role in the maintenance of the dyadic relationship. The maintenance of contact between the mother and infant monkey, for example, is largely dependent on the infant's clinging behavior. The formation of attachment in the infant nonhuman primate is presumably due to the self-reinforcing properties of such behaviors as clinging and suckling (Mason, 1971). Nonhuman primates can also develop an attachment for objects other than the mother, such as animate or inanimate surrogates, which allow the infant to cling appropriately (Harlow and Harlow, 1969; Mason and Kenney, 1974). The squirrel monkey infant has a responsive adrenal compared to the relatively inactive pituitary–adrenal system in the neonatal rat, and also reveals the high and labile levels of corticosteroids which occur normally in the adult (Brown et al., 1970). It is not surprising, therefore, that following disruption of the reflexive clinging behavior with its specific object of attachment, the infant reacts with a strong pituitary–adrenal response. Assessment of the corticoid levels following separation also indicated that the response was only ameliorated by the mother which supports previous statements that the manifestation of clinging behaviors leads to specific emotional dependence (i.e., attachment) in the primate. In most primates both the mother and infant manifest a selective preference which may be related to the fact that monkeys typically have single births and that there are several other mother–infant pairs present in the social group.

Assessment of the pituitary–adrenal responses in the squirrel monkey mothers revealed that they also responded vigorously to separation from their infants and the plasma cortisol levels were reduced only by reunion of the mother and infant. Reunion not only inhibited the pituitary–adrenal activation in the mother after brief capture and separation but also resulted in decreased levels of plasma cortisol after sustained separation. Thus, it would appear that the alteration of the mother's arousal by the infant may be an effective mechanism for inducing the attachment processes in the mother. Previous discussions have focused primarily on the role of arousal reduction in facilitating the infant's attachment (Mason, 1971). Our data would suggest that the modulation of arousal is one of the specific mechanisms through which attachment develops in both mother and infant primates.

ACKNOWLEDGMENTS

This research was supported by Biological Sciences Training Grant MH8304 from the National Institute of Mental Health to Sally Mendoza, Christopher Coe and William P. Smotherman (WPS was also supported by the C. A. Aaron Endowment Fund); NICH&HD02881 from the National Institutes of Health and MH23645 from the National Institute of Mental Health to Seymour Levine. Joel Kaplan is supported by Grant HD04905 from the National Institutes of Health. Seymour Levine is supported by USPHS Research Scientist Award K5-MH-19936 from the National Institute of Mental Health.

REFERENCES

Ainsworth, M. D. S. Attachment and dependency: A comparison. In *Attachment and Dependency,* J. L. Gewirtz, ed. V. H. Winston & Sons, Washington, D.C. (1972), pp. 97–137.

Beach, F. A. and Jaynes, J. Studies on maternal retrieving in rats. I. Recognition of young. *J. Mammology 37,* 177–180 (1956).

Bell, R. W., Nitschke, W., Bell, N. J., and Zachman, T. A. Early experience, ultrasonic vocalizations, and maternal responsiveness in rats. *Dev. Psychobiol. 7,* 235–242 (1974).

Brown, G. M., Grota, L. J., Penney, D. P., and Reichlin, S. Pituitary–adrenal function in the squirrel monkey. *Endocrinology 86,* 519–529 (1970).

Coe, C. L., Mendoza, S. P., Daividson, J. M., Smith, E. R., Dallman, M. F., and Levine, S. Hormonal response to stress in the squirrel monkey. *(Saimiri sciureus). Neuroendocrinology 26,* 367–377 (1978a).

Coe, C. L., Mendoza, S. P., Smotherman, W. P., and Levine, S. Mother–infant attachment in the squirrel monkey: Adrenal response to separation. *Behav. Biol., 22,* 256–263.

Goldman, L., Winget, C., Hollingshead, G. W., and Levine, S. Postweaning development of negative feedback in the pituitary–adrenal system of the rat. *Neuroendocrinology 12,* 199–211 (1973).

Harlow, H. F. and Harlow, M. K. Effects of various mother–infant relationships on rhesus monkey behaviors. In *Determinants of Infant Behaviour,* Vol. IV. B. M. Foss, ed. Methuen, London (1969), pp. 15–36.

Hill, S. D., McCormack, S. A., and Mason, W. A. Effects of artificial mothers and visual experience on adrenal responsiveness of infant monkeys. *Dev. Psychobiol. 6,* 421–429 (1973).

Hofer, M. A. Infant separation responses and the maternal role. *Biol. Psychiat. 10,* 149–153 (1975).

Jones, B. C. and Clark, D. L. Mother–infant separation in squirrel monkeys living in a group. *Dev. Psychobiol. 6,* 259–269 (1973).

Kaplan, J. The effects of separation and reunion on the behavior of mother and infant squirrel monkeys. *Dev. Psychobiol. 3,* 43–52 (1970).

Kaplan, J. and Russell, M. A surrogate for rearing infant squirrel monkeys. *Behav. Res. Meth. Instru. 5,* 379–380 (1973).

Kaplan, J. and Russell, M. Olfactory recognition in the infant squirrel monkey. *Dev. Psychobiol. 7,* 15–19 (1974).

Kaplan, J. and Schusterman, R. J. Social preferences of mother and infant squirrel monkeys following different rearing experiences. *Dev. Psychobiol. 5,* 53–59 (1972).

King, H. D. Life processes in gray Norway rats during fourteen years in captivity. *Am. Anat. Mem. 17,* 1–72 (1939).

Leon, M. Dietary control of maternal pheromone in the lactating rat. *Physiol. Behav. 14,* 311–319 (1975).

Levine, S., Coe, C. L., Smotherman, W. P., and Kaplan, J. Prolonged cortisol elevation in the infant squirrel monkey after reunion with mother. *Physiol. Behav. 20,* 7–10 (1978).

Levine, S., Goldman, L., and Coover, G. D. Expectancy and the pituitary–adrenal system. In *Physiology, Emotion and Psychosomatic Illness,* R. Porter and J. Knight, eds. Ciba Foundation Symposium 8, Elsevier, Amsterdam (1972), pp. 281–296.

Mason, W. A. Motivational factors in psychosocial development. In *Nebraska Symposium on Motivation, 1970,* W. J. Arnold and M. M. Page, eds. Univ. of Nebraska Press, Lincoln (1971), pp. 35–67.

Mason, W. A. and Berkson, G. Conditions influencing vocal responsiveness of infant chimpanzees. *Science 137,* 127–128 (1962).

Mason, W. A. and Kenney, M. D. Redirection of filial attachments in rhesus monkeys: Dogs as mother surrogates. *Science 183,* 1209–1211 (1974).

Mendoza, S. P., Smotherman, W. P., Miner, M. T., Kaplan, J., and Levine, S. Pituitary–adrenal response to separation in mother and infant squirrel monkeys. *Dev. Psychobiol., 11,* 169–175 (1978).

Moltz, H. The ontogeny of maternal behavior in some selected mammalian species. In *The Ontogeny of Vertebrate Behavior,* H. Moltz, ed. Academic Press, New York (1971), pp. 263–313.

Rosenblatt, J. S. The basis of synchrony in the behavioral interaction between the mother and her offspring in the laboratory rat. In *Determinants of Infant Behavior III,* B. M. Foss, ed. Methuen, London (1965), pp. 3–45.

Rosenblum, L. A. Mother–infant relations and early behavioral development in the squirrel monkey. In *The Squirrel Monkey,* L. Rosenblum and R. W. Cooper, eds. Academic Press, New York (1968), pp. 207–234.

Rosenblum, L. A. Infant attachment in monkeys. In *The Origins of Human Social Relations,* R. Schaffer, ed. Academic Press, New York (1971), pp. 85–113.

Rosenblum, L. A. Sex and age differences in response to infant squirrel monkeys. *Brain, Behav. Evol. 5,* 30–40 (1972).

Smotherman, W. P., Wiener, S. G., Mendoza, S. P., and Levine, S. Pituitary–adrenal responsiveness of rat mothers to noxious stimuli and stimuli produced by rat pups. In *Breast-Feeding and the Mother,* K. Elliott and D. W. Fitzsimons, eds. Ciba Foundation Symposium 45, Elsevier, Amsterdam (1976), pp. 5–25.

Smotherman, W. P., Brown, C. P., and Levine, S. Maternal responsiveness following differential pup treatment and mother–pup interactions. *Horm. Behav. 8,* 242–253 (1977a).

Smotherman, W. P., Mendoza, S. P., and Levine, S. Ontogenetic changes in pup-elicited maternal pituitary–adrenal activity: pup age and stage of lactation effects. *Dev. Psychobiol. 10,* 365–371 (1977b).

Smotherman, W. P., Wiener, S. G., Mendoza, S. P., and Levine, S. Maternal pituitary–adrenal responsiveness as a function of differential treatment of rat pups. *Dev. Psychobiol. 10,* 113–122 (1977c).

Stern, J. M. and Levine, S. Neuroendocrine changes during lactation in rats. *Mod. Prob. Paediatr. 15,* 106–116 (1975).

Maternal Influences and Early Behavior

11 Early Perceptual Experience and the Development of Social Preferences in Squirrel Monkeys

Joel N. Kaplan
Daniel D. Cubicciotti III

A growing body of evidence suggests that the infant primate, both nonhuman and human, is capable of processing a great deal more information about its environment within the first few days and weeks of life than was originally believed possible. Although all of the sensory systems continue to develop for some time after birth, they all seem to be responsive to environmental stimuli at birth. With regard to some modalities, young infants are capable of making acute discriminations in response to rather subtle changes in the characteristics of a sensory stimulus (Carpenter, 1974; Fantz, 1967; Johnson and Salisbury, 1975; Kaplan, 1977; Lipsitt, 1967; Macfarlane, 1975). There has not been any attempt to order the different sensory modalities in terms of their roles in perceptual development, but systems that contribute most to infant survival would be expected to be most developed and functional in the neonatal period. For example, the newborn primate is extremely sensitive to tactile stimulation, particularly around the region of the mouth. Compared to human babies, infant monkeys are probably more sensitive and responsive to tactile stimulation in general since their survival depends largely on their maintaining a firm hold of their mother as she goes about her daily activities and adjusting their posture as necessary on the mother's body to nurse. Unlike human mothers, monkey mothers provide little direct assistance to their infants in routine caretaking functions.

Olfaction and taste, which are integrally related to nursing activity, and hence to survival, might also be expected to be highly developed modalities in the neonate, and recent evidence—at least regarding the olfactory sense—certainly seems to support this view. Both human and monkey infants are capable of making rather fine discriminations between familiar and unfamiliar odors within the first few weeks of life (Kaplan, 1977; Macfarlane, 1975). Although no comparable data have been presented for gustatory stimuli, anecdotal reports indicate that human infants may be sensitive to taste changes in about the first 24 hours of life (cited by discussant in Macfarlane, 1975).

Changes in neonatal responsiveness to visual and auditory information have of course been examined more comprehensively than that of the other modalities because of the presumed dominance of these senses in primates. Recent studies indicate that as early as 2 weeks of age, human infants can differentiate their mother's face and voice from those of a strange adult female (Carpenter, 1974). Similarly, by 1 month of age, infant squirrel monkeys can identify their mother on the basis of sight alone when she is displayed adjacent to a stranger behind a one-way glass partition (Redican and Kaplan, 1978).

Although our understanding of the perceptual abilities of infant primates is being enhanced considerably by ongoing research from various laboratories, there has not been any concerted effort to determine the extent to which perceptual experiences of early life are capable of influencing socially directed behaviors at later stages of maturation. Yet such experiences would seem to play an important part in this process. For example, it is not uncommon to see humans choose mates whose physical appearance resembles that of their own parents. Moreover, some psychoanalytically oriented writers have suggested that psychosexual development in humans is influenced by odors experienced in infancy, as is the case in certain lower mammals. For example, after neonatal exposure to specific synthetic odors—typically applied to the mother, to the litter, or to both—guinea pig, mouse and rat offspring have been found subsequently to prefer the rearing odor or animals bearing that odor to other synthetic odors or animals bearing natural odors (Carter, 1972; Marr and Gardner, 1965; Marr and Lilliston, 1969; Porter and Etscorn, 1976).

The research presented here covers studies conducted in our laboratory over the last several years with the small South American squirrel monkey (*Saimiri sciureus*) and is concerned primarily with the effects of visual and olfactory experiences during the first year of life on the development of filial and subsequent peer preferences. The infant monkeys used in this research are from our own breeding colony, which contains three different varieties of squirrel monkeys that can be distinguished both on the basis of their physical appearance and on differences in chromosomal patterns (Jones and Ma, 1975; Dukelow et al., 1977). Figure 1 shows photographs of 1-year-old males of the three varieties, which are commonly referred to as Bolivian, Colombian, and Peruvian squirrel monkeys, based on the geographical regions of South America in which they are predominantly found. Primary

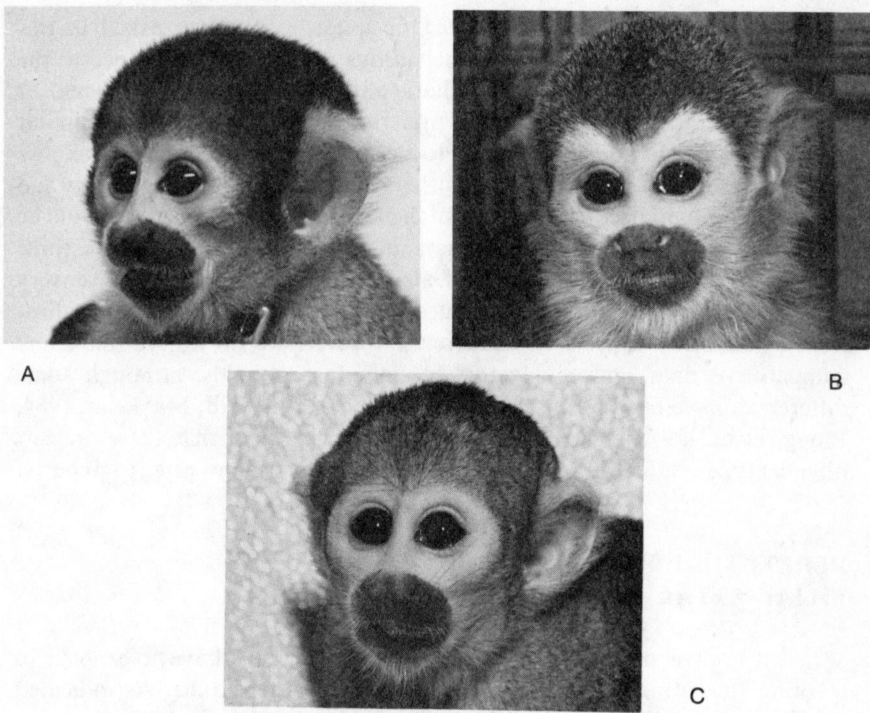

FIG. 1. Facial views of three varieties of squirrel monkeys: a) Bolivian, b) Colombian, and c) Peruvian.

distinguishing features in appearance among the three types involve their pelage coloration and the shape of the hairline around the eyes. The coats of Bolivian animals tend to be more purely yellow or orangeish than either of the other two types and the crowns of their heads are almost invariably jet black. By contrast, the head coloration of immature Colombian and Peruvian animals is a mixture of olive-green, silver-gray, and black, with Colombians appearing to have more silver-gray hairs and Peruvians more olive-green hairs. Although Peruvian females develop dark black "sideburns" as they mature, which in some cases approximates the head coloration of Bolivians, the two types can usually still be distinguished by overall body color. The shape of the hairline above the eyes of both Bolivians and Peruvians is flat and can easily be distinguished from the high peaked arch that is typical among Colombians.

The availability of these three varieties of squirrel monkeys, which—except for certain physical characteristics—appear to be remarkably similar, has helped us in our experiments dealing with the influence of specific perceptual experiences on social development. One question we have asked in this research, which will be discussed later in this present chapter, concerns the influence of particular perceptual characteristics associated with a real or surrogate mother on subsequent preferences for peers having similar attributes. One method we have used to measure this effect has been to expose young monkeys predominantly to mothers and peers of their own variety and to test their preferences for strangers of their own and other types. It should be noted that in addition to differences in physical appearance, the three varieties of squirrel monkeys could also differ in terms of other sensory characteristics (e.g., odors), communication patterns (e.g., gestures, vocalizations), and other aspects of behavior. However, we do not yet have any comparative data on such factors in immature animals, although some differences have been found in adults (Kaplan, et al., 1978; MacLean, 1964; Ploog, et al., 1975). Our general impression has been that there are few obvious type-related differences concerning these variables prior to puberty.

PERCEPTUAL PROPERTIES OF FILIAL ATTACHMENT

Infant squirrel monkeys, like other primates, generally have no problem in learning to distinguish their own mother from other adults. As indicated above, the modalities involved in accomplishing this are likely to change in importance as the infant matures. For example, it is clear that information pertaining to tactile and kinesthetic cues is acquired quite early in life, whereas details regarding the mother's visual appearance are not learned until later. This can be seen quite dramatically when an infant who is only a few days old is removed from its own mother and placed on an inanimate surrogate mother. Although infants of this age routinely maneuver about their mother's body in order to locate a nipple for suckling without any direct maternal assistance, this behavior is completely disrupted when the infant is transferred to such a surrogate, even under conditions where the dimensions of the surrogate's body and location of the nipple are similar to those of a real mother (Kaplan and Russell, 1973). Infants treated in this manner must be trained to learn how to obtain nourishment by themselves, which may take several days (Kaplan, 1974). It seems likely, therefore, that the inability of infants to make such adjustments without outside intervention is based to some extent on their ability to detect a change in the tactile and kinesthetic environment associated with the maternal figure.

The infant's ability to recognize a change in its "maternal" environment can even be observed immediately on its being placed on a surrogate after removal from its natural mother. Although an inanimate cloth-covered surrogate eventually becomes a source of attachment and comfort to the infant, the infant displays clear signs of disturbance on its initial introduction to its new "mother." Distressful vocalizations are typically emitted for an hour or more, and the infant usually refuses to stay on the surrogate until it becomes thoroughly exhausted. By the following day, however, the infant is clinging tenaciously to its surrogate mother and appears undisturbed by its new contingencies for survival. In fact, removal of the infant from the surrogate within a day or two after this initial adjustment period produces the same magnitude of disturbance found earlier on separation from the natural mother.

In addition to the apparently sophisticated detection of, and response to, tactile and kinesthetic cues early in life, infant primates also appear to be quite sensitive to the olfactory characteristics of their rearing environment, particularly those associated with the primary caretaker. For example, human neonates that are breast-fed are able to distinguish their mother's breast pad from a clean pad within the first week of life and can discriminate their own mother's pad from a different mother's by approximately 10 days of age (Macfarlane, 1975). Similar experiments on odor recognition with infant squirrel monkeys gave analogous results. Although the youngest age at which we have formally tested infant monkeys on their response to odors associated with the rearing figure has been 2 weeks, preliminary observations on even younger infants have suggested that they respond to such olfactory cues within the first few days of life.

In the first experiment to be described, 16 infants were taken from their mothers at one week of age and placed on cloth-covered surrogates. One week later they were tested under three conditions designed to assess the strength and specificity of their reactions to the accumulated odor on the surrogate. In one condition, the infant's own soiled cover remained on the surrogate; in another condition, a freshly laundered (i.e., clean) cover was substituted for the infant's own soiled cover; in a third condition, a soiled cover belonging to another like-aged infant was substituted for the infant's own soiled cover. Each condition was presented twice in separate 10-minute trials spaced a few days apart. All three conditions were tested on the same day, with a minimum of two hours between tests, and the order in which the conditions were presented was counterbalanced between infants. The procedure for all conditions consisted of removing the infant from its surrogate, placing it on the cage floor while the appropriate cover substitution was made, and then repositioning the infant on the surrogate for observation. Response measures included latency to get off of the surrogate (in seconds), duration of shrill vocalizations, and duration of sniffing the surrogate.

The results of these tests demonstrated that the infants unequivocally distinguished their own odorous cover from both the clean cover and the agemate's cover. In the own-cover condition, the infants spent virtually the entire test period clinging to or resting on their surrogates, and they rarely vocalized or sniffed the surrogate. In contrast, in both the clean-cover and agemate's-cover conditions, a significant proportion of the infants got off of the surrogate before the end of the 10-minute observation period, and levels of shrill vocalizations and sniffing the surrogate were clearly elevated (Figure 2). For all three measures, differences between the own-cover and clean-cover conditions and between the own-cover and agemate's-cover conditions were statistically significant (p's $< .01$, Wilcoxon), but differences between the clean-cover and agemate's-cover conditions were not. The results thus clearly indicate that by 2 weeks of age the infant squirrel monkey is capable of distinguishing its own surrogate from other surrogates on the basis of highly

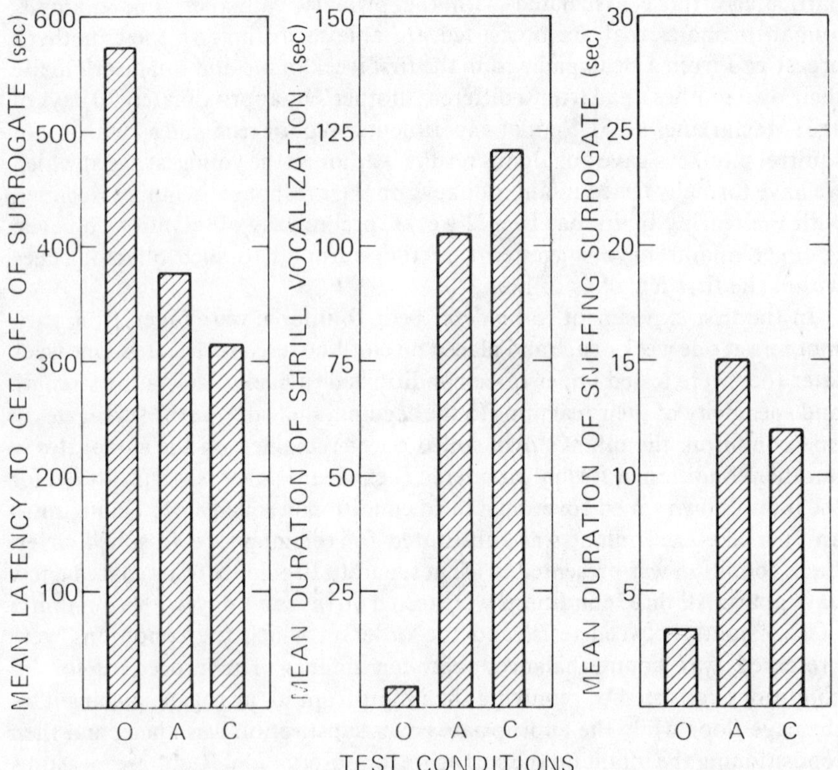

FIG. 2. Reactions of 2-week-old squirrel monkeys to olfactory attributes of the rearing surrogate. Infants were observed with three different cloth covers placed on the surrogate: *O*, their own soiled cover; *A*, an agemate's soiled cover; and, *C* a clean cover.

specific olfactory cues and that any departure from the familiar odor produces powerful tendencies for the infant to avoid the surrogate and exhibit emotional distress.

Such behavior based on olfactory cues is quite different from that observed in response to changes in the color of the surrogate's cover. When this visual dimension is manipulated so that infants are raised on a single-colored surrogate for the first six months of life and tested at monthly intervals on their preference for different-colored surrogates, surrogates of the rearing color are not preferred until about 3 months of age (Kaplan and Russell, 1974; Kaplan, 1977). In contrast, preferences for surrogates that contain the infants' own odors are present at 2 weeks of age and persist at the same high levels for several months.

This does not mean that other visual qualities either less static or more inherently attractive than color would not produce preferences at an earlier age. In fact, a recent study in our laboratory has shown that mother-reared infant squirrel monkeys as young as 1 month of age can indeed discriminate their own mothers from other mothers by sight alone (Redican and Kaplan, 1978). In that study, infants were given the opportunity to view both their own mother and another infant's mother in compartments next to each other but separated by an opaque partition. The mothers were located behind one-way glass in a sound-attenuated chamber so that they could neither see nor be heard by their infants. Under these test conditions, infants spent significantly more time directly in front of their own mother than in front of the other mother; also they contacted that section of the glass barrier both more frequently and for a longer duration than the section in front of the other mother.

The ineffectiveness of static as opposed to animate visual cues in eliciting recognition of the "maternal" figure by infants can also be found in another of our experiments in which infants were tested in the presence of their own and other anesthetized mothers (Kaplan et al., 1977). The significance of odors associated with the mother was also investigated in the same experiment so that a comparison could be made with the previously described studies that utilized inanimate surrogates and that measured the infants' responses to only their own deposited odors.

In this experiment, infants ranging in age from 8 to 24 weeks were given a choice between their own anesthetized mother and an anesthetized mother of an agemate under four conditions that systematically varied the olfactory and visual characteristics of the mothers. Both mothers could be directly contacted by the infants and were presented at opposite ends of an enclosure 120 cm long. (1) In the *Null* condition, designed to eliminate both olfactory and distinctive visual cues, mothers were washed with unscented soap and dried with warm air from a hair dryer, and their heads were covered with cloth hoods. (2) In the *Visual* condition, designed to eliminate olfactory cues and maximize visual cues, mothers were washed but were not covered with hoods. (3) In the *Olfactory* condition, designed to leave olfactory cues intact and minimize visual cues, mothers were unwashed and covered with hoods. (4) Finally, in the *Olfactory-and-Visual* condition, mothers were neither washed nor hooded. In all conditions, a circumscribed area around the nipples of each stimulus female was shave and covered with a strip of adhesive tape to prevent infants from suckling and possibly discriminating on the basis of nonolfactory cues associated with nursing. Each condition was presented in a series of six 1-minute trials in which the locations of the two mothers were alternated randomly. An interval of approximately three days elapsed between conditions, and the order in which they were presented was counterbalanced across infants. The primary dependent variables were duration of proximity and contact with each female.

The results of this experiment showed that infants of all ages clearly discriminated their own mother from the alien mother by means of olfactory cues but not by means of static visual cues, which consisted of the expressionless faces and immobile bodies of the anesthetized animals. Infants spent the most time in proximity to and in contact with their own mother in the two conditions in which olfactory cues were available (Olfactory and Olfactory-plus-Visual conditions). In contrast, in the Null and Visual conditions, the infants spent approximately equal amounts of time near their own and alien mothers, indicating that inanimate visual cues alone provided insufficient information for them to distinguish their own mother from the alien mother. These findings are clearly consistent with the results obtained on surrogate-reared infants and provide further evidence of the significance of olfactory cues in filial recognition of the maternal figure. In addition, they indicate that such recognition is not limited merely to self-deposited odors (as in the case of surrogate-reared infants), but is more broadly related to the overall complex of odors associated with the rearing figure, to which mothers and infants both contribute.

In all of the research described thus far, olfactory stimuli have consisted of odors produced by the animals themselves. To what extent such odors are prepotent in influencing preferences based on early olfactory experience has been studied in additional experiments by measuring responsiveness to arbitrary synthetic odors applied to both surrogate and real mothers (Kaplan et al., 1979; Redican and Kaplan, 1978). Because of the relative simplicity of manipulating and maintaining control over the olfactory environment, this technique permits us to directly compare the relative importance of olfactory and visual stimuli (e.g., by holding one or the other of the two modalities constant while manipulating the other).

In these experiments, synthetic clove (eugenol) and floral (geraniol) fragrances were applied on a regular basis to the surrogate covers of separate groups of infants reared on surrogates and to the natural mothers of infants reared with their own mothers. Although the test procedures differed somewhat for the surrogate-reared and mother-reared infants in these two separate studies, the results in both cases clearly showed that the clove and floral synthetic agents were much less effective than natural odors in eliciting preferential responding. Infants did not start to respond positively to the synthetic odors until about 4 months of age even though they had experienced the odors from approximately the first week of life. This contrasts markedly to the responsiveness displayed toward natural odors associated with the rearing object. As mentioned above, infants recognize and differentiate natural odors by as early as 2 weeks of age. Whether other synthetic odors, particularly those that contained chemical compounds found in natural secretions, might be more attractive would require further investigation.

The results of the synthetic odor experiment with surrogates were also interesting in other respects. In this experiment, each of the artificial odors was also associated with a surrogate cover of a particular color—green in the case of the floral fragrance and black in the case of the clove fragrance. The infants from both groups were tested monthly for 6 months in three different conditions that presented a choice between two surrogates situated next to each other and differing in color, odor, or both.

Although there was no *a priori* reason to expect differences between the two rearing groups, they clearly differed in their responses to both the odors and colors of the surrogates. Infants reared on green/floral surrogates (N=6) displayed somewhat stronger and earlier preferences for their rearing odor than those in the black/clove group (N=6), whereas the latter showed the reverse effect for color. Specifically, infants in the green/floral group reliably identified surrogates scented with the rearing odor by Months 4–6, and in some cases as early as Month 3, but infants in the black/clove group showed no clear-cut recognition of their rearing odor throughout the entire 6-month test period. In contrast, the black/clove infants developed an exceptionally strong preference for the rearing color, which was clearly evident as early as Month 2, but the green/floral infants responded only minimally to their rearing color.

Although more than one interpretation of these results is possible, we believe that the eugenol solution, used as the clove fragrance, reduced the infants sensitivity to olfactory stimuli, which in turn produced a heightened attraction to the surrogate's color. This conclusion is supported by information that we obtained after the experiment was completed indicating that eugenol has mild topical anesthetic properties and is often used by dentists for such purposes. Furthermore, the difference in responsiveness to color cues found in infants reared with black/clove or green/floral surrogates cannot be explained in terms of greater attractiveness of the black color per se since we have previously found no difference in preference scores for naturally scented black and green surrogates.

DEVELOPMENT OF PREFERENCE FOR PEERS

Under normal circumstances, the strong bond between an infant nonhuman primate and its mother is gradually replaced by close affiliations with peers. These alliances are largely influenced by prior association with particular individuals and can generally be seen in the greater attraction to and positive social interaction between familiar—as opposed to unfamiliar—peers (Hansen, 1966; Rosenblum and Lowe, 1971). Familiarity with a given individual is not the sole determinant of social preference, however, and other less obvious factors, such as the type of rearing or mere physical appearance of an individual, may also play a role in social attraction. For example, juvenile rhesus monkeys raised for the first 18 months of life under widely differing conditions of social contact have been found to prefer like-reared peers even in the absence of previous social experience with them (Pratt and Sackett, 1967).

In our laboratory we have attempted to assess the relative contributions of perceptual and social experiences to the development of social preference. To begin with, we asked whether mother-reared juveniles who had contact with only animals of their own subtype would prefer such animals to those of another subtype. As mentioned earlier, one distinguishing characteristic of the different subtypes of *Saimiri* has to do with their visual appearance, and on this basis alone it might be expected that animals would develop a preference for their own type. Although little is known about behavioral differences among the different subtypes, particularly with respect to immature animals, if such differences did exist they could also serve as a basis for subtype preferences in much the same way as physical appearance. For example, there might be type-specific facial expressions or vocalizations that elicit unlearned approach responses in like-type animals, as has been hypothesized to explain the finding that infant rhesus monkeys raised in the absence of all adults, including their mother, show a preference for adult females of their own species over those of other macaque species (Sackett, 1970). Clearly, then, if a general preference for own type was found in squirrel monkeys who had been reared with animals of that type, it would be impossible to determine the exact cause of such preference. Nevertheless, such information would provide a foundation on which to design additional experiments that would specify the source of the effect in greater detail.

To determine whether young squirrel monkeys do in fact prefer peers of their subtype, we compared social attractions to unfamiliar peers of like- and opposite-subtypes. Furthermore, to provide some indication of the strength of this effect relative to a determinant of social attraction that has already been established as important, the same experiment also compared attractions to a like-subtype familiar peer vs. a like-subtype stranger. Ten immature Bolivian and 10 immature Colombian animals served as subjects. All of the monkeys were housed with their biological mothers for approximately seven months; they were then housed in like-subtype pairs for approximately eight weeks.

The test apparatus was a 30 × 40 × 120 cm straight enclosed alleyway made of wood framing and wire mesh. A small Plexiglas-fronted cage containing either the cagemate, a like-subtype, or an opposite-subtype stranger was abutted against one end of the apparatus and an identical empty cage was abutted against the opposite end. All stimulus animals were within 1 month of age of the subject. A single runway traversed the entire length of the alleyway and was divided into five sections numbered from 0, nearest the empty cage, to 4, nearest the stimulus animal. A quantitative measure of the subject's attraction to the stimulus, an approach score, was obtained by noting its numbered location on the runway during 25 consecutive 12-second intervals in a 5-minute test. The minimum score obtainable by this method was zero (the subject remaining near the empty cage throughout the test), and the maximum score obtainable was 100 (the subject continuously remaining in close proximity to the agemate). Each stimulus condition was presented for three 5-minute trials, occurring on separate days, and the order of presentation was counterbalanced across days.

The results of this experiment showed that Bolivian and Colombian infants both displayed highest attraction to the cagemate, intermediate attraction to the same-subtype stranger, and lowest attraction to the opposite-subtype stranger (Figure 3). Differences in approach scores toward these three stimulus animals were statistically significant for each subtype considered separately, as well as for the combined subtypes (p's $< .01$, Friedman). Further comparisons showed that the mean approach score toward the same-subtype stranger was significantly higher than toward the opposite-subtype stranger and significantly lower than toward the cagemate (p's $< .01$, Wilcoxon). Thus, although cagemates were clearly preferred to strangers, strangers of the same-subtype were clearly preferred to those of the opposite subtype.

Preference Based on Visual Experience

Although the subtype preferences found in the preceding experiment could not be attributed to a single factor, it seems likely that such preferences develop largely as a consequence of the particular perceptual attributes of the

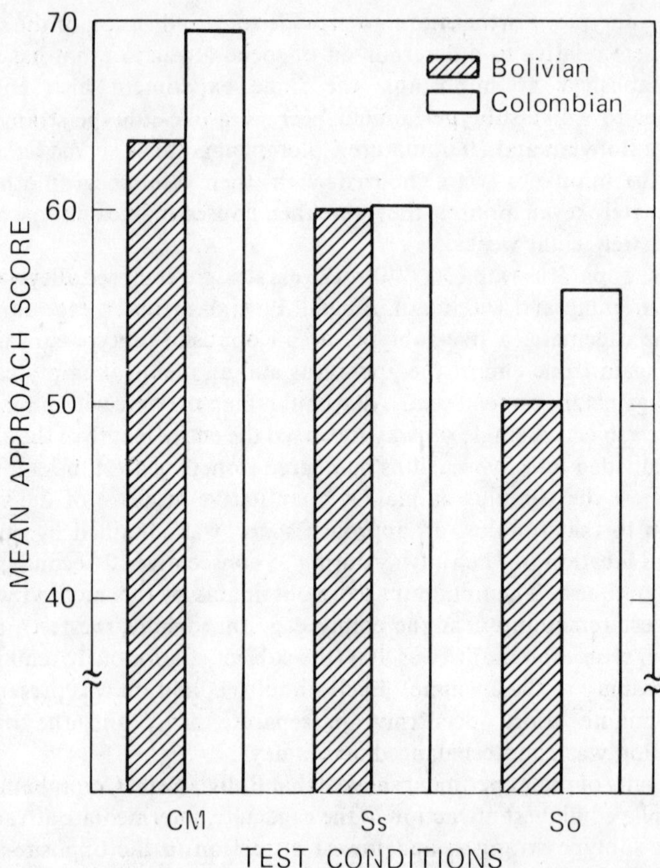

FIG. 3. Attraction of juvenile Bolivian and Colombian squirrel monkeys to peers varying in familiarity and subtype (*CM*, cagemate; *Ss*, stranger of same subtype; *So*, stranger of opposite subtype).

infant's first object of attachment. According to this hypothesis, the infant develops a "perceptual schema" of its principal rearing figure and this "schema" continues to influence the animal's attraction to different available social partners for some time thereafter. As an initial test of this hypothesis, it occurred to us that the infants that had been reared in our laboratory with colored surrogates offered a unique opportunity to investigate the effect of one conspicuous "maternal" attribute, color, on subsequent social attractions.

As discussed earlier, infants reared with distinctively colored surrogates generally develop a specific preference for a surrogate of the rearing color by 3 or 4 months of age. To determine whether such differentiation of the maternal figure as an object having specific color characteristics might persist beyond the sphere of filial attachment and influence the infant's subsequent preferences for particular agemates as well, we conducted a two-phase experiment that assessed the infant's attractions to peers clothed with either surrogate-colored or alien-colored cloth jackets. In Phase I of the experiment, infants were tested prior to weaning, while they were still housed with their colored surrogates. In Phase II, the same infants were tested after they had been weaned from their surrogates and housed for approximately two months with agemates wearing jackets of the rearing color.

The infants used in this study were the same 12 who had been raised on green and black surrogates containing synthetic odors. In addition, 12 like-aged mother-reared infants that had had no previous experience with the experimental rearing colors were tested in the same conditions. It was anticipated that in contrast to the surrogate-reared infants, the mother-reared group would show no differential attraction to peers on the basis of their colored jackets. Both groups of infants consisted of Peruvian and Colombian animals. In order to limit the extent to which visual cues other than the colors of the jackets could influence preferential responding, the subtype of the stimulus animal was randomized in both phases of the experiment, and no attempt was made to segregate the two subtypes when peers were housed together during Phase II.

Phase I: Social Attractions Prior to Weaning

The first phase of the experiment, prior to weaning, began when the infants were approximately 7 months old. Three different conditions presented a same-sex, unfamiliar agemate wearing either a green jacket, a black jacket, or no jacket. Each infant received three trials in each condition over a 3-week period, and the same unfamiliar agemate was used as the stimulus for a given subject in all three conditions. The test apparatus and scoring procedures were identical to those used in the previous experiment on subtype preferences.

Although we expected that the surrogate-reared infants would show higher approach scores toward peers wearing jackets of the rearing color than to those clad in the alien color, the results of this phase of the experiment indicated that neither surrogate- nor mother-reared animals differentiated the various jacket conditions. The mean approach score for the surrogate-reared infants over all conditions was 41.4 and varied less than 2 points (5%) between conditions. The comparable mean for the mother-reared infants was 49.9 and likewise did not vary significantly as a function of the jacket conditions. Although the mean approach score was somewhat higher for the mother-reared infants than for the surrogate-reared infants, the difference between groups was not statistically significant, suggesting that surrogate-rearing per se produced no substantial reduction in attraction to social stimuli in this situation.

Phase II: Social Attractions Following Peer-Group Formation

The above results were somewhat discouraging in that a highly discrete visual cue that was a salient part of the early rearing environment did not appear to influence the infant's attraction to a social stimulus that bore some resemblance to that cue. It is conceivable, however, that the lack of the anticipated effect was due largely to the fact that the familiar-colored jacket differed substantially in size and contour from the surrogate figure and was encountered in a very novel context (on a live and unfamiliar animal). Therefore, to reduce some of these elements of novelty, we decided to expose both surrogate- and mother-reared animals to jacket-clad cagemates for a period of time and then determine whether such additional exposure to the familiar color would reveal an increased sensitivity or attraction to it. Thus, following the completion of Phase I, all of the infants were weaned from their surrogate or real mothers and outfitted with green or black jackets. The 24 infants were then housed in eight visually isolated groups of three identically clothed peers. In the case of surrogate-reared infants, the jacket color corresponded to the color of the surrogates on which they had been reared. Surrogate-reared and mother-reared infants were intermixed and cagemates were of the same sex. To allow infants to form stable social relationships, the groups were left undisturbed (except to exchange soiled jackets for clean ones) for eight weeks prior to testing. The average age of infants at the end of this period was approximately 9 months.

Each infant was tested in six conditions. As in phase I, three conditions presented a same-sex unfamiliar peer outfitted with either a familiar-colored jacket, an alien-colored jacket, or no jacket. Three additional conditions presented a familiar cagemate with the same changes of jackets. Each subject received two 5-minute trials in each condition over a 4-week period, using the same apparatus and test procedures that were used in Phase I.

The results of Phase II showed that although surrogate-reared and mother-reared infants both differentiated cagemates from unfamiliar peers, only surrogate-reared infants distinguished the stimulus animals on the basis of the jacket colors (Figure 4). Consider first the results for the surrogate-reared group. This group showed the strongest attraction to a cagemate presented with the familiar-colored jacket and relatively weaker attractions when the

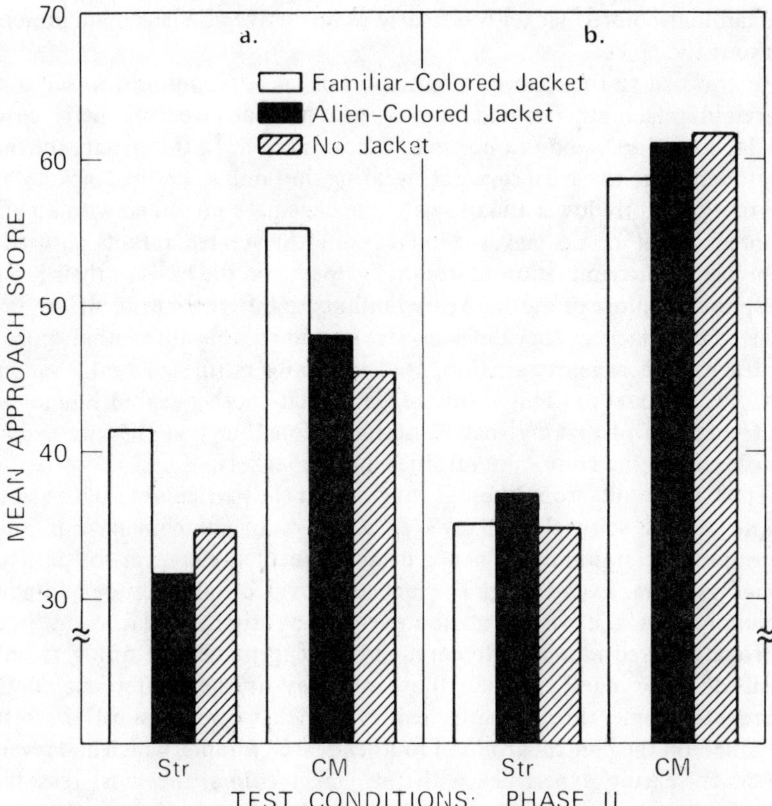

FIG. 4. Jacket experiment, Phase II: Attraction of a) surrogate- and b) mother-reared juveniles to familiar (CM) and unfamiliar (Str) peers wearing either a familiar-colored jacket, an alien-colored jacket, or no jacket. For eight weeks prior to testing, both groups of monkeys were housed with cagemates clothed with like-colored jackets. In the case of surrogate-reared monkeys, the jacket color corresponded to the original rearing color. Mother-reared monkeys had no experience with the jacket colors during rearing.

cagemate was presented with either an alien-colored or no jacket. The difference among these conditions was statistically significant ($p < .02$, Friedman). Similarly, when the stimulus animal was a stranger, surrogate-reared infants again clearly differentiated the various jacket conditions, displaying highest approach scores toward a stranger wearing a familiar-colored jacket. The effectiveness of the various jacket conditions in altering the infants' attractions to social incentives is perhaps best illustrated by noting that despite the strong differentiation of familiar from unfamiliar peers (mean approach scores = 49.5 vs. 35.9, $p < .02$, Wilcoxon), a strange peer wearing the familiar-colored jacket was nearly as attractive as a cagemate presented without the jacket.

In contrast to the clear differentiation of jacket conditions in surrogate-reared infants, mother-reared infants—who had had no early experience with the jacket colors—showed no such discrimination. In this group, the mean approach score toward a cagemate wearing the familiar-colored jacket was, if anything, slightly lower than toward the cagemate presented with an alien-colored jacket or no jacket. Similarly, mother-reared infants showed no appreciable discrimination of unfamiliar peers on the basis of their jackets. Despite the failure of mother-reared infants to differentiate agemates on the basis of their jackets, they did show strong and reliable differential approach scores toward cagemates as opposed to strangers (means = 60.6 vs. 35.6, $p < .01$, Wilcoxon). This result suggests that mother-reared infants were quite capable of making social discriminations but that they were simply indifferent to the color cues afforded by the jackets.

Thus, the results from Phase II suggest that the particular visual attributes of an infant squirrel monkey's first object of attachment can, under appropriate conditions, influence its subsequent preferences for particular social partners. Even though the jackets provided only a crude and partial simulation of the visual attributes of the original attachment figure, surrogate-reared infants differentiated both cagemates and strangers on the basis of color cues in much the same way as they differentiated their surrogates some three months earlier. When viewed against the results obtained on the control group of mother-reared infants, which had received no prior rearing experience with the jacket colors, the most reasonable interpretation of these findings is that established attractions to the rearing color in surrogate-reared infants persisted beyond weaning and continued to be expressed with respect to new objects of attachment (peers) that, by our intervention, had some of the same visual attributes as the original attachment figure.

SUMMARY AND CONCLUSION

The studies that have been presented here on infant squirrel monkeys clearly demonstrate that certain types of early perceptual experience can influence both the reactions to a rearing figure and subsequent responses to familiar as well as unfamiliar individuals. In comparing olfaction and vision, we found that although both modalities were effective sources of information for discriminating the mother, the former was operative at an earlier age. This result is consistent with that reported recently for the human neonate.

However, to what extent other species of nonhuman primates would also respond in such a manner has yet to be determined.

Our results involving the persistent influence of early visual experience on subsequent social attraction are the first of this sort reported in a primate and consequently must be intepreted with caution until studies have been conducted on other primates. How much of an impact visual or other perceptual experiences will have on social development will likely depend on several factors, including the inherent attractiveness of a given stimulus, length of exposure to the stimulus, when in development it occurs, and the contingencies of reinforcement associated with its presence. Clearly, our own work with the squirrel monkey has just begun to scratch the surface of a relatively new area of research, one that should provide insight into the significance of specific aspects of early experience that heretofore either have not been considered to be influential in primate development or have been too difficult to study empirically.

ACKNOWLEDGMENTS

This research was supported by Grant No. HD04905 from the National Institute of Child Health and Human Development.

REFERENCES

Carpenter, G. Mother's face and the newborn. *New Sci.* 21st March, 742–745 (1974).

Carter, C. S. Effects of olfactory experience on the behavior of the guinea-pig (*Cavia porcellus*). *Anim. Behav. 20,* 54–60 (1972).

Dukelow, W. R., Ariga, S., Kuehl, T. J., and Burke, D. B. Application of karyological techniques to reproductive studies with the squirrel monkey (*Saimiri sciureus*). Paper presented at the meeting of the American Society of primatologists, Seattle, April 1977.

Fantz, R. L. Visual perception and experience in early infancy: a look at the hidden side of behavior development. In *Early Behavior: Comparative and Developmental Approaches,* H. W. Stevenson, E. H. Hess, and H. L. Rheingold, eds. John Wiley & Sons, Inc., New York (1967), pp. 181–224.

Hansen, E. W. The development of maternal and infant behavior in the rhesus monkey. *Behaviour 27,* 107–149 (1966).

Johnson, P. and Salisbury, D. M. Breathing and sucking during feeding in the newborn. In *Parent-Infant Interaction.* Ciba Foundation Symposium 33. Elsevier, Amsterdam (1975), pp. 119–135.

Jones, T. C. and Ma, N. S. F. Cytogenetics of the squirrel monkey (*Saimiri sciureus*). *Fed. Proc. 34,* 1646–1650 (1975).

Kaplan, J. Growth and behavior of surrogate-reared squirrel monkeys. *Dev. Psychobiol. 7,* 7–13 (1974).

Kaplan, J. Perceptual properties of attachment in surrogate-reared and mother-reared squirrel monkeys. In *Primate Bio-social Development,* S. Chevalier-Skolnikoff and F. E. Poirier, eds. Garland Publishing, Inc., New York (1977), pp. 225–234.

Kaplan, J. N., Cubicciotti III, D., and Redican, W. K. Olfactory and visual differentiation of synthetically scented surrogates by infant squirrel monkeys. *Dev. Psychobiol., 12,* 1–10, (1979).

Kaplan, J. N., Cubicciotti III, D., and Redican, W. K. Olfactory discrimination of squirrel monkey mothers by their infants. *Dev. Psychobiol. 10,* 447–453 (1977).

Kaplan, J. and Russell, M. A surrogate for rearing infant squirrel monkeys. *Behav. Res. Meth. Instru. 5,* 379–380 (1973).

Kaplan, J. and Russell, M. Olfactory recognition in the infant squirrel monkey. *Dev. Psychobiol. 7,* 15–19 (1974).

Kaplan, J. N., Winship-Ball, A., and Sim, L. Maternal discrimination of infant vocalizations in squirrel monkeys. *Primates 19,* 187–193 (1978).

Lipsitt, L. P. Learning in the human infant. In *Early Behavior: Comparative and Developmental Approaches,* H. W. Stevenson, E. H. Hess, and H. L. Rheingold, eds. John Wiley & Sons, Inc., New York (1967), pp. 225–247.

Macfarlane, A. Olfaction in the development of social preferences in the human neonate. In *Parent–Infant Interaction,* Ciba Foundation Symposium 33. Elsevier, Amsterdam (1975), pp. 103–117.

MacLean, P. D. Mirror display in the squirrel monkey, *Saimiri sciureus. Science 146,* 950–952 (1964).

Marr, J. N. and Gardner, L. E. Early olfactory experience and later social behavior in the rat: preference, sexual responsiveness, and care of young. *J. Gen. Psychol. 107,* 167–174 (1965).

Marr, J. N. and Lilliston, L. G. Social attachment in rats by odor and age. *Behaviour 33,* 277–282 (1969).

Ploog, D., Hupfer, K., Jurgens, U., and Newman, J. D. Neuroethologic studies of vocalizations in squirrel monkeys with special reference to genetic differences of calling in two subspecies. In *Growth and Development of the Brain,* M. A. B. Brazier, ed. Raven Press, New York (1975), pp. 231–254.

Porter, R. H. and Etscorn, F. A sensitive period for the development of olfactory preference in *Acomys cahirinus. Physiol. Behav. 17,* 127–130 (1976).

Pratt, C. L. and Sackett, G. P. Selection of social partners as a function of peer contact during rearing. *Science 155,* 1133–1135 (1967).

Redican, W. K. and Kaplan, J. N. Effects of synthetic odors on filial attachment in infant squirrel monkeys. *Physiol. Behav. 20,* 79–86 (1978).

Rosenblum, L. A. and Lowe, A. The influence of familiarity during rearing on subsequent partner preferences in squirrel monkeys. *Psychon. Sci. 23,* 35–37 (1971).

Sackett, G. P. Unlearned responses, differential rearing experiences, and the development of social attachments by rhesus monkeys. In *Primate Behavior: Developments in Field and Laboratory Research, Vol. 1,* L. A. Rosenblum, ed. Academic Press, New York (1970), pp. 111–140.

12

Effects of Parental Characteristics and Prenatal Factors on Pregnancy Outcomes of Pigtail Macaques

Gene P. Sackett
Richard A. Holm

The importance of genetic, prenatal, and intergenerational influences on postnatal development has been identified for a number of mammalian species, and prenatal factors have been shown to affect many dimensions of behavioral development (e.g., Joffe, 1969). In mice (Fuller and Herman, 1974; Henderson, 1976), and dogs (Scott and Fuller, 1965) effects of a variety of rearing conditions appear to depend on which species (and even which strain) is being studied. Premating stress applied to females may also interact with genetic and prenatal variables to determine some adult behaviors in rats (Joffe, 1965). Prenatal influences may involve factors related to sexual differentiation of the fetus (e.g., Levine, 1966; Greenough, et al., 1977). Another set of prenatal influences on development may arise from a nongenetic intergenerational mechanism in which environmental effects on mothers during their own infancy are passed on to offspring via fetal growth disturbances or other intrauterine abnormalities (e.g., Denenberg and Whimbey, 1963). This literature illustrates the complexity inherent in understanding the behavioral development. It also underscores the truism taught in introductory psychology classes that behavior is an interactive function of genetic and environmental factors.

Although the genetic-environment interaction model has been taken very seriously by investigators of infraprimate species, it has played only a minor role in laboratory research on development of nonhuman primates. Most primate research has focused on maternal and infant rearing variables. Little direct experimental consideration has been given to genetic or prenatal factors that might interact with these postnatal variables. This chapter will briefly review a series of studies on social isolation rearing in rhesus and pigtail macaques, showing that the effects depended on the sex and species of the infant monkey. These data lead us to conclude that, as with infraprimates, an understanding of primate development depends on the study of genetic, prenatal, and perhaps even intergenerational variables. We follow this review with a description of an experimental model that we are currently using to study the effects of such variables on primate development.

EFFECTS OF SOCIAL ISOLATION REARING

Most contemporary laboratory research on primate behavioral development stems from the well known pioneering work of Harlow and his colleagues on rhesus monkeys (*Macaca mulatta*). This work began with studies of infants reared on cloth or wire surrogate mothers (Harlow, 1958), and was quickly expanded to investigate effects of total social isolation at different periods during infancy (Harlow and Harlow, 1965). Other studies assessed developmental effects of rearing infants with peers but no mothers, rearing in partial social isolation, and rearing with "motherless mothers" who were themselves raised under isolation conditions during infancy (Harlow and Harlow, 1966; Arling and Harlow, 1967). Total social isolation rearing involved placing the newborn monkey in a completely enclosed chamber, thereby depriving it of all sensory contact with species members. It also involved perceptual deprivation, as the infant's own actions provided the only source of varied stimulation. Partial social isolation involved rearing in wire cages from which other monkeys could be seen and heard, but not physically contacted.

This work led to the following conclusions: 1) Total isolation rearing from 6–12 months following birth produces abnormal personal behaviors such as stereotyped and repetitive motor behaviors, self-clutching, rocking, huddling, and self-mouthing actions. Total isolates also seem uninterested in or unwilling to explore novel or complex stimuli. They exhibit little or no positive social behavior with agemates, and are extremely deviant in sexual and maternal behavior. Isolates often display bizarre actions such as suddenly peering at an arm or leg, then grabbing the offending limb and violently biting it. In short, this rearing condition appears to eliminate many species-typical behaviors permanently, replacing them with bizarre and deviant actions. Interestingly, when compared with either wild-born or other laboratory-born monkeys raised with mothers or peers, total social isolates did not appear to be intellectually abnormal (Harlow et al., 1969). 2) Rearing in partial social isolation without peer contact early in infancy also produces deviant behavior. However, many of the behavioral abnormalities seen in partial isolates are not as extreme either quantitatively or qualitatively as those produced by total isolation. Further, some partial isolates show some normalization following one or two years of post-isolation social experience. 3) Monkeys reared with agemates or with mothers and agemates do not develop the deviant behaviors seen in total or partial isolates. Thus, for rhesus monkeys, physical contact during infancy appears to be a necessary condition for the development of species-typical behavior.

Attempts to ameliorate the effects of total social isolation (reviewed by Sackett, 1972a) by long-term social interaction with agemates and by specific therapy regimens involving operant conditioning failed to produce any noticeable positive effect. However, subsequent studies by Suomi and Harlow (1972) and Suomi et al. (1974) apparently identified at least one condition that could reverse total isolate deficits. The treatment consists of placing isolates in contact with much younger "therapist" monkeys shortly after they emerge from isolation. Thus, it may be possible to reverse rhesus isolate behavior deficits, although probably only when "treatment" is applied immediately after the end of isolation.

Sex Differences in the Effects of Isolation

Harlow and Lauersdorf (1974) summarized a number of studies on mother–peer raised rhesus monkeys which revealed developmental and adult sex differences. Male–female differences were especially prominent in the quality of infant play, in aggression, and of course in sexual behavior. On other behavioral dimensions such as exploration and learning, sex differences were not found or were inconsistent from study to study. However, in groups subjected to isolation rearing, large sex differences appeared on each dimension characteristic of the basic isolation rearing syndrome. Sex differences were found in exploratory behavior at 2 (Sackett, 1974) and at 5 years of age (Sackett, 1972b); in amount of abnormal personal behaviors such as stereotypy, body rocking, and huddling (Sackett, 1974; Pratt, 1969); in self-directed aggression (Gluck and Sackett, 1974); in the extent of adult sexual behavior abnormalities (Harlow et al., 1966); and in amount of positive social behavior (Sackett, 1972a). Although animals raised in total isolation from 9–12 months from birth consistently showed large differences from controls, even in this extremely deprived group females were less deviant than males. Sex differences were especially prominent in partial isolates. On many measures partial isolate females were not very different from female controls, while partial isolate males behaved much more like total social isolates.

These studies suggest that rhesus females are relatively buffered against the detrimental effects of stimulus deprivation during rearing while rhesus males are much more vulnerable to developing persistent abnormal behavior. The reasons for this sex effect are unclear. One hypothesis is that the factors determining this differential risk relate to anatomical or biochemical differences which develop at the time of sexual differentiation in utero. For rhesus monkeys this maturational period is probably about 40–60 days in the total gestation period of 165–170 days (Eaton et al., 1973; Resko, 1970). If this hypothesis is valid, an understanding of the effects of deprivation rearing would depend on studying how prenatal factors relate to variability in risk for developing abnormal behavior. Prenatal factors causing sex differences in susceptibility to abnormal rearing may also contribute to variability between members of the same sex on these measures.

Species Differences in the Effects of Isolation

Between 1970 and 1974 we attempted to replicate the total social isolation phenomena described for rhesus macaques in a closely related species, the pigtail macaque (*M. nemestrina*). These experiments duplicated the rhesus monkey rearing and testing conditions as closely as possible. On postrearing social behavior tests pigtail isolates exhibited high levels of nonsocial exploratory behavior and had less than half the amount of deviant personal behavior exhibited by rhesus isolates on comparable tests (Sackett et al., 1976). Pigtail isolates had at least some positive social behaviors on these tests, while rhesus isolates almost without exception displayed no positive behaviors. Some of the pigtail isolates were housed together in pens until they were 4 years old. Without any special therapy such as pairings with younger immature monkeys, these isolates all developed a full repertoire of species-typical social interactive behaviors. However, they did continue to exhibit some personal idiosyncracies such as motor stereotypies and self-clutching. The sex differences which were so prominant between rhesus isolates failed to appear in our pigtail monkeys (Sackett et al., 1976). In fact, the only statistically reliable sex differences for pigtail monkeys occurred in nonsocial exploration, where male isolates scored higher than females.

In sum, these between-species comparisons failed to replicate either the extreme and persistent effects of total social isolation or the sex differences found for rhesus monkeys. We believe that the findings identify a genetic difference in vulnerability to abnormalizing effects of deprivation rearing. Rhesus monkeys appear to be a high-risk species, while pigtail monkeys appear to be relatively buffered against the detrimental effects of total social isolation. This conclusion suggests that an understanding of rearing condition effects must include study of genetic or other predisposing factors that make individuals at relatively high or low risk for developing abnormal behavior.

AN EXPERIMENTAL MODEL FOR THE STUDY OF PRIMATE DEVELOPMENT

The Infant Primate Research Laboratory at the University of Washington maintains a neonate care facility which is staffed 24 hours a day. Besides caring for newborn monkeys serving as subjects in a variety of studies, the nursery receives newborns from a pigtail monkey breeding colony containing about 600 animals. These newborns are ones who cannot be cared for by their mothers owing to illness, low birthweight or prematurity, or have been rejected or injured while with their mother in a social housing group. These animals are studied for physical and behavioral development during the first year of life. Measures taken to date show that many of these animals are slow to develop reflex behaviors, maintain low growth rates during infancy, take over three times as many days to achieve the developmental milestone of complete self-feeding, and exhibit quantitative deficits in the development of social behavior at 3–4 months of age (Sackett et al., 1974). This is especially true for low birthweight and/or premature animals, who also exhibit deviant patterns of activity state, respiration, heart rate, and temperature diurnal cycles during the first 30 days of life. In many respects these monkeys present behavioral and growth deficits which resemble those reported for human premature and very low birthweight babies (e.g., Illingsworth, 1967; Saint-Anne Dargassies, 1966).

These observations suggested to us that factors producing poor pregnancy outcomes might also be related to the factors that produce differential risk for abnormal behavioral development. To pursue this idea we did statistical studies on the 12-year computerized breeding and health records maintained on pigtail monkeys at the Washington Regional Primate Research Center. Our goal was to determine whether we could identify any factors that would characterize female or male breeders who produced an excess of poor pregnancy outcomes such as abortion, still birth, low birthweight, or neonatal death. Employing a discriminant analysis procedure, we found that a history of bad pregnancy outcomes, maternal age and parity, birth order, days the female was in her current social group prior to conception, and number of treatments received for bite wounds, were all factors related to producing poor pregnancies (Sackett et al., 1974). When tested on the pregnancy outcomes of 100 conceptions that were not included in the data used to obtain the discriminant function, a success rate of better than 90% for breeders at the high and low extremes of expected risk was obtained. Many of the factors that allowed us to make these predictions were the same as those found to be correlated with bad pregnancy outcomes in humans (Kelly et al., 1976).

A particularly interesting finding concerned the bite wound factor. Females who were bitten in the six months prior to conception showed an excess of offspring neonatal death relative to animals not bitten during this period. Females bitten during pregnancy had an excessive abortion rate. In monkeys groups, bite wounds can be considered a crude index of social stress. Females receiving bite wounds severe enough to require treatment are often either new to the social group or are at the very low end of the group dominance hierarchy. Thus, these data suggested that social stress either before or during pregnancy could be a major factor in determining bad pregnancy outcomes and possibly even risk for abnormal or deviant development in surviving offspring. We next designed a study to validate our statistical study for predicting breeders at risk for poor pregnancy outcomes and to assess the effects of stress during pregnancy on pregnancy outcomes and offspring development.

The basic design of our experimental plan was a 2 × 2 factorial study. The first factor, pregnancy outcome risk, concerned mating together male and female breeders who were at very high or very low predicted risk for abortion, still birth, low birthweight, or neonatal death of their next offspring. The second factor, stress during pregnancy, concerned whether the female would receive a physical stressor involving daily capture by an animal technician on an unpredictable schedule versus maintaining pregnancy under as low stress as possible. The physical capture stressor was chosen because we knew that our breeders do not adapt to the procedure even after years of handling, and the procedure produces obvious overt signs of disturbance. In fact, the females housed in the high stress room quickly learn the characteristics of the capture technician, and explode into intense locomotor activity and vocalization whenever he appears at the door to the room.

HIGH VERSUS LOW RISK BREEDER CHARACTERISTICS

Breeders were selected from the overall colony on the basis of their past pregnancy outcomes. Among females, potential candidates included only those who had three or more prior conceptions in the colony. Among males, potential candidates were selected from animals siring at least 25 prior offspring with many different females. Table 1 presents data summarizing the breeding outcomes of high- and low-risk females prior to grant assignment compared with all other female breeders at or beyond their third colony conception. Low-risk breeders produced 93.2% viable offspring who survived the neonatal period, compared with 66.0% for the intermediate breeders. High-risk females produced only 35.7% viable surviving offspring, with excesses in each of the poor pregnancy outcome categories and in the percentage of low birthweight deliveries.

TABLE 1
Pregnancy Outcome Patterns for High, Low, and Intermediate Risk Multiparous Female Breeders Prior to Assignment to Experimental Matings

		Pregnancy Outcome					
Risk		*Viable*	*Abort*	*Stillborn*	*Neonatal Death*	*Total*	*Low Birth Weight*
High	N Conceptions	66	51	38	30	185	62
(n = 37)	Mean	1.8	1.4	1.0	0.8	5.0	1.7
	%	35.7	27.6	20.5	16.2		33.5
Low	N Conceptions	150	6	1	4	161	6
(n = 29)	Mean	5.2	0.2	0.0	0.1	5.6	0.2
	%	93.2	3.7	0.6	2.5		3.7
Inter-	N Conceptions	376	86	54	54	570	58
mediate	Mean	3.4	0.8	0.5	0.5	5.2	0.5
(n = 110)	%	66.0	15.1	9.5	9.5		10.0

TABLE 2

Pregnancy Outcome Patterns among High Risk Female Breeders Prior to Assignment to Experimental Matings. High Risk Females are Categorized into One of Four Risk Types and Outcomes for Each Group are Displayed.

		Pregnancy Outcome					
Type of Risk		*Viable*	*Abort*	*Stillborn*	*Neonatal Death*	*Total*	*Low Birth Weight*
Abortion	N Conceptions	6	28	6	4	44	6
(n = 10)	Mean	0.6	2.8	0.6	0.4	4.4	0.6
	%	13.6	63.6	13.6	9.1		13.6
Perinatal-	N Conceptions	4	0	8	9	21	12
Neonatal	Mean	0.7	0.0	1.3	1.5	3.5	2.0
Death	%	19.0	0.0	38.1	42.9		57.1
(n = 6)							
Low Birth	N Conceptions	29	3	5	0	37	19
Weight	Mean	4.1	0.4	0.7	0.0	5.3	2.7
(n = 7)	%	78.4	8.1	13.5	0.0		51.4
Mixed	N Conceptions	27	20	19	17	83	25
(n = 14)	Mean	1.9	1.4	1.4	1.2	5.9	1.8
	%	32.5	24.1	22.9	20.5		30.1

Table 2 presents a breakdown for four general types of high-risk breeders. It can be seen that the high-risk breeders are actually a heterogeneous group, some of whom had a history of only certain types of bad pregnancy outcomes. Ten of these breeders had an excess of abortions. Six others had an excess of late term or neonatal deaths, and also had a high percentage of low birthweight deliveries. Seven high-risk breeders did not actually have a deficiency in delivering live offspring, but did have a high incidence of low birthweight babies. Fourteen others presented a mixed picture, having very low viable offspring rates with a mixture of the four types of bad pregnancy outcomes. Data on humans suggest that this mixed group might be likely candidates for chromosomal abnormalities, so their offspring should be of major interest with respect to possible genetic mechanisms involved in risk for abnormal development (Jacobs et al., 1975).

Table 3 presents the pregnancy outcome patterns for three high and three low-risk male breeders who served as sires in the selective breeding experiment. The low-risk breeders had 74.5% viable offspring while the high-risk animals managed only 28.9%. Excesses can be seen in each poor pregnancy outcome category for the high-risk males. This finding takes on special importance in light of the fact that these males were bred in a large and randomly selected set of females who were not themselves biased toward bad pregnancy outcomes. Thus, males seem to contribute to bad outcomes independently of female breeder variables. Potential mechanisms mediating the male effect are under study. It is possible that the effect lies in genetic factors related to mismatching of chromosomes or blood types. It is also possible that the male effect is behavioral. Colony breeding is performed in harem groups containing a single male and up to 16 females. These high-risk males may stress their females during pregnancy through excessive aggression or some other behavioral mechanism. Thus, the effect could actually be mediated by prenatal factors resulting from the behavioral interactions of females with high-risk breeder males.

FINDINGS

To date we have studied 13 low-risk and 8 high-risk females with a pregnancy under each stress condition. We have studied an additional five low-risk and seven high-risk females during the first experimental pregnancy, about half under each stress condition. Table 4 displays the outcomes of these 53 pregnancies by risk group and stress. The mixing of paired and independent subjects in this table makes significant testing difficult; however, some trends do stand out. The high-risk group has a higher incidence of abortion than the low-risk group. Stress appears to have no effect on the high-risk females, while dramatically increasing abortion in the low-risk breeding.

TABLE 3
Pregnancy Outcome Patterns for High and Low Risk Male Breeders Prior to Assignment to Experimental Matings

		Pregnancy Outcome					
Risk		*Viable*	*Abort*	*Stillborn*	*Neonatal Death*	*Total*	*Low Birth Weight*
High	N Conceptions	28	28	16	25	97	25
(n = 3)	Mean	9.3	9.3	5.3	8.3	32.3	8.3
	%	28.9	28.9	16.5	25.8		25.8
Low	N Conceptions	73	12	5	8	98	5
(n = 3)	Mean	24.3	4.0	1.7	2.7	32.7	1.7
	%	74.5	12.2	5.1	8.2		5.1

TABLE 4
Pregnancy Outcomes During the Study for High and Low Risk Breeders by Stress Condition

	High Risk				*Low Risk*			
	Stress		*No Stress*		*Stress*		*No Stress*	
Abort	42%	(5)	55%	(6)	35%	(5)	6%	(1)
Breech-Stillborn	8%	(1)	9%	(1)	7%	(1)	0%	(0)
Liveborn	50%	(6)	36%	(4)	60%	(9)	94%	(15)
N =		12		11		15		16

The latter point is better illustrated in Table 5, which presents the matched outcomes under each stress condition for females who have completed the study. Abortions, stillborns and breech deaths have all been pooled as fetal loss. None of the high-risk females changed the type of pregnancy outcome from one stress condition to the other. The five low-risk females whose outcomes were different under the two conditions all had liveborns in the low stress condition and fetal losses under the high stress. A one-tailed binomial test suggests that this is a reliable effect (for 0 out of 5, $p = .031$).

These findings clearly indicate that we have identified groups of breeders at high and low risk for a variety of bad pregnancy outcomes. The interaction of the risk and stress conditions is of considerable interest. Live borns from each cell in the research design are currently being studied. Measures taken on these individuals deal with growth, reflex development, learning, and social behavior. All of these offspring have daily social interactions with peers, a procedure which results in very normal animals. When study is completed we

TABLE 5
Pregnancy Outcomes of the High and Low Risk Breeders Who Have Had a Conception Under Both Stress Conditions.

	High Risk No Stress		*Low Risk No Stress*	
	Fetal Loss	*Live*	*Fetal Loss*	*Live*
Stress				
Fetal Loss	5	0	0	5
Live	0	3	0	8

will begin breeding for a study of the effects of isolation rearing on offspring resulting from the four combinations of parental risk and prenatal stress.

ACKNOWLEDGMENTS

The research reported in this paper was supported by NIH grants HD-08633 from NICHD Mental Retardation Branch, RR-00166 from Animal Resources Branch, and HD-02274.

REFERENCES

Arling, G. L. and Harlow, H. F. Effects of social deprivation on maternal behavior of rhesus monkeys. *J. Comp. Physiol. Psych. 64,* 371–377 (1967).

Denenberg, V. H. and Whimbey, A. E. Behavior of adult rats is modified by the experiences their mothers had as infants. *Science 142,* 1192–1193 (1963).

Eaton, G. G., Goy, R. W., and Phoenix, C. H. Effects of testosterone treatment in adulthood on sexual behavior of female pseudohermaphrodite rhesus monkeys. *Nature 242,* 119–120 (1973).

Fuller, J. L. and Herman, G. H. Effect of genotype and practice upon behavioral development of mice. *Dev. Psychobiol. 7,* 21–30 (1974).

Gluck, J. and Sackett, G. P. Frustration and self-aggression in social isolate rhesus monkeys. *J. Abnorm. Psychol. 83,* 331–334 (1974).

Greenough, W. T., Carter, C. S., Streerman, C., and DeVoogd, T. J. Sex differences in dendritic patterns in hamster preoptic area. *Brain Res.* in press (1977).

Harlow, H. F. The nature of love. *Am. Psychol. 13,* 673–685 (1958).

Harlow, H. F. and Harlow, M. K. The affectional systems. In *Behavior of Nonhuman Primates,* Vol. 2, A. H. Schrier, H. F. Harlow, and F. Stollnitz, eds. Academic Press, New York (1965).

Harlow, H. F. and Harlow, M. J. Learning to love. *Am. Scient. 54,* 244–272 (1966).

Harlow, H. F., Joslyn, W. D., Senko, M. G., and Dopp, A. Behavioral aspects of reproduction in primates. *J. An. Sci. 25,* 49–67 (1966).

Harlow, H. F., Schiltz, K. A., and Harlow, M. K. Effects of social isolation on the learning performance of rhesus monkeys. In *Proceedings of the 2nd International Congress of Primatology,* Vol. 1, C. R. Carpenter ed. Karger, New York (1969).

Harlow, H. F. and Lauersdorf, H. E. Sex differences in passion and play. *Persp. Biol. Med. 17,* 348–360 (1974).

Henderson, N. D. Short exposures to enriched environments can increase genetic variability of behavior in mice. *Dev. Psychobiol. 9,* 549–553 (1976).

Illingsworth, P. *The Development of the Infant and Young Child: Normal and Abnormal.* Livingston, Ltd., London (1967).

Jacobs, P., Frackiezwicz, A., Law, P., Hilditch, C. J., and Morton, N. E. The effects of structural aberrations of the chromosomes on reproductive fitness in man. II. Results. *Clin. Genet. 8,* 169–178 (1975).

Joffe, J. M. Genotype and prenatal and premating stress interact to affect adult behavior in rats. *Science 150,* 1844–1845 (1965).

Joffe, J. M. *Prenatal Determinants of Behavior.* Pergamon Press, New York (1969).

Kelly, S., Hook, E., Janerich, D., and Porter, I. *Birth Defects: Risks and Consequences.* Academic Press, New York (1976).

Levine, S. Sex differences in the brain. *Scientific American* 76–81 (1966).

Pratt, C. L. The developmental consequences of variations in early social stimulation. Unpublished doctoral dissertation, University of Wisconsin (1969).

Resko, J. A. Androgen secretion by the fetal and neonatal rhesus monkey. *Endocrinology 87,* 680–687 (1970).

Sackett, G. P. Isolation rearing in monkeys: Diffuse and specific effects on later behavior. In *Animal Models of Human Behavior,* R. Chauvin, ed. Paris: Colloques Internationaux du C.N.R.S., (1972*a*).

Sackett, G. P. Exploratory behavior of rhesus monkeys as a function of rearing experiences and sex. *Dev. Psychol. 6,* 260–270 (1972*b*).

Sackett, G. P. Sex differences in rhesus monkeys following rearing experiences. In *Sex Differences in Behavior,* R. M. Richart and R. L. Vandewiele, eds. John Wiley & Sons, Inc., New York (1974).

Sackett, G. P., Holm, R. A., Davis, A. E., and Fahrenbruch, C. E. Prematurity and low birth weight in pigtail macaques: Incidence, prediction, and effects on infant development. In *Symposia of 5th Congress of the International Primatological Society,* S. Kondo, M. Kawai, A. Ehara, and S. Kawamura, eds. Japan Science Press, Tokyo (1974).

Sackett, G. P., Holm, R. A., and Ruppenthal, G. C. Social isolation rearing: Species differences in behavior of macaque monkeys. *Dev. Psychol. 12,* 283–288 (1976).

Sackett, G. P., Holm, R. A., Ruppenthal, G. C., and Fahrenbruch, C. E. The effects of total social isolation rearing on behavior of rhesus and pigtail macaques. In *Advances in Behavioral Biology,* Vol. 17, R. N. Walsh and W. T. Greenough. *Environments as Therapy for Brain Dysfunction.* Plenum, New York (1976).

Saint-Anne Dargassies. Neurological maturation of the premature infant: 28–41 weeks gestational age. In *Human Development,* F. Falkner, ed. Saunders, Philadelphia (1966).

Scott, J. P. and Fuller, J. L. *Genetics and the Social Behavior of the Dog.* University of Chicago Press, Chicago (1965).

Suomi, S. J. and Harlow, H. F. Social rehabilitation of isolate-reared monkeys. *Dev. Psychol. 6,* 487–496 (1972).

Suomi, S. J., Harlow, H. F., and Novak, M. A. Reversal of social deficits produced by isolation rearing in monkeys. *J. Human Evol. 3,* 527–534 (1974).

Maternal Influences and Early Behavior

13

Infant Development and Maternal Behavior in Captive Chimpanzees

Janice R. Horvat
Christopher L. Coe
Seymour Levine

Extensive study of mother–infant relations in infrahuman primates has revealed that the mother plays a primary role in the infant's emotional and social development (Harlow and Harlow, 1969; Mason, 1970), in laying the groundwork for the infant's later dominance status (Koyama, 1967) and in the learning of the species' social organization and traditions (Lancaster, 1973; McGrew, 1977). If one looks across the Primate Order, from the prosimians to the monkeys and finally to the apes there is a trend towards prolongation and intensification of the mother–infant relationship. This prolongation is extremely accentuated in the apes, the chimpanzee (van Lawick-Goodall, 1968), the gorilla (Fossey, in press; Schaller, 1963) and the orangutan (Horr, 1977), since the mother–infant bond in these species usually lasts between three to eight years. Several studies describing aspects of chimpanzee mother–infant relations and indicating the extent of the mother–infant attachment have been completed under laboratory and field conditions (e.g., Clark, 1977; McGrew, 1977; Nicolson, 1977; Rogers and Davenport, 1970; Savage et al., 1973; Savage and Malick, 1977; Silk and Kraemer, 1978; Yerkes and Tomilin, 1935; and van Lawick-Goodall, 1967, 1968).

The first major study was by Yerkes and Tomilin (1935), and described primarily postparturient behavior in mother–infant dyads which were housed alone. The infants were subsequently separated after the first year of life. This study indicated the supportive role of the mother, her capacity for complex interactions with the infant and the wide range of individual differences in maternal behavior. The authors also observed differences between primiparous and multiparous mothers and emphasized the important role of experience in the manifestation of competent maternal care. A more recent study by Rogers and Davenport (1970) has indicated further that the mother's own rearing has an effect on her postparturient behaviors. Female chimpanzees who had spent less than 18 months with their own mothers were significantly less proficient in caring for neonates than were females who had received longer maternal rearing.

More detailed descriptions of the mother–infant relations have appeared in the last decade, derived primarily from observations of wild chimpanzees at the Gombe Research Center, Tanzania. Van Lawick-Goodall (1967, 1968) has characterized the period of infancy as lasting 3.5–4.0 years based on the length of suckling, being transported by the mother and sleeping in the mother's nest. The early mother–infant relations are affectionate and intensive. The mother is extremely protective of the young infant, typically supporting and cradling the neonate on her ventrum. The infant continues to remain in the ventral position while the mother travels for most of the first year. After 6 months of age, however, there is a gradual transition to a dorsal riding position which becomes the predominant mode of traveling during the second year of life. During this period the infant engages in independent excursions and social interactions with increasing frequency. Weaning is a gradual and usually gentle process, often beginning in the second year of life and extending over a 2-year period. The weaned offspring continue to associate with their mothers and under conditions of high arousal they may return to their mothers for reassurance or protection. The maintenance of long-term, extended family relations are also evident in the types of affiliative interactions between older family members.

A more recent study on the mother–infant relations of Gombe chimpanzees has related the occurrence of weaning behaviors to the female reproductive pattern (Clark, 1977). Clark reports that initial maternal rejections are subtle (e.g., blocking access to the nipple, avoiding the infant or restricting infant movement) and gradually intensify over a 2- to 3-year period. However, she reports that these weaning behaviors increase in frequency and intensity when the mother resumes cycling and subsequently becomes pregnant. The infant, who may stop suckling at this point, responds to the altered relationship with higher levels of distress behaviors (e.g., whimpering and screaming vocalizations, emotional tantrums, and occasionally depression).

The extended length of the mother–infant relationship permits a wealth of information to be conveyed to the infant. The complexity and the time course of the transmission of learning skills has been studied by McGrew (1977), who has observed the socialization of certain food-getting behaviors and related aspects of imitative and observational learning. For example, the development of "termite-fishing" techniques, which involve tool-making and using, takes several years. "Ant-dipping," which requires more sophisticated tool-using abilities in order to avoid painful bites, is not acquired until a few years later. This study indicates an important functional relationship between the acquisition of food-getting abilities and the extended mother–infant relationship.

Despite the availability of this information on the mother–infant relations in the chimpanzee, a quantitative evaluation of the behavioral dynamics of the mother–infant relationship has been difficult because the data are of necessity based primarily on cross-sectional rather than longitudinal studies. In most of the field work on apes, it has not been possible to follow the same infant continuously throughout the period of infancy. It is critical to our understanding of the mother–infant relationship that we document the sequence of events from parturition onward. Thus, we at the Stanford Outdoor Primate Facility (SOPF) began longitudinal studies of captive mother–infant pairs of chimpanzees to establish a basic behavioral profile using spatial measurements and interactional and maintenance behaviors. We have attempted to balance two important considerations, the need for a complex social and living environment as well as the importance of regular observations and a reliable data collection system. We have restricted this present chapter to a discussion of the ontogeny of infant independence in terms of the following behaviors: spatial relations between mother and infant, travel, suckle and feed, food sharing, mother–infant play, distress, rejections, independent motor activity, and social play.

SUBJECTS AND METHODS

The major portion of data presented in this chapter is based on three mother–infant pairs of chimpanzees (*Pan troglodytes*). The mothers were primiparous and all the infants were female. Pertinent information on the dates and locations of infant births are presented in Table 1. The mothers were imported from the wild as infants between 1–3 years of age and were later established in a juvenile group which has remained essentially intact for the last 10 years (see McGinnis and Kraemer, 1977; Menzel, 1972; Merrick, 1977). The three mother–infant pairs lived in a freely-interacting social group which also contained three adult males. These males were also wild born and imported between 1–3 years of age.

The chimpanzee group lived initially in a 0.4 hectare (1 acre) outdoor enclosure at the Delta Regional Primate Research Center (Louisiana) where the oldest infant (DL) was born (see Table 1). Subsequently, the group was transferred to a small island (0.1 hectare) at Lion Country Safari Park

TABLE 1
Birth Dates and Locations of Observation for the Chimpanzees of the Present Study. Note that the Data on the Male Infant (BA) are Presented Separately in the Chapter.

Mother	*Infant*	*Born*	*Observation Months and Location**		
			DRPRC	*LCS*	*SOPF*
Gigi (GY)	Delta (DL)	May 1, 1972	1–4	5–25	26–36
Polly (PO)	Palita (PA)	January 15, 1974		1–5	6–36
Bido (BO)	Betty (BY)	September 5, 1974			1–36
Bashful (BS)	Bahati (BA)	July 7, 1976			1–12

*DRPRC—Delta Regional Primate Research Center
LCS—Lion Country Safari
SOPF—Stanford Outdoor Primate Facility

(California) for 1.8 years where the second infant (PA) was born. Since June 1974, the group has lived at the Stanford Outdoor Primate Facility (California). DL was 26 months of age and PA was 6 months of age when the group was established at SOPF. The youngest infant (BY) was born three months after the group arrived.

The chimpanzee facility is located on a secluded 9.7 hectare tract of oak-savanna grassland at Stanford University (see Fig. 1). The chimpanzee living area is enclosed by a 4.9 m high semicircular wall and a second wall divides the area into two 0.6 hectare (1.5 acre) outdoor enclosures. The vegetation within each area consists primarily of grasses and herbaceous plants. There are also three large, but now dead oak trees in each area. Artificial structures have been added, including a large and complex wooden sleeping structure (8 m × 5 m × 6 m high), two large concrete culverts and smaller movable objects such as automobile tires and empty oil drums.

The chimpanzees are observed from an observation deck in the laboratory building which overlooks the outdoor enclosures. Observations are presently made through one-way vision windows, and 7 × 35 mm binoculars are used to facilitate the data collection. Behaviors are recorded on standardized checksheets and the short-term timing of the observations is regulated by an electronic timer audible to the observers.

Each mother–infant pair has been observed from parturition onward and the data presented on the first three years of life are based on over 1000 total hours of observation. Some changes in the methods of data collection have been made during the five years of observation. The first 15 months of observations on DL involved continuous recording but all subsequent observations on DL and the other infants have utilized a time-sampling procedure (all graphs for DL except Spatial Relations include "through-the-

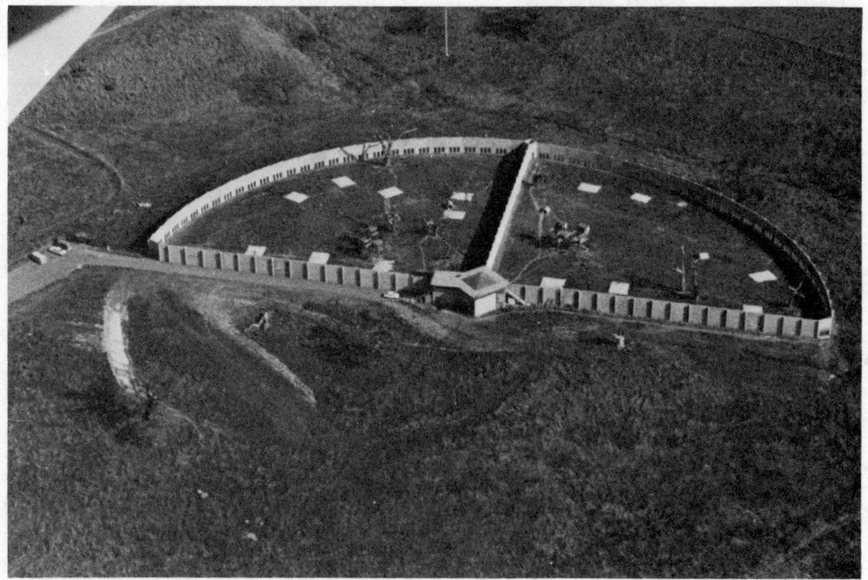

FIG. 1. Aerial view of the Standard Outdoor Primate Facility, showing the two chimpanzee enclosures and the laboratory building.

minute"—Hansen frequency—data up to and including month 15). Several parameters of mother–infant interactions are recorded simultaneously at minute intervals during a 30-minute recording session. The predefined behaviors, based on Goodall's behavior glossary (van Lawick-Goodall, 1968), characterize the social interactions and spatial relations between mother and infant, and the social interactions and association patterns of both the mother and infant with others. The frequency and context of infant distress and maternal rejection as well as the responses to these behaviors have also been recorded, initially in narrative form and subsequently on checksheets. Since January 1975 each mother–infant pair has been observed for three 30-minute sessions a week during a morning, midday, and afternoon period (Kraemer et al., 1978).

Although numerous behaviors have been recorded, only those most representative of the ontogeny of independence are presented in this chapter. Most behaviors have been presented as the percent of observation per month during which the specific behavior occurred. For graphic presentation, a "smoothed" average for each month was determined by sequential averaging of three months of data in order to more clearly illustrate the developmental trends (Kendall, 1955, p. 372).

SPATIAL RELATIONS BETWEEN MOTHER AND INFANT

Contact

During the first 6 months, the mother-infant dyads were almost continuously in contact. The three mothers showed typical maternal responsiveness, carrying and cradling the young infants on their ventrum (Figure 2). As can be seen in Figure 3, despite the shifts in group location and the different ages of the infants, a consistent developmental progression emerged. The percent of the observation during which the mother and infant were in contact is illustrated in Figure 3A. During the first six months of life, the dyads were almost continuously in contact. The lower initial values for PA were due to the relative difficulty of observation at the island habitat and reflect periods when contact could not be observed rather than an individual difference. After 6 months of age there was a rapid decline in the contact time, decreasing most precipitously between 6–18 months of life. The amount of contact decreased further during the next 1.5 years but at a more gradual rate and at 3 years of age the infants were still maintaining low levels of contact. Although not graphically protrayed, DL who is now 5 years of age continues to maintain contact with GY during 10–25% of the observation.

There are several points on each infant's curve when the gradual decline in contact was interrupted. Environmental or social changes accounted for most of these alterations, resulting in a reassertion of higher levels or a sudden decline in contact between the mother and infant. An evaluation of the contact levels maintained between GY and DL, for example, revealed transitory changes following the group move to SOPF, a subsequent shift between the two SOPF enclosures, and also after the other infants were born. Another variable which appeared to have had an effect on the mother–infant relationship was the resumption of sexual cycles in the females. Both GY/DL and PO/PA revealed lower contact levels after the occurrence of sexual cycles and BO/BY manifested heightened levels (GY, PO and BO resumed cycling in Months 37, 28, and 32 respectively). Thus, there appeared to be an overriding tendency for a progressive decline in contact which could be accelerated or slowed by environmental and social changes, depending in part upon the infant's age at the time of occurrence.

Near

The overall decline in the affiliative aspects of the mother–infant relationship was also reflected by two complementary measures of dyadic spatial relations. The time each dyad spent in the *Near* (less than 5 m travel

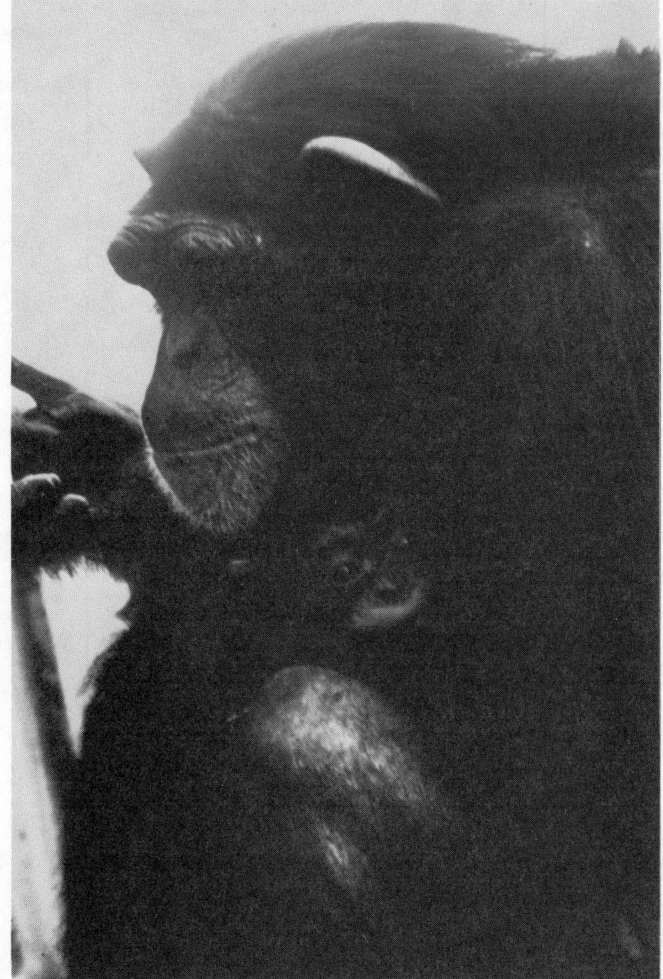

FIG. 2. An adult female (PO) cradling her young infant (PA) on her ventrum.

distance) and *Far* (greater than 5 m travel distance) categories was determined at minute intervals throughout the observations. These measures are also presented in Figure 3 as the percent occurrence per observation month. An evaluation of the time spent in Near distances clearly reflected the movement of the mother and infant away from each other, occurring concomitantly with the decline in the levels of contact (see Fig. 3B). Beginning at around 6 months of age, the mothers and infants were increasingly observed away from each other and the occurrence of Near distances rose sharply during the following months. During the third year the time spent in Near distances appeared to

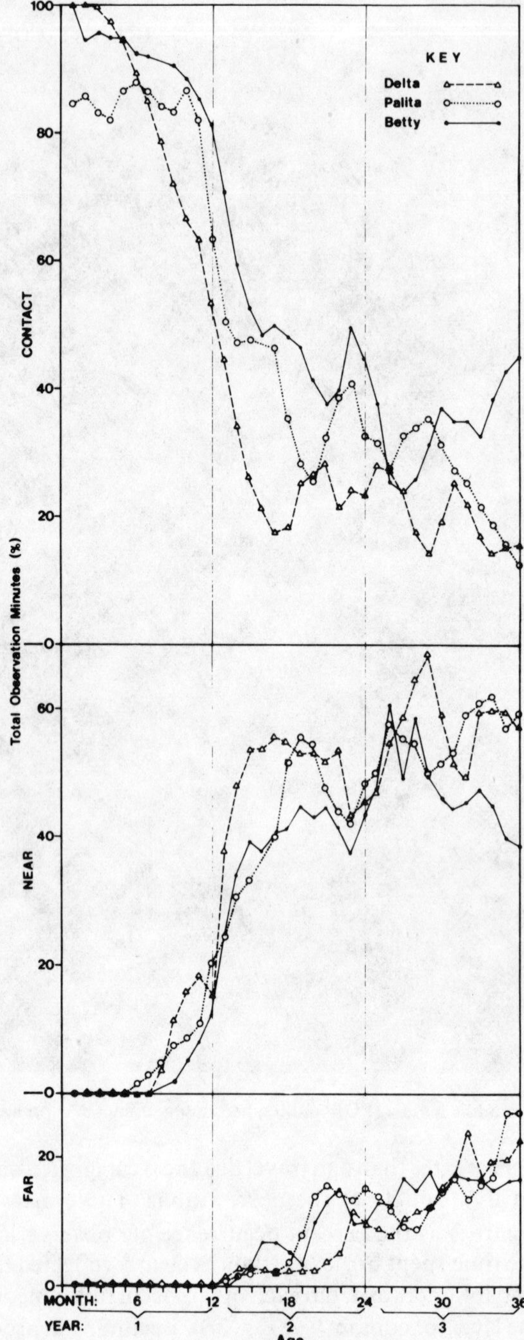

FIG. 3. Spatial relations between the mother and infant chimpanzees. Percent of observations spent in contact (upper graph, A), in Near (middle graph, B) and Far distances (lower graph, C). The total occurrence of these measures is equal to the total of good observation time.

stabilize between 40–60% of the observation. However, further observations of DL have indicated that the time spent in close proximity actually declined in subsequent months as she and her mother continued to spend more time at greater distances from each other.

Far

A look at the time spent in the Far category reveals that a spatial separation of this magnitude required longer to develop (see Fig. 3C). Although the dyads were occasionally observed more than 5 m apart during the first year, this greater spatial separation did not occur regularly until the second year of life. Thereafter, these greater separations were often observed, occurring during 6% of the observation time by 2 years of age and during 15% by 3 years of age. DL, at 5 years of age, now spends nearly 45% of the observation time at these greater distances from her mother.

These progressive changes in the mother–infant relationship are in keeping with descriptive reports of chimpanzee development in the wild and under other captive settings. Van Lawick-Goodall (1967) has reported that infant chimpanzees at Gombe begin to break contact with their mothers between 4–6 months of age and readily move away from their mothers during the second year of life. The continued maintenance of lower levels of contact and proximal distances until 5 years of age has also been reported (Clark, 1977). More detailed analyses comparing SOPF infants with those at Gombe have indicated that captive infants shifted to proximal distances a few months later and at a slightly faster rate than wild infants (Silk and Kraemer, 1978). At present it is not possible to explain this difference since it may reflect a complex interaction of the age and parity status of the SOPF mothers, the sex of the infants, and the different environmental conditions. However, as will be discussed, the overall similarity in the development and sequence of behaviors is more striking than the temporal differences in mother–infant proximity.

MOTHER–INFANT TRAVEL AND THE ONTOGENY OF INDEPENDENT TRAVEL

Ventral Travel

Similarities between SOPF and Gombe infants can be seen in an evaluation of the SOPF infants' shift to different modes of travel: ventral, dorsal and lone travel. During the first 10 months of life the SOPF infants were almost exclusively in the ventral position while traveling with their mothers (see Fig. 4A), which is similar to field reports of ventral travel occurring for the first

6–9 months (van Lawick-Goodall, 1968). Thereafter, the amount of ventral travel declined, dropping from an average 74% of the travel time at 1 year of age to an average of 15% by the end of the second year. By 3 years of age, the SOPF infants rarely assumed this position while traveling. The occasional occurrence of heightened levels of ventral travel in older infants was often related to an environmental or social change, as in the relationship between overall contact levels and disturbance. During times of social excitement or aggression the infant may return to the ventral position for reassurance or protection.

Dorsal Travel

The transition to dorsal travel, which was related to the decline in ventral travel, also was affected by environmental conditions (see Fig. 4B). Van Lawick-Goodall (1968) reports from field observations that it is the mother who initiates the position change and that it usually begins between 5–7 months of age when the infant has more coordination and muscle control. Dorsal travel becomes the predominant mode during the second year of life and allows the mother more ease and comfort in travel. The occurrence of dorsal travel for PA and BY appeared between 10–11 months of age and within a few months it accounted for more than 50% of the travel time. DL differed from this pattern in that she did not travel in the dorsal position until the end of the second year of life. Moreover, DL's manifestation of dorsal travel peaked at only 35% and then declined to 12% at the end of the third year. The delay in the appearance of DL's dorsal travel and its abbreviated occurrence reflects the two environmental shifts which occurred during her development. The fact that GY and DL were living on a relatively small island during the period when we would have expected to see the inception of dorsal travel most probably inhibited its occurrence. DL did ride dorsal, although infrequently, just prior to the move to SOPF. After the move, she traveled in the dorsal position with increased regularity in the succeeding months. It is also noteworthy that despite the individual differences in the onset of dorsal travel, it began to decline in all the infants during the third year of life as independent travel occurred more frequently.

Independent Travel

In Figure 4C the percent of the infant's time spent traveling when out of contact with the mother is portrayed. This form of independent (lone) travel was often done in association with the mother and other animals, occurring as a type of group travel. The developing infants first began to travel out of contact with their mother at the end of the first year and progressively spent

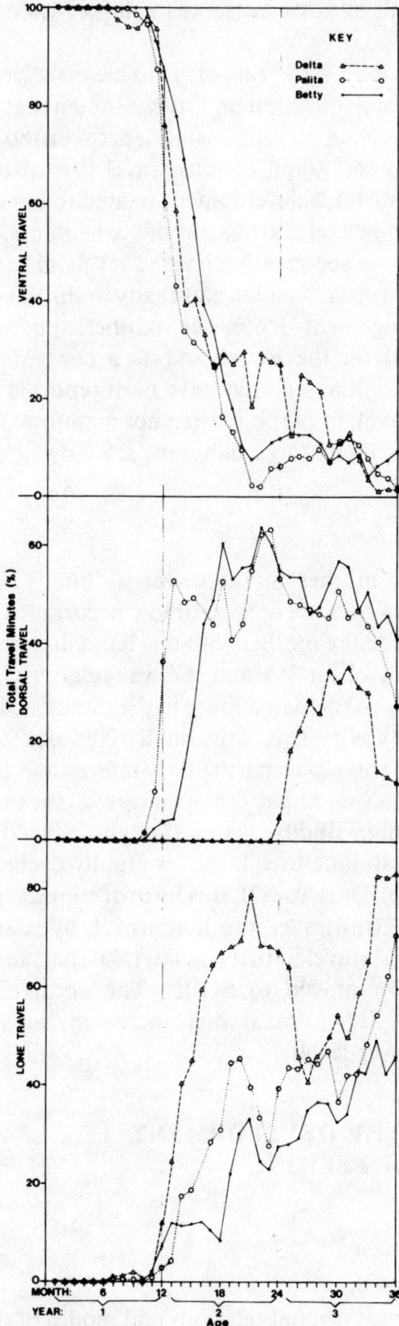

FIG. 4. Types of mother-infant travel and independent travel. Percent of total travel time spent in ventral (upper graph, A), dorsal (middle graph, B) and lone travel (lower graph, C).

more time traveling alone. At 3 years of age, a mean 67% of the travel was lone travel. Subsequent data collection on DL has shown that during the fifth year of life, she was traveling in this fashion between 80–99% of the travel observation time. In the graph of lone travel it is also possible to see an idiosyncratic aspect of DL's development related to her delay in the onset of dorsal travel. During her second year of life, when dorsal travel would have typically developed, we see greatly elevated levels of lone travel. Although speculative, it would appear that DL was ready to shift to dorsal travel but did not receive encouragement from her mother, possibly because travel distances were small on the island and as a consequence DL shifted to independent travel. Similar findings have been reported for monkey species that utilize dorsal travel, in that it is often not manifested under the confined conditions of captive living (e.g., baboons; see Rowell, 1972, p. 142).

Buddy Walk

Another mode of mother–infant travel is "buddy walk," which is not illustrated graphically because of its sporadic occurrence. In buddy walk, the infant travels alongside the mother with one hand on the mother's waist. The frequency of such travel for PA and BY was relatively low (less than 8%), when it occurred. DL participated more in the buddy walk during her second year, again most likely as a result of the small island size. The manner in which she used this form of travel was particularly interesting. Her buddy walk and lone travel exhibited a similar pattern of increase at the same time that ventral travel was decreasing. Buddy walk, though, peaked at 20% and was manifested earlier than lone travel; then it rapidly declined while lone travel continued to increase. Thus, for DL this form of contact travel appeared to be a transition from ventral travel into lone travel, bypassing temporarily the usual pattern of dorsal travel until much later. DL had another peak of buddy walk after the group moved to SOPF. The occurrence of buddy walk continued to increase as her dorsal travel increased, but after a few months it declined to much lower levels.

SUCKLING AND THE DEVELOPMENT OF INDEPENDENT FEEDING

Suckling

These shifts in the dyads' spatial relations and modes of travel paralleled the changes in the infants' nutritional dependence on their mothers. Clark (1977) reports that nipple contact in Gombe infants was highest during the first six months of life, bouts occurring 2.7 times per hour, and then declined to stable levels of once per hour during the second and third year of life. Suckling by the SOPF infants, based on the observation of nipple contact, was highest during the first six months of life (see Fig. 5A). The low levels of suckling indicated for PA during her first few months were due to difficulty of observation on the island. Between Months 7 and 15, the levels of suckling decreased and then plateaued at a low level. These low levels were maintained until the end of the third year of life when there was a small but consistent increase in nipple contact for all infants apparently related to the onset of their mother's sexual cycles. The increase in nipple contact may have occurred because of decreased milk production by the mothers. However, another contributing factor may be that the increase in nipple contact occurred because of the higher incidence of maternal rejection and infant distress occurring at this time (portrayed later in Fig. 7). GY did not conceive after she resumed cycling and DL continued to manifest the higher levels of nipple contact during the fourth year of life (an IUD was inserted in GY when DL was 42 months old and removed during Month 61). In contrast, nipple contact for PA declined sharply after her mother conceived in Month 34 and six months later PA had virtually stopped suckling. BY, at 36 months, continues to show the higher incidence of suckling which began after BO resumed cycling.

Feeding

Paralleling the decline in suckling there was a progressive increase in eating of solid foods and drinking (see Fig. 5B). Independent feeding started to occur between Months 4–6 and increased rapidly with age. The infants developed their feeding habits through the manipulation of foodstuffs while with their mothers and through observational learning, and appeared to use begging as a transition from suckling to foraging for their own food (McGrew, 1975, 1977). The occurrence of infants begging or taking food from their mothers and from other chimpanzees increased along with the development of independent feeding (Fig. 6). Begging involves the infant peering into another animal's face, mouth, or hands. The infant may then be offered some food, allowed to take some, or the infant may snatch some away from the other animal. The frequency of this behavior increased during the infant's first three years, but as it did, there was also a tendency for the frequency of unsuccessful begs to increase. Generally during the second year, the infant started to beg more often from individuals other than the mother, although the begs from the mother were usually more successful than those from others. Individual differences can be seen in the amount of begging, and the success or failure of the begging bouts. These results are in agreement with those obtained by Silk (1978) from the chimpanzees at the Gombe National Park. She also states that after 3 years of age, the frequency of food sharing decreases.

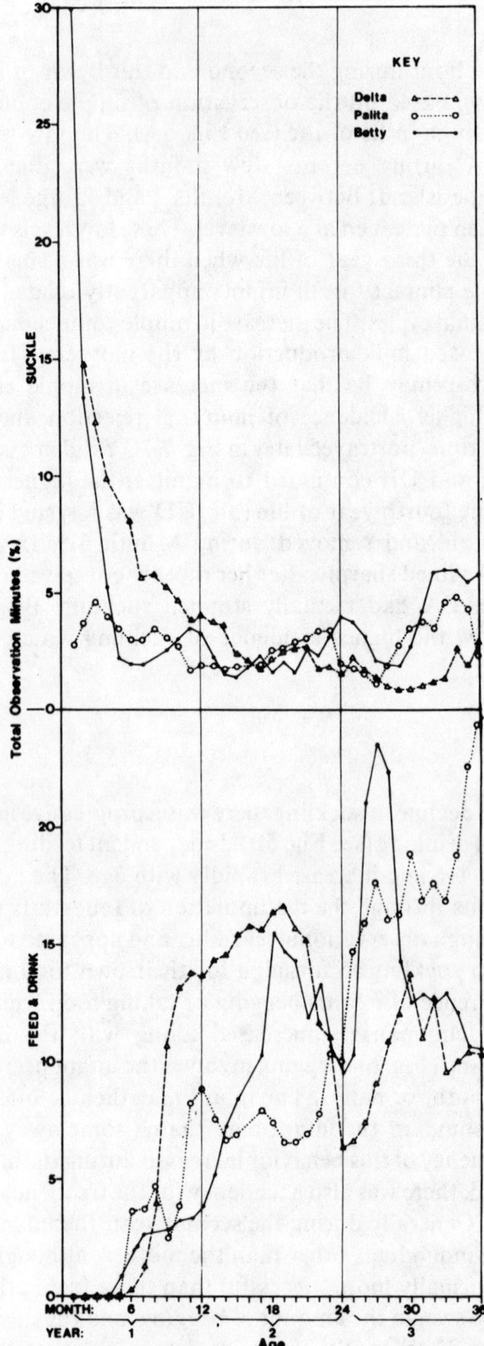

FIG. 5. Percent of the observations that the infants spent suckling (upper graph, A) and in feeding and drinking (lower graph, B).

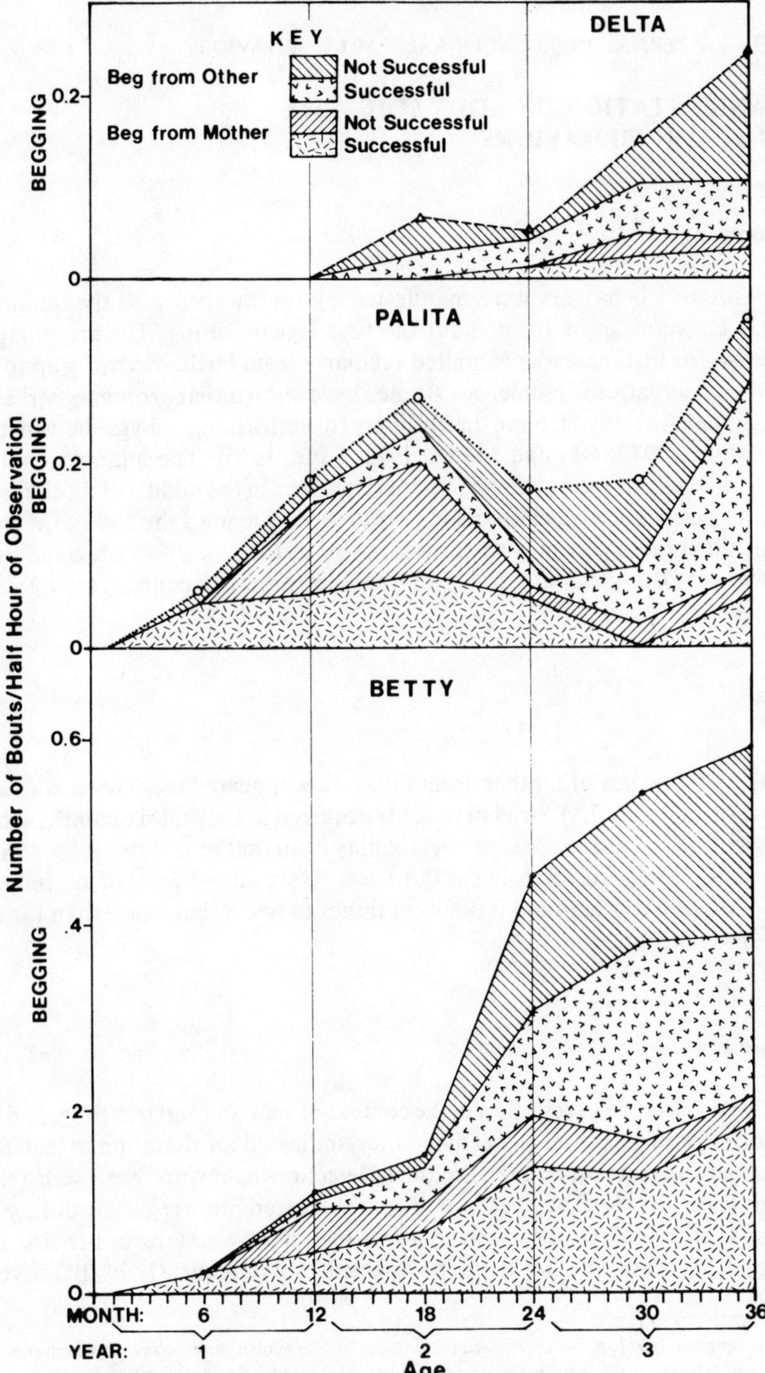

FIG. 6. Frequency of infant begging for food from the mother and other chimpanzees. The data have been presented as the number of begging bouts per 30-minute observation at 6-month intervals and also indicate the level of successful food-sharing.

MANIFESTATION OF ADDYADIC AND ABDYADIC BEHAVIORS[1]

Grooming

Affiliative behaviors were manifested by the mothers and the infants at fairly constant levels throughout the first 3 years of life. The grooming of infants, for instance, was exhibited regularly from birth, occurring up to 7% of the observations. Numerous studies have shown that grooming serves to strengthen the social bond in addition to performing a hygienic function (Lindburg, 1973; Oki and Maedi, 1973; Sade, 1965). The infants were first seen to briefly and clumsily groom their mothers in the middle of the first year but its occurrence was infrequent. From that time until the end of the third year, the infants groomed their mothers for less than 1.0% of observed time. However, DL's grooming of her mother increased in frequency after 3 years of age.

Play

The occurrence of mother–infant play also appeared to serve an addyadic function (see Fig. 7A). Brief play bouts occurred in the first six months. There was a trend toward increasing levels of play from that time through the second year and decreasing levels in the third year. Data after 3 years of age indicate play between mothers and infants continues to occur, but at less than 1.0% of the observed time.

Rejections

The occurrence of rejection in the context of suckling and traveling, and the occurrence of active maternal avoidance, indicated an alteration in maternal responsiveness toward older infants. Rejection behaviors were seen infrequently during the first 2 years of life and occurred more regularly during the third year (Fig. 7B). BY received a few scattered rejections in her first and second year but she began to be rejected more frequently by BO several

[1]Rosenblum (1971, p. 346) proposed these terms to distinguish those behaviors which enhance and maintain the mother-infant bond from those which reduce and disrupt it.

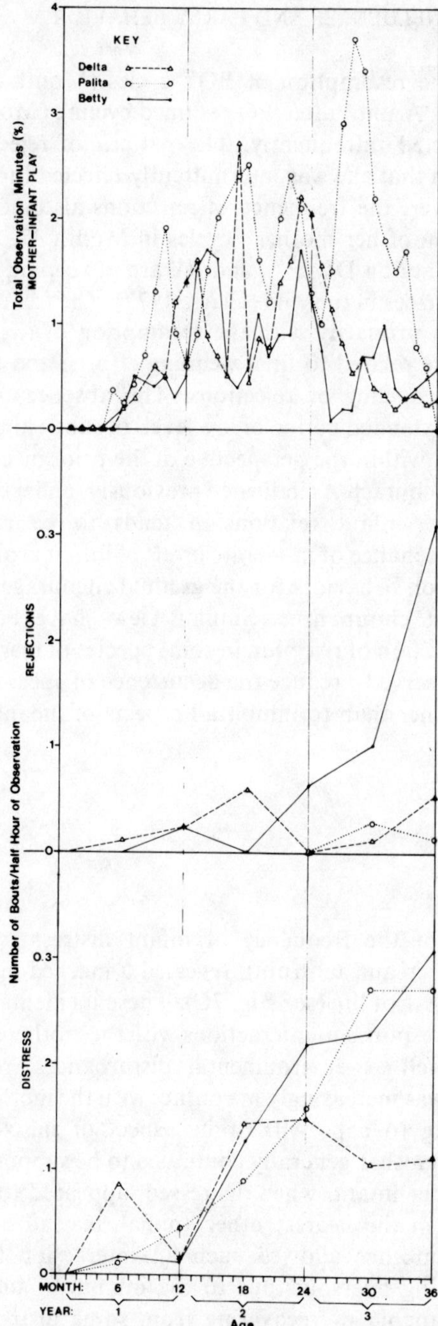

FIG. 7. Percent of observations during which play occurred between mother and infant (upper graph, A). The frequencies of maternal rejection (middle graph, B) and infant distress (lower graph, C) per 30-minute observation are also indicated at 6-month intervals.

months prior to the resumption of BO's cycles (Month 32). PO was not observed to reject PA until after PO resumed cycling (Month 28) and even then PA was rejected infrequently. The pattern of rejections which DL received differed, in that she was intermittently rejected throughout the first three years. However, the frequency of rejections also increased markedly after the resumption of her mother's cycles in Month 37.

These rejection data on DL, PA, and BY are in keeping with the study of weaning in chimpanzees in the wild (Clark, 1977). The frequency of rejection behaviors increases primarily with the resumption of the mother's sexual cycle, they are more related to final weaning efforts, and the mothers vary greatly in their frequency of rejections. The absence of overt punitive behaviors and the extended period of low levels of subtle and active rejections may be understood within the perspective of the prior discussion of arousal and mother–infant contact. As indicated previously, under conditions of high arousal the mother–infant relationship tends to be reestablished and therefore, the maintenance of moderate levels of infant arousal may be more critical than rejection behaviors for the gradual encouragement of independenc in the infant chimpanzee. Similar views have been expressed in interpreting the function of rejection in some species of macaque and suggest that rejection may serve to reduce the occurrence of specific components of infant behavior rather than to inhibit all aspects of the infant's attachment (Rosenblum, 1971).

Distress

An evaluation of the frequency of infant distress (seek reassurance, whimper, squeak, scream, tantrum), revealed a marked increase during the second and third year of life (see Fig. 7C). These incidents of infant distress which occurred in response to interactions with the mother and also the other chimpanzees as well as environmental disturbances, revealed that the developing infant was increasingly in conflict with the mother or increasingly found itself having to cope with some aspect of the social or physical environment. The mother generally continued to be supportive and reassure the infant. The older infant, when distressed, appeared to be soothed by a reassuring hug from the nearest other animal, instead of seeking out the mother, and the mother allowed such an interaction to occur without interfering and being oversolicitous to the infant. In addition, the infant appeared to be capable of recovering from some distress bouts without reassurance during years 2 and 3.

ONTOGENETIC CHANGES IN THE INFANT

Independent Motor Activity

A large component of the ontogeny of independence appeared to be due to a change in the infant's attention away from the mother and toward the environment and other social partners. As the infant's physical capabilities developed, it expressed a greater interest in the environment. This progression can be seen in Figure 8A which shows the time spent in independent motor activity which includes object exploration and play, lone locomotor play, and general activity. General activity includes that portion of the infant's time when the infant is squirming, aimlessly wandering around, or amusing itself with no apparent purpose. Independent motoric activity appeared in the first few months of life, developed progressively during the second year of life, and plateaued at a mean 23% during the third year. Although the levels differed between infants, the pattern of progressive development remains clear. Some of the differences between infants may be accounted for by a revision in definitions in Month 33, 13 and 5 for DL, PA and BY respectively, which may have elevated the levels of independent motor activity.

Social Play

In addition to the development of lone activities, the infants became more attracted to and responsive to other animals. Although a full discussion of these interactions is beyond the scope of the present chapter, a presentation of the development of social play reveals the major point (Fig. 7B). As the infant develops, an increasing percentage of its day is spent in interaction with others. Play, as in most mammalian young, becomes a common behavior pattern. It occurred frequently after the infant was able to make independent excursions and by 3 years of age it was occurring during 12% of the observations, further facilitating the shift away from the mother.

COMPARISON WITH A DEVELOPING MALE INFANT

A year of observation has been completed on a male infant, reared under similar conditions in the second enclosure at SOPF. Observations were begun at parturition and are continuing. The data collection was identical to that

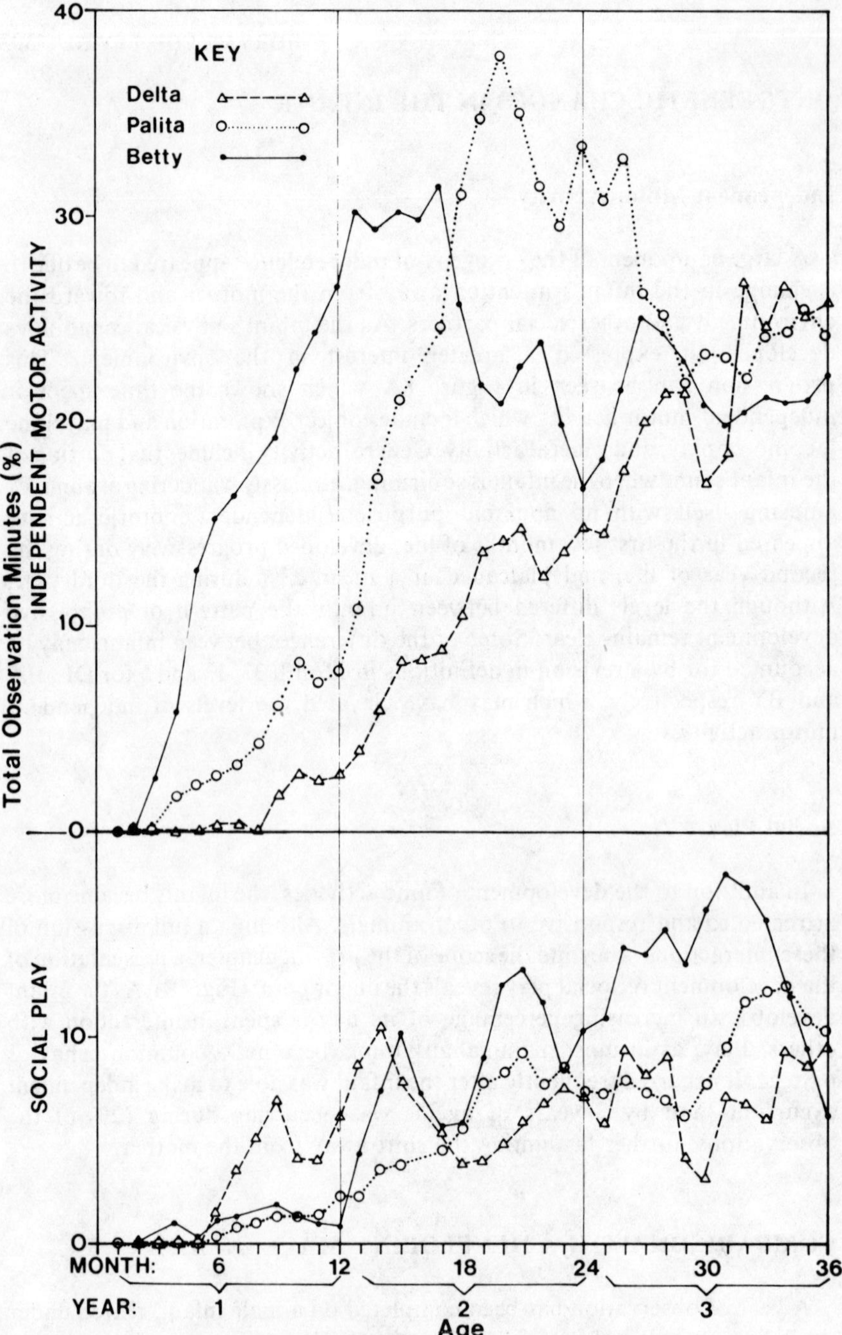

FIG. 8. Development of independent infant behaviors. The percent of the observations that the infants spent in object exploration and play, lone locomotor play, and general activity is indicated in the upper graph (A). The percent occurrence of infant social play with chimpanzees other than their mother is indicated in the lower graph (B).

described previously. The mother, Bashful (BS) had a similar rearing to the other mothers in that she was imported from the wild between 1-2 years of age and was reared in a captive social group. Her first infant, Bahati (BA) was born at SOPF on July 7, 1976. Their social group consisted of one adult male, two adult females, two adolescent males and two juvenile males. (Prior to the birth of BA, BS displayed some aspects of maternal behavior to two infant males—now juveniles—when they were introduced as orphans to BS's social group. Therefore, BS should possibly be considered as having prior "maternal experience.")

Although one must be cautious in making comparisons at this point, there were several striking differences in this infant's developmental pattern that are worthy of note. The entire developmental sequence was accelerated when compared to the other SOPF infants. Although the decline in mother-infant contact was not overtly different, BA was first seen in the Near category in Month 4, which was earlier than the female infants. After 6 months of age, he and his mother were spending more time away from each other in each succeeding month than did the female infants. Similarly, this precocious pattern was evident in the shift to further distances. BA began to be in the Far category shortly after 6 months of age and by 10 months he was manifesting levels not seen by the female infants until they were 1.5 years of age.

The different modes of travel also revealed a marked acceleration of his development when compared with the other infants. The decline in ventral travel began in Month 4 rather than in Month 7 as had been previously observed, and he continued to manifest lower levels of ventral travel during his first year. It was not surprising therefore to see an accelerated appearance of dorsal travel, occurring regularly after Month 4, and a more rapid development of lone travel. Also, BA did not engage in any buddy walk with his mother. An evaluation of maternal rejections and infant distress also reflected the more rapid developmental pattern of BA. He received rejections throughout his first year, and they occurred at a greater frequency between Months 6–12 than they did for any of the other infants. His frequency of distress also occurred at levels above that of DL, PA or BY for the same time period.

The differences in the social rearing environment do not permit a postulation of sex differences as the underlying cause of BA's early development of independence, even though there is some evidence to support a conjecture of this sort (Jensen et al., 1968; Mitchell, 1968; Nicolson, 1977; Rosenblum, 1974; Sackett, 1972; Silk and Kraemer, 1978). It is of more general interest, however, to consider the interrelationship of the developing behaviors. The early appearance of one behavior seemed to lead sequentially into the accelerated development of other behaviors. Thus, the pattern of BA's development also portrays the set of spatial and interactive behaviors as an integrated behavioral system.

DISCUSSION

The data presented on the SOPF mothers and infants indicate that under some captive conditions there appears to be a normal unfolding of the chimpanzee mother-infant relationship. The developmental patterns of the mother-infant spatial relations, modes of travel, suckling and interactional behaviors were similar to those reported for wild chimpanzees (Clark, 1977; van Lawick-Goodall, 1967, 1968). This finding is encouraging for the further study of mother-infant relations under captive conditions because it qualifies previous reports of aberrant maternal behaviors manifested in captivity (Nicholson, 1977; Rogers and Davenport, 1970; Yerkes and Tomilin, 1935). The presence of a freely-interacting social group and relatively enriched living environment provided at SOPF seems to facilitate the more species-typical development of mother-infant relations. This point is especially interesting in light of the fact that all the mothers were primiparous and had been reared in captivity. Although the patterns of infant development at SOPF were similar to those known for chimpanzee infants in the wild, one might expect that the levels of occurrence of specific behaviors would be different due to ecological pressures and social factors. In the wild, the mother-infant pairs are often alone (Halperin, in press), whereas at SOPF they are members of a relatively constant social group. Therefore, the levels of mother-infant behaviors, such as groom and play, may be lower at SOPF than at Gombe, and similarly social interactions with others may occur at greater frequency than in the wild. However, systematic comparisons, other than of mother-infant spatial proximity (Silk and Kraemer, 1978) have not been made.

This chapter represents only a portion of the data collected on these mother-infant pairs. We plan further analysis of the remaining data and also additional studies of the more subtle aspects of the mother-infant relationship. This chapter, though, indicates that the progression toward independence during the first three years is due in large part to ontogenetic changes in the infant rather than due to rejection by the mother. The infants revealed a steady increase in independent activities (e.g., feeding, environmental exploration, and social interactions) during this period whereas maternal rejections did not appear regularly until the end of the third or early in the fourth year of life. These data suggest that the mother encourages the development of independence through supportive behaviors and that the infant's readiness for independent activities is facilitated by maintenance of moderate levels of arousal (Mason, 1970, 1971). The increased frequency of rejection behaviors appeared to be related to the onset of sexual cycles in the mother and to the final weaning efforts, as has been suggested by Clark (1977). This temporal association is suggestive of a hormonal influence on the manifestation of maternal behavior; however a causal relationship has not been established.

Although the mother-infant relationship in the chimpanzee is greatly extended, the underlying developmental progression appears to be similar to that observed in other simian primates. The concepts of "contact comfort" (Harlow and Zimmerman, 1959) and the "approach-withdrawal" dichotomy (Hinde and Spencer-Booth, 1967; Schneirla, 1959), for example, appear to have general applicability to chimpanzee development. As observed in other primates there appears to be an extended period of maternal support followed by a transitional stage of maternal rejection related to weaning (Harlow et al., 1963). These shifts in the mother's behavior are paralleled by ontogenetic changes in the infant. A decrease in the infant's dependence on the mother occurs concomitantly with an expansion in its social and environmental spheres and results finally in diminished levels of mother-infant contact and interaction.

SUMMARY

Developmental changes in the chimpanzee mother-infant relationship were studied in four captive dyads at the Stanford Outdoor Primate Facility. The occurrences of the following behaviors were analyzed for the first 3 years of life: spacial relations between mother and infant, travel, suckle and feed, food sharing, mother-infant play, maternal rejections, infant distress, independent motor activity and social play. The unfolding of the developmental sequence for the SOPF infants was similar to that reported for infants in the wild although differences in the frequencies of the behaviors undoubtedly exist.

ACKNOWLEDGMENTS

This chapter is the result of over five years of observations on these chimpanzee mothers and infants. Such a long-term study is possible only with the combined efforts of many people, a list far too long to name each person here. We warmly thank each of them. Special thanks are due: Byron Alexander, Cathy Clark, Debi Hamburger, Janet Hoare, Nancy Merrick, and Pal Midgett. Most importantly, it was the foresight and cooperation of Drs. Jane Goodall, David A. Hamburg, Helena C. Kraemer and Patrick R. McGinnis that made SOPF a reality. Funds were provided by the Grant Foundation and NIH Grant No. MH 23645. Finally, we express our appreciation of the mothers and infants, not only for what we have learned from them, but also for the pure pleasure they have given us all.

REFERENCES

Clark, C. B. A preliminary report on weaning among chimpanzees of the Gombe National Park, Tanzania. In *Primate Bio-Social Development: Biological, Social and Ecological Determinants*, S. Chevalier-Skolnikoff and F. E. Poirier, eds. Garland Publishing, Inc., New York (1977), pp. 235–260.

Fossey, D. Development of the mountain gorilla (*Gorilla gorilla beringei*) through the first thirty-six months. In *Perspectives on Human Evolution, Vol. 5: The Great Apes*, D. A. Hamburg and E. R. McCown, eds. W. A. Benjamin Press, Menlo Park, California (in press).

Halperin, S. D. Temporary association patterns in free ranging chimpanzees: An assessment of individual grouping preferences. In *Perspectives on Human Evolution, Vol. 5: The Great Apes*, D. A. Hamburg and E. R. McCown, eds. W. A. Benjamin Press, Menlo Park, California (in press).

Harlow, H. F. and Harlow, M. K. Effects of various mother-infant relationships on rhesus monkey behaviors. In *Determinants of Infant Behaviour, Vol. 4*, B. M. Foss, ed. Methuen, London (1969), pp. 15–36.

Harlow, H. F. and Zimmerman, R. R. Affectional responses in the infant monkey. *Science 130*, 421–432 (1959).

Harlow, H. F., Harlow, M. K., and Hansen, E. W. The maternal affectional system of rhesus monkeys. In *Maternal Behavior of Mammals*, H. L. Rheingold, ed. John Wiley & Sons, Inc., New York (1963), pp. 254–281.

Hinde, R. A. and Spencer-Booth, Y. The behavior of socially living rhesus monkeys in their first two and a half years. *Anim. Behav. 15*, 169–196 (1967).

Horr, D. A. Orang-utan maturation: Growing up in a female world. In *Primate Bio-social Development: Biological, Social and Ecological Determinants*, S. Chevalier-Skolnikoff and F. E. Poirier, eds. Garland Publishing, Inc., New York (1977), pp. 289–321.

Jensen, G. D., Bobbitt, R. A., and Gordon, B. N. Sex differences in the development of independence of infant monkeys. *Behaviour 30*, 1–14 (1968).

Kendall, M. G. *The Advanced Theory of Statistics.* Volume II, Charles Griffin and Co., Ltd., London (1955), p. 372.

Koyama, N. On dominance rank and kinship of a wild Japanese monkey troop in Arashiyama. *Primates 8*, 189–216 (1967).

Kraemer, H. C., Alexander, B., Clark, C., Busse, C., and Riss, D. Empirical choice of sampling procedures for optimal research design in the longitudinal study of primate behavior. *Primates, 18,* 825–833 (1978).

Lancaster, J. B. In praise of the achieving female monkey. *Psychol. Today 7*, 30–37 (1973).

Lindburg, D. G. Grooming behavior as a regulator of social interactions in rhesus monkeys. In *Behavioral Regulation of Behavior in Primates*, C. R. Carpenter, ed. Bucknell University Press, Lewisburg (1973), pp. 124–148.

Mason, W. A. Chimpanzee social behavior. In *The Chimpanzee, Vol. 2*, G. H. Bourne, ed. S. Karger, Basel (1970), pp. 265–288.

McGinnis, P. R. and Kraemer, H. C. The Stanford Outdoor Primate Facility: A new laboratory for biobehavioral research in chimpanzees. Laboratory of Stress and Conflict Technical Report Series #114 (Stanford Univ.) (1977).

McGrew, W. C. Patterns of plant food sharing by wild chimpanzees. In *Proceedings of the Vth Congress of the International Primatological Society*, Nagoya, Japan. Karger, Basel (1975).

McGrew, W. C. Socialization and object manipulation of wild chimpanzees. In *Primate Bio-social Development: Biological, Social and Ecological Determinants*, S. Chevalier-Skolnikoff and F. E. Poirier, eds. Garland Publishing, Inc., New York (1977), pp. 261–281.

Menzel, E. W. Spontaneous invention of ladders in a group of young chimpanzees. *Folia Primatol. 17*, 87–106 (1972).

Merrick, N. Social grooming and play behavior of a captive group of chimpanzees. *Primates 18*, 215–224 (1977).

Mitchell, G. D. Attachment differences in male and female infant monkeys. *Child Dev. 37*, 781–791 (1968).

Nicolson, N. A. A comparison of early behavioral development in wild and captive chimpanzees. In *Primate Bio-social Development: Biological, Social and Ecological Determinants.* S. Chevalier-Skolnikoff and F. E. Poirier, eds. Garland Publishing, Inc., New York (1977), pp. 529–560.

Oki, J. and Maedi, Y. Grooming as a regulator of behavior in Japanese macaques. In *Behavioral Regulation of Behavior in Primates*, C. R. Carpenter, ed. Bucknell University Press, Lewisburg (1973), pp. 149–163.

Rogers, C. M. and Davenport, R. K. Chimpanzee maternal behavior. In *The Chimpanzee*, Vol. 3, G. H. Bourne, ed. S. Karger, Basel (1970), pp. 361–368.

Rosenblum, L. A. The ontogeny of mother-infant relations in macaques. In *The Ontogeny of Vertebrate Behavior*, H. Moltz, ed. Academic Press, New York (1971), pp. 315–367.

Rosenblum, L. A. Sex differences, environmental complexity, and mother-infant relations. *Arch. Sex. Behav. 3*, 117–128 (1974).

Rowell, T. *Social Behavior of Monkeys.* Penguin Books, London (1972).

Sackett, G. P. Exploratory behavior of rhesus monkeys as a function of rearing experiences and sex. *Dev. Psychol. 6*, 260–270 (1972).

Sade, D. S. Some aspects of parent-offspring and sibling relations in a group of rhesus monkeys, with a discussion of grooming. *Am. J. Phys. Anthropol. 23*, 1–17 (1965).

Savage, E. S. and Malick, C. Play and socio-sexual behaviour in a captive chimpanzee (*Pan troglodytes*) group. *Behaviour LX*, 1–2 (1977).

Savage, E. S., Temerlin, J. W., and Lemmon, W. B. Group information among captive mother-infant chimpanzees (*Pan troglodytes*). *Folia Primatol. 20*, 453–473 (1973).

Schaller, G. B. *The Mountain Gorilla: Ecology and Behavior.* University of Chicago Press, Chicago (1963).

Schneirla, T. C. An evolutionary and developmental theory of biphasic processes underlying approach and withdrawal. *Nebraska Symposium on Motivation*, University of Nebraska Press (1959), pp. 1–43.

Silk, J. B. Patterns of food sharing among mother and infant chimpanzees at Gombe National Park, Tanzania. *Folia Primatol. 29,* 129–141 (1978).

Silk, J. B. and Kraemer, H. C. Comparison of mother-infant proximity among wild and captive chimpanzees, in *VIth Congress of the International Primatological Society*, Cambridge. Karger, Basel (1978).

van Lawick-Goodall, J. The behavior of free-living chimpanzees in the Gombe Stream Reserve. *Anim. Behav. Monogr. 1*, 161–311 (1968).

van Lawick-Goodall, J. Mother-offspring relationships in free-ranging chimpanzees. In *Primate Ethology*, D. Morris, ed. Aldine Publishing Company, Chicago (1967), pp. 365–436.

Yerkes, R. M. and Tomilin, M. I. Mother-infant relations in chimpanzee. *J. Comp. Psychol. 20*, 321–359 (1935).

Maternal Influences and Early Behavior

14

Maternal Separation Studies in Children and Nonhuman Primates

Lynda M. McGinnis

Over the last twenty years or so, considerable research has been carried out on the response of infant non-human primates and children to brief loss of the mother-figure (Bowlby, 1951; Jensen and Tolman, 1962; Heinicke and Westheimer, 1965; Seay, Hansen and Harlow, 1962; Bowlby, 1973; Kaufman and Rosenblum, 1969; Spencer-Booth and Hinde, 1971; Hinde and Davies, 1972; Rutter, 1972; Schlottman and Seay, 1972; and Hinde and McGinnis, 1977). The findings on children and monkeys have complemented one another and have added considerably to our understanding of the dynamics of the mother-infant relationship. These studies have gone a long way in helping to assess the importance of the mother-figure in infancy and have indicated the importance of the quality of interaction between mother and infant.

HISTORICAL REVIEW

Controversy still rages over the importance of the mother *per se*. Bowlby (1951) claimed that "... mother love in infancy and childhood is as important for mental health as are vitamins and proteins for physical health." Rutter (1972) claimed that it may not be loss or lack of mother that is wholly responsible for the extreme emotional distress in young children separated from their mothers, but that factors arising from loss or lack of mother may in part also be responsible such as: less attention and care given the infant, exposure to unfamiliar surroundings and persons, and lack of adequate substitutes for the mother. Rutter argued that if these factors could be controlled in maternal separations, then extreme adverse effects may be reduced. He quoted, as an example, the work of Robertson and Robertson (1971) in which young children exposed to temporary loss of mother were cared for by relatively familiar caretakers in familiar surroundings during the mother's absence. These infants were less distressed than infants left in completely unfamiliar places with strangers. The Robertsons also took special care to follow the mother's routine in caretaking behaviors, so that the infants suffered minimal degree of change in care and attention received. There is contrary evidence from other studies, however, that children were still distressed during mother's absence, even if they were left at home with familiar caretakers (Deutsch, 1919; Spiro, 1958). These latter findings imply that it is loss of mother per se that is responsible for the infants' distress. The mother-figure does have many stress-reducing properties for young children exposed to extremely alarming situations. Fagin (1966) showed that the distress produced by hospitalization was much reduced if mothers were admitted with their children, and Rheingold (1969) found that distress in strange environments was reduced when the infants' mothers were present. A study by Vernon et al. (1967), however, suggested that mothers had only a small effect in reducing infant distress on hospitalization, indicating that other factors may be operative. These studies were reviewed by Rutter (1972).

The findings from these different studies are often conflicting and confusing, and yet some answer needs to be reached. In this day and age, when young mothers have many other interests outside home activities and day-care centers are flourishing, one needs to be able to assess the effects of these brief separations on young children, not only for the child's healthy development, but also for the reassurance of anxious mothers who have to work, or who have to suffer separations from their young children as a result of necessary travel or hospitalization. Bowlby's findings implied that maternal deprivation in infancy was responsible for a variety of maladaptive behaviours such as: dwarfism, affectionless psychopathy, mental retardation, deliquency, and depression. Rutter (1972) emphasised that some distinction should be made between the effects of loss of mothering (or deprivation) and lack of mothering (privation), and that factors operating in each situation should be analyzed and the separate effects of each determined.

PRIVATION STUDIES

Extreme syndromes such as dwarfism and affectionless psychopathy and mental retardation have been shown to result from complete lack of any kind of mothering in infancy. Dwarfism has been found to be a result of malnutrition that accompanies extreme neglect (Rutter, 1972). Mental retardation is also a result of extreme neglect and possibly poor nutrition as well. Brossard and Décarie (1972) found that if children in institutions were given some form of sensory stimulation in infancy, their mental development was much improved. In the old style orphanages and creches, the infants were often left during their waking hours in their cots without any form of suitable sensory or social stimulation. It is now thought that this accounted for mental retardation and affectionless psychopathy seen in these children as they developed. Although sensory stimulation in infancy seems to improve mental functioning, there is no evidence to support the view that it enables infants to form social attachments. Rheingold (1956) showed that extra mothering in institutionalized infants did help them to form attachments, however, and in more modern orphanages children have been shown to form attachments when mothered, even though they may have multiple mother-figures (Stevens, 1971). Thus some form of mothering seems to help in the development of social attachments in children who have no experience of normal mothering.

In connection with these privation studies on children, research has been carried out on infant rhesus monkeys by Harlow and his colleagues at Wisconsin. They have subjected newborn rhesus infants to various forms of privation rearing, to test the importance of the different affectional systems (Harlow and Harlow, 1972). Infant monkeys reared in total or partial social isolation were totally inept as socially functioning individuals. They did not show adequate social, play, sexual or maternal behaviors, and their behavior was remarkably similar to that of psychotic humans.

Harlow did show that infant rhesus monkeys could be reared successfully without mothering, however, if they were reared in peer groups. These infants reared together without mothers formed intense attachments to each other, which retarded the development of normal play behaviors; but once the pattern of intense clinging behavior was broken, the infants played normally and developed adequate social behaviors. The latter case is similar to that described for six refugee children by Freud and Dann (1972). These children also formed intense attachments to each other that were broken only with difficulty and they related poorly to others at first. Later they began to develop adequate social responses. Thus, peers can compensate for mothers in social development.

In monkeys, however, it must be borne in mind that such a system would not work in the wild. Infant monkeys could not survive without their mothers' milk, or without maternal protection from predators and maternal transport in keeping up with the troop (Harlow and Harlow, 1972).

The severe effects of lack of mothering, therefore, do not seem to be due to lack of mother per se, but to complete rejection or neglect, resulting in malnourishment and total lack of adequate sensory and social stimulation. In young children and monkeys, where the period of dependency is so extended, it seems unlikely that some safeguard does not exist to ensure normal social development, since loss of mother is possible and, therefore, other figures should be able to compensate somewhat for the loss of mother (Harlow and Harlow, 1972).

DEPRIVATION STUDIES

The characteristic responses to loss of mother (to whom attachment has already been formed) are the depression or despair reaction and, in children, but not usually monkeys, the rejection response on reunion with the mother (Robertson and Bowlby, 1952). The depression response may predispose individuals to depression at later stages of development and, therefore, impair mental health. It is possible that a maternal separation in infancy may be the child's first distressful experience in development and may be the child's first encounter with a threat to personal security. It is a new situation in most cases, and one in which the child has to learn new ways of coping. The following factors have been found to affect the response of young children and monkeys to brief loss of mother.

Experience with Substitute Caretakers Before Separation

If others with whom the child has formed attachments and with whom the child feels secure are present during separation, they may help considerably in the child's ability to cope with loss of mother. Evidence for this comes from the studies by the Robertsons cited previously, and from studies on monkeys by Kaufman and Rosenblum (1969). In the latter, it was found that bonnet macaque infants were less affeced by maternal separation than pigtail macaque infants. The former had experienced a much greater degree of interaction with group companions in the course of development than the pigtail infants. When the bonnet mothers were removed, their infants were cared for by others, whereas the pigtail infants were rebuffed by their companions in their mothers' absence and received no care. The pigtail infants became exceedingly depressed, while the bonnet infants, although distressed initially, did not show depressed behavior.

The reasons for these species differences in response to loss of mother were attributed to differences in social organization. Bonnet macaque adults spend a great deal of time in close proximity to each other and bonnet females allow others to handle and take their infants, even in the early stages of development. Pigtail mothers, on the other hand, keep apart and prevent others' access to their infants. The latter tends to give rise to more exclusive attachment to the mother, which may produce greater distress at separation.

Species differences in infant response to separation have to be taken into account in separation experiments with monkeys, therefore, and the fact that these experiments are also performed in artificial groupings that occur in laboratories is another important aspect to be considered. In their natural conditions in the wild, there is evidence that pigtails live in kin groups, in which they do spend more time in closer proximity to each other than in unrelated groupings in captivity (Rosenblum, 1973).

These findings on monkeys are similar to those emphasized for different human societies by Mead (1962). Mead pointed out that in certain human societies infants are cared for by a number of individuals as well as their mothers, and these infants do not seem to be distressed by maternal separations. These findings do not rule out the possibility that there may be a limit to the number of caretakers to whom the child can relate in a meaningful and more permanent way.

The Effects of Age, Sex and Duration of the Separation Period

Other important factors that have to be considered in cases of maternal separation are the age and sex of the child and the duration of the separation experience. It is difficult to set age limits on a child's response to loss of mother, because individual differences in response at each age are vast. Presumably, the separation syndrome of protest, despair, and rejection are not seen before the child is able to distinguish mother from others, and there may be a great deal of individual variation in the age at which this occurs. Characteristically, distress at separation is not usually seen in infants under 6 months of age (Rutter, 1972). Distress at separation may be less marked once a child is able to use and understand language effectively and has developed other social ties such as peer companionships. However, there is individual variation in the upper age limit (Rutter, 1972).

In monkeys and apes, upper age limits are also subject to individual variation. Infant monkeys are not usually affected by maternal separations after 1 year of age. Spencer-Booth and Hinde (1971) report that from 20 to 30 weeks of age the response of infant rhesus monkeys to separation was similar, but that younger infants recovered faster on reunion with their mothers, since these mothers were usually more attentive and less rejecting than mothers of older infants. There are indications from studies of chimpanzees in the wild that even when the older juveniles are approaching the stage of travelling apart from their mothers, they may indicate some distress at their mothers' reluctance to follow them or they are distressed if they temporarily lose their mothers (Pusey, 1977). One 8-year-old chimp became exceedingly depressed on the loss of his elderly mother, and in this weakened state became susceptible to infection and died. However, this was an unusually prolonged and close association between mother and son (Goodall, 1975).

Orphaned chimps, whose mothers have died after their infants can fend for themselves as far as food-getting is concerned, have a very high mortality rate unless cared for by elder siblings. These orphaned chimps show extreme depression and withdrawal from social activities (Goodall, 1975).

Kaufman and Rosenblum (1969) noted that in pigtail monkeys, elder siblings became depressed on the birth of younger offspring, and in many species of monkey, infants withdraw from social play activities and stay nearer mother at stages of active weaning (Hinde, 1971). These periods of depression are not long-lasting, however, and are not as marked as the distress and depression seen in infant monkeys (about 4 to7 months of age) as a result of maternal separation.

There is evidence in humans that boys are more susceptibel to social stress than girls (Rutter, 1970). In rhesus monkeys, Spencer-Booth and Hinde (1971) report that infant males are more adversely affected by separation than infant females.

The duration of the separation experience is an important factor in the response of children and monkeys to maternal separation; the longer the period of continuous separation, the greater the distress (Heinicke and Westheimer, 1965 for children; Spencer-Booth and Hinde, 1971, for rhesus monkeys).

Although factors such as age, sex, duration of separation, presence of suitable caretakers, maintenance of care and attention, and experience with conspecifics other than the mother have been shown to be important in affecting children's and infant monkeys' responses to maternal separation, there still may exist further individual variation in distress. This variation indicates that other more pertinent factors may be operating, as well. Hinde and colleagues have provided evidence that the nature of the mother-infant relationship plus the nature of the infants' relationships with other familiar companions may also be important determinants in the response to separation. The roles played by both mother and infant in determining the nature of their relationship have been studied in detail in the rhesus by Hinde (1969) and several important measures have been devised which may indicate important areas of study in determining the course of mother-infant relations in humans (Hinde and Atkinson, 1970; Hinde and White, 1974).

Factors Affecting the Ease with Which the Mother-Infant Relationship is Reestablished on Reunion

Spencer-Booth and Hinde (1971) showed that infant rhesus monkeys that had disturbed relationships with their mothers before separation occurred were the most distressed during separation and were slower to recover following reunion. The infants' recovery from separation following reunion with the mother depended upon the ease with which the mother-infant relationship was reestablished. This recovery, in turn, depended upon the nature of the mother-infant relationship before separation and upon factors operating to affect the relationship at reunion, such as the mothers' need to reestablish social relationships with group companions, if the mothers had been removed from their social groups for separation. In a series of four separation experiments, Hinde and his colleagues illustrated these points further, and were able to assess the importance of the mother figure in influencing not only the infants' response to separation but also the infants' responses to group companions. Hinde et al. also showed how the infants' behavior affected the mothers' interactions with group companions. The four separation experiments were of the following kind:

Spencer-Booth and Hinde

Spencer-Booth and Hinde (1971) separated six 30- to 32-week-old rhesus monkeys from their mothers for 13 days. The infants were left in their social groups while their mothers were removed for the separation period. The social groups consisted of one fully adult male, three to four adult females and their young of varying ages. There were six social groups in all, each group living in an outdoor cage 548 × 243 × 246 cms which connected with an inside cage 185 × 133 × 239 cms. (Fig. 1). The monkeys were locked outside for observations. The mothers were taken to the monkey room about 50 meters from the main colony for separation and housed alone in cages 82 × 74 × 103 cms. The separations were performed one at a time so that there was no overlap of mothers in the monkey room. After 13 days, the mothers were returned to their infants within the social group. During the mothers' absence, the infants had shown an initial phase of protest, lasting roughly 24 hours, which was followed by a period of withdrawal from social activities, in which the infants assumed hunched postures, huddled in corners and looked depressed. They were looked after by others, in some cases, but the care given was transitory in nature, and certainly not of the quality given by the infants' mothers. Caretaking behaviors by others did not seem to alleviate the infants'

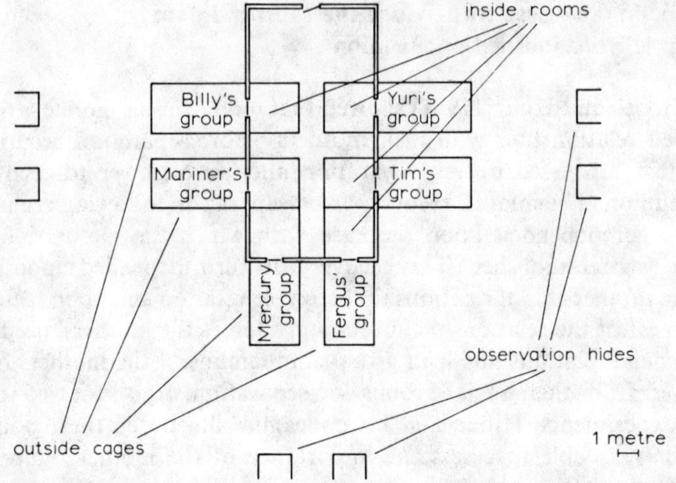

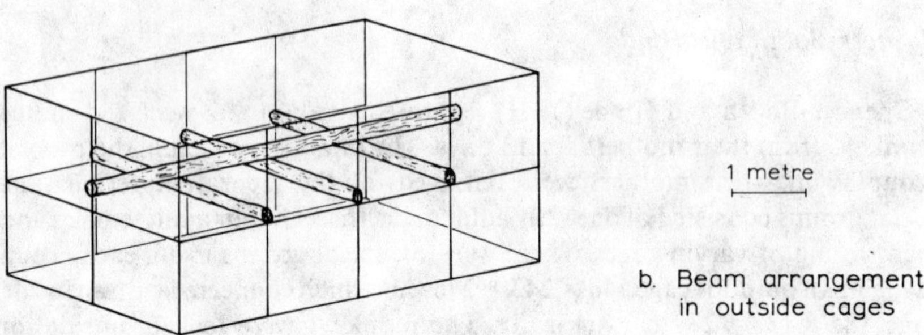

FIG. 1. The monkey colony

distress in those cases where it occurred. The infants remained withdrawn until their mothers' return. On reunion, mother and infant immediately related to each other and, in most cases, the infants stayed on their mothers' ventrum for the rest of the day. As the post-reunion period progressed, however, it soon became apparent that there was a degree of tension in the mother-infant relationships. The mothers had to reestablish social relationships and wanted their infants off them. The infants, however, were highly dependent on their mothers and reluctant to get off. The mothers became rejecting, the infants more clinging, and the mother-infant relationship suffered marked disturbance. These infants required well over one month to resume normal social and play activities.

Hinde and Davies

Hinde and Davies (1972) altered the procedure by removing five 30- to 32-week-old rhesus infants from the group for 13 days, but this time leaving their mothers with social companions. In this case, the infants responded to loss of mother and exposure to unfamiliar surroundings with prolonged protest lasting five days, which was followed by periods of quiet, subdued behavior, interspersed with bouts of hyperactivity and distress vocalizations. In later separation stages these infants also assumed hunched postures and appeared depressed. After 13 days the infants were returned to their mothers in their social groups. Mothers and infants related to one another immediately. On reunion and in later reunion stages, the mothers were very attentive to their infants (the mothers in this case did not have to reestablish social relationships) and the infants recovered within 24 hours of their return and began playing with their peers the next day. They were neither clinging nor overly dependent on their mothers.

Two suggestions were formulated to explain these differences:

1) The mothers were more attentive in the Hinde and Davies study and the mother-infant relationship was reestablished with greater ease, because the mothers did not have to reestablish social relations on reunion as well as the mother-infant relationship. Thus, disturbance to the mothers may affect the ease with which mother-infant relations are restored and hence the infants' recovery from maternal separation.

2) The infants that had been left in their social groups for separation in the Spencer-Booth and Hinde study may have been adversely conditioned to their surroundings during separation and home was no longer a pleasant place for them. They were highly dependent on their mothers on reunion, therefore, and their mothers were consequently more rejecting. The infants in the Hinde and Davies study had suffered the ill effects of separation away from the home group and so home may still have been a pleasant place for them on reunion. They may also have experienced a sense of "relief" at being home again. This may have made them less clinging and less dependent on their mothers. The attentiveness on the part of the mothers may have assisted in reestablishing the "normal" state for these infants (it also may have been an improvement over preseparation conditions for these infants) and consequently these infants recovered faster than those in the Spencer-Booth and Hinde study. It is possible that both suggestions apply and that mothers and infants may have influenced the course of their relationship on reunion.

McGinnis

To determine which influences the infants' response and recovery rate in separation experiments—disturbance to the mothers by removal from the group or infants' surroundings during separation—McGinnis (1978; 1979) carried out two experiments: the first involved removing both mothers and infants from their social groups and then separating them from each other for 13 days; the second involved removing mothers and infants from their social groups but housing them together for 13 days. The latter did not involve maternal separation and, therefore, is not strictly speaking a separation experiment.

In the first experiment (involving removal from the social group and maternal separation), the infants' response to separation was similar to that described for the infants in the Hinde and Davies study. On reunion with their mothers (in the social group), the infants and mothers readily related to one another; in later reunion stages the mothers in the McGinnis study proved to be more attentive to their infants than the mothers in the Spencer-Booth and Hinde study, despite the fact that, like the mothers in Spencer-Booth and Hinde study, they also had to reestablish social relations on reunion as well as the mother-infant relationship. The mothers in the McGinnis study were not quite as attentive as the mothers in the Hinde and Davies study. However, the latter did not have to also reestablish social relations on reunion.

At first glance it seems difficult to account for the greater attentiveness of the mothers in the McGinnis study since, to all intents and purposes, their experiences were similar to the mothers' in the Spencer-Booth and Hinde study. It is possible that differences in infants' behavior were responsible for differences in the mothers' behavior. In the McGinnis study, as in the earlier one by Hinde and Davies, the infants that were returned to their groups following separation were more subdued and quiet than infants left at home for separation. The latter were clinging and dependent on their mothers. The subdued behaviour of the "removed" infants may have made their mothers more attentive to them. The resultant ease with which the mother-infant relationship was reestablished may have enabled the mothers in the McGinnis study to reestablish social relations with greater ease than the mothers in the Spencer-Booth and Hinde study, and so the mothers did not have to reject their infants to the same extent as the mothers in the Spencer-Booth and Hinde study. The infants in the McGinnis study recovered faster than those in the Spencer-Booth and Hinde study, implying that the infants' behavior on reunion, which was probably influenced by their separation experiences, affected the ease with which the mother-infant relationship was reestablished.

The mothers in the McGinnis study, however, were not as attentive as the mothers in the Hinde and Davies study, although their infants behaved in similar ways upon reunion. The infants in the McGinnis study also took longer to recover than the infants in the Hinde and Davies study. In the latter study the mothers were not removed from their groups for separation and did not have to reestablish social relations upon reunion. These findings implied that disturbance to the mothers on reunion also influenced the ease with which the mother-infant relationship was reestablished. The McGinnis study, therefore, showed that the infants' behavior and the mothers' behavior determine the nature of the mother-infant relationship on reunion and hence the infants' recovery from separation.

In McGinnis' second experiment where mother-infant pairs were removed from their social groups, but not separated from one another, the infants were not distressed during the separation period, despite their unfamiliar surroundings. They were frightened initially and stayed on their mothers, but later they readily moved around and seemed at ease. Their mothers appeared restless, however. These findings were similar to those reported earlier for children in strange surroundings with their mothers. In both monkey and human infants, mothers had calming effects under unfamiliar conditions. On reunion with the social group, the nonseparated mothers and infants immediately went their separate ways. The mothers reestablished social relations and paid scant attention to their infants, while the infants readily interacted with their peers, but also kept a watchful eye on mother. In later reunion stages, these infants began to seek out their mothers once more and, if their mothers were inattentive and preoccupied with social relations, the infants began to withdraw from social activities and became more dependent on their mothers. Although these nonseparated infants never appeared to be as depressed and dependent upon their mothers as separated infants, they were disturbed to a degree by their mothers' preoccupation with social companions. Thus, disturbance to the mothers by removal from the group can affect their relationships with their infants without a maternal separation experience. Where disturbance to mothers and separation occur together, the effects on the infants are more profound and distressing. There is an indication, therefore, that in rhesus monkeys at least, the mother may play a greater role than the infant in determining the nature and course of the mother-infant relationship before and following a separation experience.

The findings from these four experiments are summarized in Table 1. The least distressed infants were those that had not experienced maternal separation. This indicates that it was loss of mother per se that produced marked distress in infant rhesus monkeys. Of the separated infants, the infants of the Hinde and Davies study, whose mothers were not disturbed by removal from the group and were the most attentive to their infants upon reunion, were the least distressed. Thus disturbance to the mothers, resulting in their relative inattentiveness to the infants upon reunion, was an important

TABLE 1
Summary of Separation Experiments on Rhesus Monkeys

Experiment	*Maternal Separation Occurred*	*Removal of Mother from Group Occurred*	*Removal of Infant from Group Occurred*
A. Spencer-Booth & Hinde (1971)	Yes	Yes	No
B. Hinde & Davies (1972)	Yes	No	Yes
C. McGinnis (1978)	Yes	Yes	Yes
D. McGinnis (1979)	No	Yes	Yes

If A and C are compared, the effects of the infants' surroundings during separation could be assessed.
If B and C are compared, the effects of disturbance to the mothers' behavior may be assessed.
If D and C are compared, the effects of maternal separation may be assessed.

Ranks based on the infants' rates of recovery from a maternal separation experience on reunion with their mothers:

A. were the most distressed of all infants in the post-reunion period and took longer to recover from separation. Their mothers were disturbed by removal from the group, and these infants were clinging and demanding on reunion, suggesting they had been adversely conditioned to their home surroundings during separation.
B. which involved removal of the infant only from the group for separation, were the next least distressed of all the infants in the reunion period, and recovered the fastest after maternal separation.
C. which involved maternal separation, removal of mother and infant from the group, were the next least distressed of all the infants in the reunion period. They took longer to recover than B, but recovered faster than A, suggesting the infants' surroundings during separation affected the mothers' responses to them on reunion, by affecting the infants' behavior on reunion.
D. which involved no maternal separation experience, were the least distressed of all the infants in all periods.

factor affecting infants' response to and recovery from maternal separation. Of the two remaining studies, the most adversely affected infants were those of the Spencer-Booth and Hinde study that had experienced maternal separation in their home groups while their mothers had been removed. Adverse conditioning to their surroundings during separation may have influenced the infants' behaviour upon reunion making the infants more clinging and dependent on their mothers. These findings are described in greater detail in Hinde and McGinnis (1977).

Findings from human studies indicate that mothers' preoccupation with personal relations do affect the course of the mother-infant relationship (Robertson, 1965), but in the study by Robertson and Robertson (1971) infants left with familiar caretakers were less distressed by separation. This is contrary to findings on rhesus monkey infants above, and is more in agreement with the findings of Kaufman and Rosenblum (1969) on bonnet macaque infants and Kaplan on squirrel monkey infants (1970). However, the rhesus infants in the above experiments received very little care from companions in their mothers' absence. There is evidence from recent studies on the plasma cortisol response of infant squirrel monkeys to separation that, even though these infants were cared for by others in their mothers' absence, they were under considerable physiological stress (Coe et al. 1978). These biological measures may serve as more sensitive indicators of stress than behavioural measures used alone. The response to loss of mother may be more overt under conditions of extreme stress such as when infants are exposed to unfamiliar places and unfamiliar caretakers during separation, but the stress response may be just as great, albeit covert, when infants are left with familiar caretakers in familiar surroundings. We do not understand the response to loss of the primary caretaker sufficiently to assume that such a loss is easily compensated for by care from others. The fact that extreme behavioural manifestations of distress such as depression are prevented by adequate substitute care does seem beneficial in cases where maternal separation is unavoidable.

The findings on rhesus monkeys support the view that it is absence of mother that is mainly responsible for distress seen in maternal separations. There are indications, however, that it is the nature of the mother-infant relationship that determines in part the degree of distress seen and the rate of recovery on reunion.

Social Context of Mother-Infant Separations

In most studies to date on children and monkeys, the emphasis has been on the mother-infant pair, as distinct from the companions that make up their social environment. This is somewhat artificial, as the mother-infant relationship is only one in a whole complex network of social relationships, changes in any part of which affect all relationships (Hinde, 1972). In the two experiments described by McGinnis (1978; 1979) which the rhesus monkey mother-infant pairs were removed from their groups and separated , and where they were removed and not separated, detailed analyses were made of the mothers' and the infants' social interactions as well as mother-infant interactions. This revealed further factors affecting individual differences in response within each group.

In the separated group, it was found that infants that had disturbed relations with their mothers before separation, tended to be infants of low-rank females (i.e., females that spent most of their time alone and were threatened by others more than they threatened others and avoided others more than they were avoided). It seemed, therefore, that mothers that had disturbed social relations had disturbed mother-infant relations also. Their infants were the most distressed and most dependent on their mothers and also avoided social interactions. Mothers that spent the most time with others and that engaged in more friendly behaviors with others, had the most sociable and playful infants. Correlations between measures showed that infant distress was closely related to high locomotor activity levels on the part of the mothers. Low-rank females were the most active in avoiding social encounters and may, therefore, have provided a less secure base to which the infants coud refer when necessary. Infants of these low-rank females were the most distressed during separation and following reunion took longer to recover from maternal separation.

In the nonseparated group there was a tendency for low-rank infants to be disturbed before removal and upon reunion with the group, but in this group the infants whose mothers were of insecure high rank were the most distressed in all periods. The high-rank mothers in the separated group had been of secure high rank. In the nonseparated group the mothers of insecure high rank were preoccupied with social relations before removal and following reunion. Their inattentiveness to their infants produced marked disturbance to the mother-infant relationship and in one case an infant whose mother lost her high social rank became as depressed and withdrawn as separated infants, even though she had not experienced maternal separation. Rosenblum (1973) reports a similar decrease in play activities and social interactions in bonnet macaque and pigtail macaque infants whose mothers lost social rank. The changes in the infants' behavior were attributed in these cases to increased tension and restrictiveness in the mothers.

Summary

To summarize, low-rank females usually have more tense social relations. This tension is exacerbated upon reunion following a period of absence from the group. Returning group members are the focus of attention and this may prove extremely stressful for low-rank females that usually avoid social interactions. The social situations for these females is more predictable, however, than that for those high-rank females whose social status is insecure. Low-rank females quickly settle back into their groups, but females of insecure rank have a much longer period of resettlement, and even then may find their social relationships greatly changed. This latter situation was found to produce marked tension in the mother-infant relationship. It was not social status as such (which at its best is only an abstract concept) but, rather, the nature of the mothers' social relations that influenced the nature of the mother-infant relationship. Smotherman et al. (1979) found that rhesus monkey infants of high-rank females showed a higher plasma cortisol response to short, repeated separations from mother and group than infants of low-rank females. Here again the high-rank females were very active and appeared tense in social interactions.

Comparison between nonseparated and separated mothers and between nonseparated and separated infants on measures of social interactions are given in Figure 2, 3, and 4, and Figures 5, 6, and 7, respectively. Separated mothers and infants gave priority to reestablishing the mother-infant relationship upon reunion with the group, and only later reestablished social relationships. Nonseparated mothers and infants, on the other hand, gave priority to reestablishing social relationships upon reunion with the group. They did not have to reestablish the mother-infant relationship. The separated mothers and infants were much less active than the nonseparated mothers and infants, and this greater passivity enabled the separated mothers to reestablish social relations with their companions with greater ease than the nonseparated mothers; i.e., they were threatened less by their companions. The important issue here, however, was that even in cases where the mothers' social relations were greatly disrupted by removal from the social group, the mothers still gave priority to reestablishing the mother-infant relationship if this had also been disrupted by separation.

DISCUSSION

There is a great deal of individual variation in the response to maternal separation in children and nonhuman primates. Some are extremely adversely affected, while others show hardly any ill effects. In monkeys there are species differences in the severity of response seen (Kaufman and Rosenblum, 1969) based upon the social organization of the group studied and the degree of interaction with companions in infancy. Similar differences in response exist in human societies, in which infants are exposed to more than one caretaker in the course of their development (Mead, 1962). The age and sex of children and infant monkeys are important in determining their response to separation from the mother, but it is possible that emotional maturity at a particular age may depend on other factors such as the experiences of the child or monkey up to that age, and the nature of their relationships with their primary caretakers throughout development. The differences in response shown by males and females in response to separation may, in part, depend on the different attitudes of mothers to offspring of different sexes; this factor may, therefore, affect the nature of their relationship with these offspring and, hence, give rise to differences in susceptibility to distress at maternal separation.

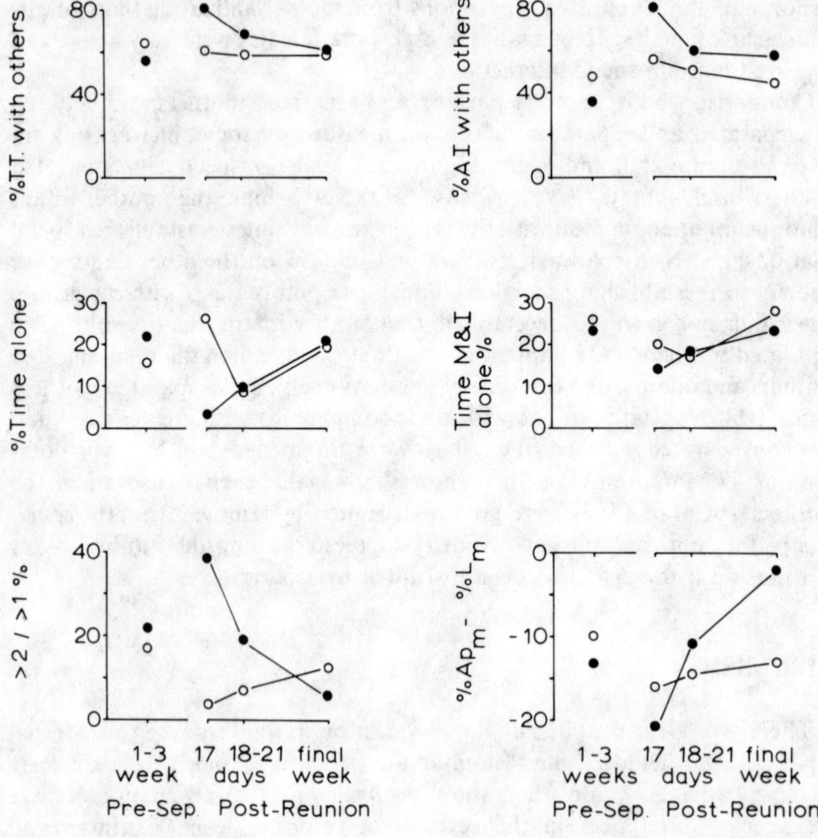

FIG. 2. The intensity of the mothers' social interactions before and after separation/removal; top left, the time the mothers spent within 60 cm of others; top right, the time spent by the mothers in interactions with others when within 60 cm of them; middle left, time spent alone, i.e. more than 60 cm from anybody; middle right, time the mother and infant pair spent more than 60 cm from others; bottom left >2/>1%, sociable when sociable measure, i.e. the number of half minutes the mothers were with more than two others as a percentage of the number of half minutes they were with more than one other; bottom right, the mothers' role in maintaining proximity to others.

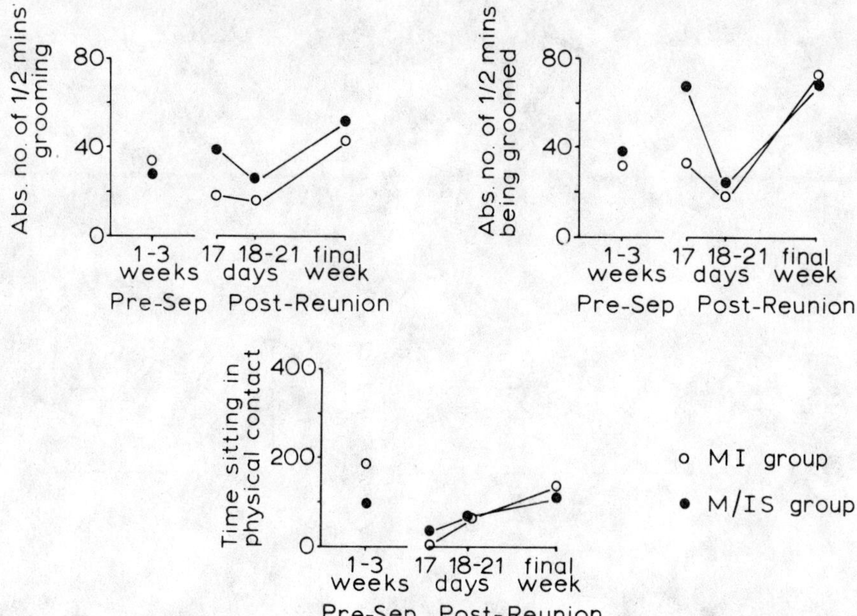

FIG. 3. The mothers' "friendly" interactions before and after separation/ removal. Top left, mothers groom others; top right, mothers are groomed by others; bottom center, time spent huddling.

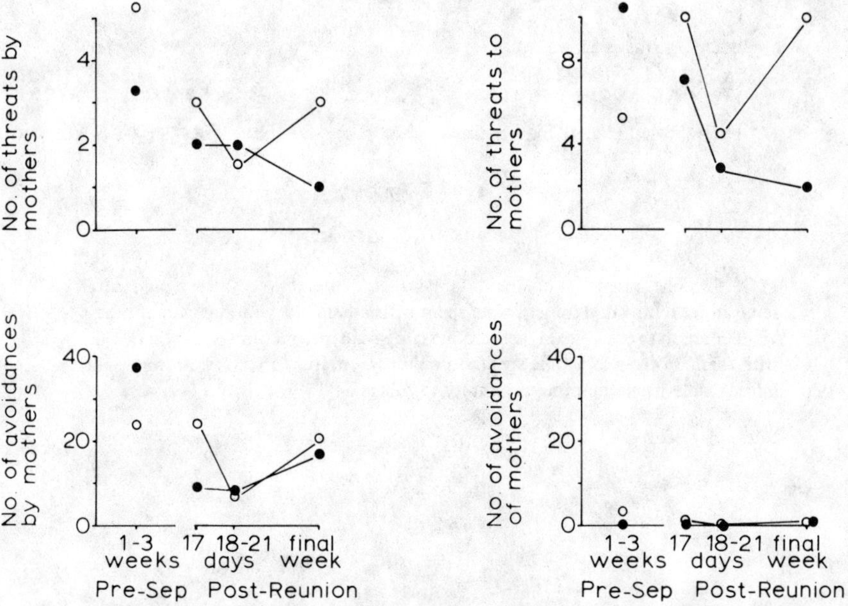

FIG. 4. The mothers' "agonistic" interactions before and after separation/ removal. Top left, mothers threaten others, top right, mothers are threatened by others; bottom left, mothers avoid others; bottom right, mothers are avoided by others.

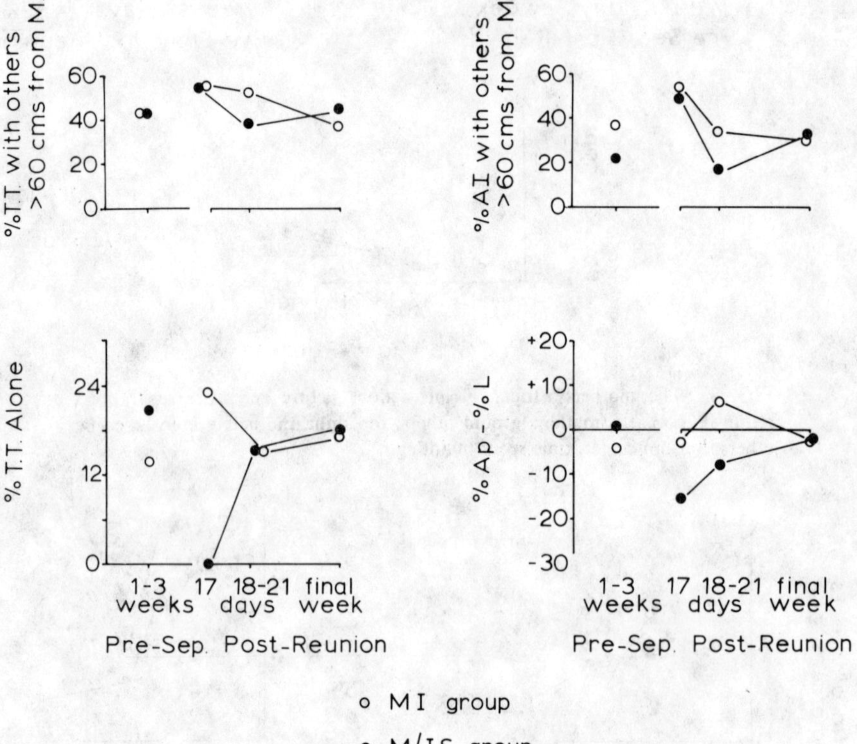

FIG. 5. The intensity of the infants' social interactions before and after separation/removal. Top left, time spent with others, i.e. within 60 cm of others while more than 60 cm from their mothers; top right, interactions with others when with them; bottom left, time spent more than 60 cm from anybody; bottom right, infants' role in maintaining proximity to others.

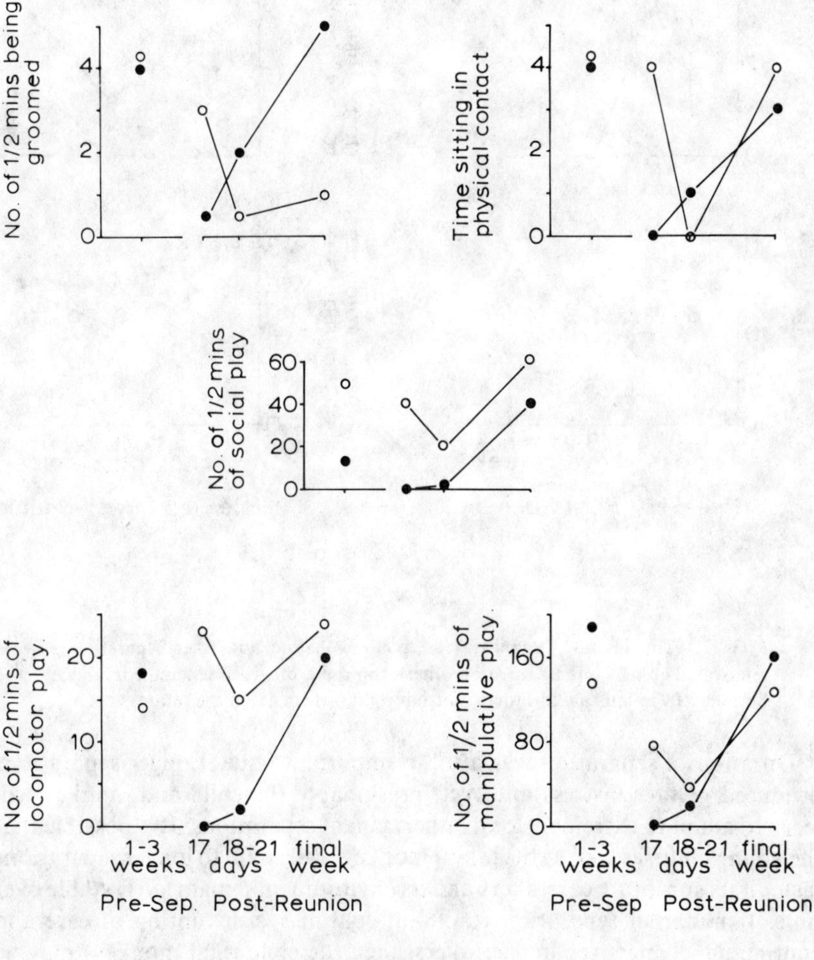

FIG. 6. The infants' "friendly" interactions and play behaviour before and after separation/removal. Top left, infants are groomed by others; top right, infants huddle to others; Center, amount of social contact and non-contact play engaged in by the infants; bottom left, amount of solitary locomotor play engaged in by the infants; bottom right, the amount of solitary manipulative play engaged in by the infants.

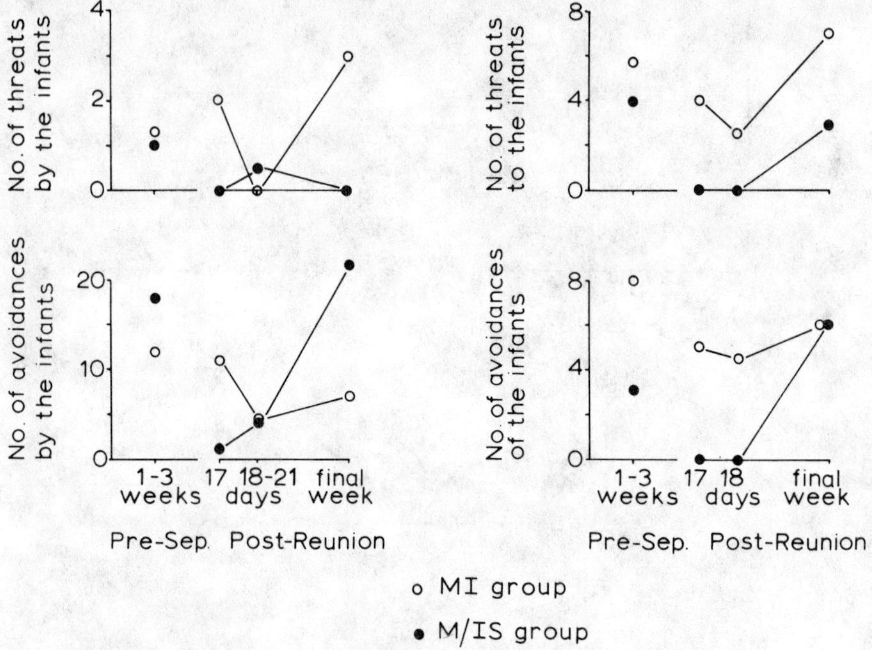

FIG. 7. The infants' "agonistic" interactions before and after separation/ removal. Top left, infants threaten others; top right, others threaten the infants; bottom left, infants avoid others, bottom right, others avoid the infants.

Duration of separation was also an important issue. Longer separations produced greater distress and, yet, presumably the child and monkey will learn to adapt to extremely long or permanent separations. It is possible that the young child, as well as the infant monkey, will adapt to longer separations faster if its substitute caretakers and its environment remain fairly stable over time. If maternal separation results in continuous disruption of care and continuous changeover in caretakers, then the child (and monkey) may be more severely affected and find great difficulty in learning to adjust. The nature of the child's or monkey's relationships with their caretakers during maternal separations may also be important in affecting the period of adjustment.

By taking all these factors into consideration, it may be possible to alleviate the marked distress shown by young children and nonhuman primates to loss of mother, but we still have a long way to go before we can accurately assess how the loss of mother actually affects the infant. We may alleviate the severe behavioral symptoms of distress, but we cannot know what the child or infant monkey may be covertly experiencing in terms of emotional and physiological stress.

In our human social structure, as well as that of nonhuman primates, the mother has taken full responsibility for caring for the infant throughout its early development. Others may assist in caretaking, but the mother is the most constant source of care and social stimulation.

There is some debate as to whether mother is the primary source of the child's ability to form social attachments (Kohlberg, 1969). We have reviewed monkey studies in which normal social development can occur without mothering (Harlow and Harlow, 1972); we have also seen in studies on human children that they do develop social attachments even when raised by multiple caretakers (Stevens, 1971).

There is more to being a social individual than is indicated by the normal give-and-take interactions of social exchange, however, particularly in humans. The mother provides a secure base from which the child may then attempt social interactions with other companions. Once the child begins relating to others, he learns new forms of social exchange that are not as loving and secure as the mother-infant experience, but which require more sophisticated techniques of asserting oneself, such as sometimes giving-in to others in order to ultimately get one's own way.

It is possible that children may learn the difference between "self" and "others" in social exchanges with peers. Children may learn to modify their own needs in order to accommodate those of others in interactions with individuals aside from their mothers. In such exchanges, however, there may be an element of competitiveness not present to the same degree in exchanges between mother and child. When peers interact, each interactant may not be concerned directly with the welfare of the other, and they are both aware of this to some extent. In mother-infant interactions, on the other hand, although each may be asserting their needs over one another, there is a well-established basis of trust and loving care built up between them in the very early stages of the mother-infant relationship. The child's sense of "personal security" may be provided by the mother's loving care, for even if they disagree the child learns that such discord is not permanent, and that love and care persist. In this way the child may learn that he can be assertive with the mother, without threatening their relationship.

If a child does not experience a loving or caring relationship in development (or if such a relationship is disrupted at a sensitive stage of development) the child may be deprived of a secure base from which to begin learning other forms of social interaction. It may help a child to know that if early attempts at forming peer relationships prove difficult, they still have the warm reassurance of their relationship with their mother. Learning not to be too assertive in social interactions or too self-denying may be acquired from peer interaction, however.

These suggestions imply that the mother figure is of extreme importance in early social development, but the relationship provided by the mother may not be exclusive to the mother. Other family members, as well as foster mothers, may provide a warm, loving relationship for the child and separation from these individuals may also produce distress in children (Rutter, 1972). It is not the biological mother that is important, but the secure, loving relationship. Mothers, on the other hand, are ideally suited to provide this kind of interaction, and there may be a greater risk of the child not having this kind of relationship without a mother, or there may be a greater risk of this type of relationship being thwarted when mother-infant relationships are disrupted by separations. The marked distress shown by children and infant monkeys when the mother-infant relationship is disrupted by separation (without being replaced by some sort of secure care during the mother's absence) indicates that our evolutionary or biological heritage may predispose us to expect some kind of loving, continuous care up to a certain stage of development, once we have had some initial experience with such a relationship.

In our human society social norms are rapidly changing. Increasingly more women want careers as well as families; many more women must have careers in order to support families, and hence, day-care centers are thriving. If we place less emphasis on the importance of maternal care in infancy, then we have to be able to assess the importance of the mother-figure and the early mother-infant relationship.

Separation studies have provided a way of beginning to assess these problems, but the results are often conflicting possibly because the contexts of maternal separations vary in each individual case and are therefore far from comparable, especially in humans. From studies on monkeys it does seem that the nature of the early mother-infant relationship is important in determining the infant's response to brief loss of mother, and if the mother-infant relationship is rapidly and easily reestablished on reunion, the infant recovers faster. In monkeys the mother plays a large role in determining the course of mother-infant relations, and she in turn is influenced by the nature of her relations with her social companions. As infant monkeys mature within their social groups, they assume ranks just below that of their mothers (Koyama, 1967; Sade, 1967).

In McGinnis' studies (1978; 1979) it was seen that the infants' patterns of social interactions followed closely those of their mothers. It may be that an infant monkey's relations with its mother, plus the responses of group companions to the mother-infant pair, shape the future social position taken by the infants as they grow up in the social group (Nagel and Kummer, 1974).

Long-term studies are needed on humans to determine the roles played by mother and infant in their early interactions with each other. The effects of the mother's relations with those that form her social environment on her relations with her infant, and the effects of cultural and socioeconomic standards on the mother's behavior such that they may influence her expectations for the infant and her standards of what is acceptable behavior from her infant,also need to be determined.

Caudill and Weinstein (1969) have studied the influences of different cultures on early mother-infant relations and Kagan and Tulkin (1971) have studied mother-infant relations in different socioeconomic classes within the same culture. Maternal and infant personalities may provide more sensitive areas for study. If a mother is constantly tense and unresponsive, an infant might try to form a more stimulating relationship with other individuals. If these are not available, then the infant may be influenced more by maternal mood. Mothers that are happy with their situation, whether they stay at home or go to work, may form better relationships with their infants than mothers that are unhappy with their lot.

ACKNOWLEDGMENTS

The author's study was supported by a scholarship awarded by the Medical Research Council of Great Britain. I wish to thank my supervisor, Professor Robert A. Hinde, Dr. Helena Kraemer, and Dr. Michael Rutter for all their helpful comments and advice. Thanks also go to all the people at Madingley, who were engaged in work on the monkey colony, especially Lilyan White and Messrs, Jock Jolley, Bob Seekings and Tom Goss.

REFERENCES

Bowlby, J. *Maternal Care and Mental Health.* World Health Organization, Geneva (1951).

Bowlby, J. *Attachment and Loss: II. Separation*, Basic Books Inc., New York (1973).

Brossard, M. and Décarie, T. G. The effects of three kinds of perceptual-social stimulation on the development of institutionalized infants: preliminary report of a longitudinal study. In *Readings in Child Behavior and Development, Third Edition*, C. Standler Lavatelli and F. Stendler, eds. Harcourt Brace Jovanovich, Inc. (1972), pp. 173–183.

Caudill, W., and Weinstein, H. Maternal care and infant behavior in Japan and America. *Psychiatry 32*, 12–43 (1969).

Coe, C. L., Mendoza, S. P., Smotherman, W. P., Miner, M. T., Kaplan, J., and Levine, S. Mother-infant attachment in squirrel monkeys: Adrenal response to separation. *Behav. Biol. 22*, 256–263 (1978).

Deutsch, H. A two-year-old boy's first love comes to grief. In *Dynamic Psychopathology in Childhood*, L. Jessner and E. Pavenstedt, eds. Grune and Stratton (1919), (cited in Rutter, 1972).

Fagin, C. M. R. N. *The Effects of Maternal Attendance during Hospitalization on the Post-Hospital Behavior of Young Children: A Comparative Study*, F. A. Davis (1966).

Freud, A., with the collaboration of Sophie Dann. An experiment in group upbringing. *In Readings in Child Behavior and Development, Third Edition*, C. Stendler Lavatelli and F. Stendler, eds. Harcourt Brace Jovanovich, Inc. (1972), pp. 472–489.

Harlow, H. F., and Harlow, M. K. Effects of various mother-infant relationships on rhesus monkey behaviors. In *Readings in Child Behavior and Development Third Edition*, C. Stendler Lavatelli and F. Standler, eds. Harcourt Brace Jovanovich, Inc. (1972), pp. 202–209.

Heinicke, C. M., and Westheimer, I. J. *Brief Separations*. New York: International University, New York; Longman, London (1966).

Hinde, R. A. Analyzing the roles of the patners in a behavioural interaction-mother/infant relations in rhesus macaques. *Ann. N. Y. Acad. Sci. 159*, 651–667. (1969).

Hinde, R. A. Development of social behaviour. In *Behavior of Nonhuman Primates: Modern Research Trends, Vol. 3*. A. M. Schrier and F. Stollnitz, eds. Academic Press, London; New York (1971), pp. 1–68.

Hinde, R. A. *Social Behaviour and its Development in Subhuman Primates*, Condon Lectures, Oregon State System of Higher Education, Eugene, Oregon (1972).

Hinde, R. A. and Atkinson, S. Assessing the roles of social partners in maintaining mutual proximity, as exemplified by mother-infant relations in rhesus monkeys. *Anim. Behav. 18*, 169–176 (1970).

Hinde, R. A. and Davies, L. M. Removing infant rhesus from mother for 13 days compared with removing mother from infant. *J. Child. Psychol. Psychiatr. 13*, 227–237 (1972).

Hinde, R. A. and McGinnis, L. M. Some factors influencing the effects of temporary mother-infant separation-some experiments with rhesus monkeys. *Psychol. Med. 7*, 197–212 (1977).

Hinde, R. A. and White, L. The dynamics of a relationship: Rhesus monkey ventroventral contact. *J. Comp. Physiol. Psychol. 86*, 8–23 (1974).

Jensen, G. D. and Tolman, C. W. Mother-infant relationship in the monkey *Macaca nemestrina*: The effect of brief separation and the mother-infant specificity, *J. Comp. Physiol. Psychol. 55*, 131–136 (1962).

Lawick-Goodall, J. van. The chimpanzee, In *The Quest for Man*, V. Goodall, ed. Praeger Publishers, New York (1975), pp. 131–169.

Kagan, J. and Tulkin, S. R. Social class differences in child rearing during the first year. In *Origins of Human Social Relations*, H. R. Schaffer, ed. Academic Press (1971), pp. 165–183.

Kaplan, J. The effects of separation and reunion on the behavior of mother and infant squirrel monkeys. *Develop. Psychobiol. 3*, 43–52 (1970).

Kaufman, I. C., and Rosenblum, L. A. Effects of separation from mother on the emotional behavior of infant monkeys. *Ann. N. Y. Acad. Sci. 159*, 681–695 (1969).

Kohlberg, L. Stage and sequence: the cognitive-developmental approach to socialization. In *Handbook of Socialization: Theory and Research*, D. A. Goslin, ed. Chicago Rand McNally (1969).

Koyama, N. On dominance rank and kinship of a wild Japaneses monkey troop in Arashiyama. *Primates 8*, 189–216 (1967).

McGinnis, L. M. Maternal separations in rhesus monkeys within a social context. *J. Child Psychol. Psychiatr. 19*, 313–327 (1978).

McGinnis, L. M. Maternal separation vs. Removal from group companions in rhesus monkeys. *J. Child Psychol. Psychiatr. 20*, 15–27 (1979).

Mead, M. A cultural anthropologists's approach to maternal deprivation. In *Deprivation of Maternal Care; A Reassessment of Its Effects*. World Health Organization, Geneva. (1962).

Nagel, U., and Kummer, H. Variation in cercopithecoid aggressive behavior. In *Primate Aggression, Territoriality, and Xenophobia: A Comparative Perspective*, R. L. Holloway, ed. Academic Press New York; London (1974). pp. 159–184.

Pusey, A. E. *The Physical and Social Development of Wild Adolescent Chimpanzees* (*Pan Troglodytes Schweinfurthii*), Unpublished Ph.D. thesis, Stanford University (1977).

Rheingold, H. L. The modification of social responsiveness in institutional babies, *Monogr. Soc. Res. Child Devel.*, Vol. 21, suppl. 63 (1956).

Rheingold, H. L. The effect of a strange environment on the behavior of infants. In *Determinants of Infant Behaviour*, vol. 4, B. M. Foss (ed.) Methuen (1969), pp. 137–166.

Robertson, J. Mother-infant interaction from birth to twelve months; Two case studies. In *Determinants of Infant Behaviour*, vol. 3, B. M. Foss, ed. Methuen London (1965), pp. 111–127.

Robertson, J. and Bowlby, J. Responses of young children to separation from their mothers. *Courr. Cent. Int. Enf. 2*, 131–142 (1952).

Robertson, J., and Robertson, J. Young children in brief separation: A fresh look. *Psychoanal. Study Child. 26*, 264–315 (1971).

Rosenblum, L. A. Maternal regulation of infant social interactions. In *Behavioral Regulators of Behavior in Primates*, C. R. Carpenter, ed. Bucknell University Press (1973), pp. 195–217.

Rutter, M. Sex differences in children's responses to family stress. In *The Child in His Family*, E. J. Anthony and C. M. Koupernik, eds. Wiley New York: London (1970).

Rutter, M. *Maternal Deprivation Reassessed*, Penguin Science of Behaviour Baltimore (1972).

Sade, D. S. Determinants of dominance in a group of free-ranging rhesus monkeys. In *Social Communication Among Primates*, S. A. Altman, ed. University of Chicago Press (1967) pp. 99–114.

Schlottman, R. S. and Seay, B. Mother-infant separation in the Java monkey (*Macaca irus*). *J. Comp. Physiol. Psychol. 29*, 334–340 (1972).

Seay, B., Hansen, E., and Harlow, H. F. Mother-infant separation in monkeys. *J. Child. Psychol. Psychiatr. 3*, 123–132 (1962).

Smotherman, W. P., Hunt, L. E., McGinnis, L. M., and Levine, S. Mother-infant separation in group-living rhesus macaques: A hormonal analysis. *Develop. Psychobiol. 12* (3), 211–217 (1979).

Spencer-Booth, Y. and Hinde, R. A. The effects of 13 days maternal separation on 30–32 week-old rhesus monkeys compared with those of shorter and interrupted separations. *Anim. Behav. 19*, 595–605 (1971).

Spiro, M. E. *Children of the Kibbutz*, Oxford University Press (1958).

Stevens, A. G. Attachment Behaviour, separation anxiety, and stranger anxiety in polymatrically reared infants. In *The Origins of Human Social Relations*, H. R. Schaffer, ed. Academic Press London; New York (1971), pp. 137–146.

Vernon, D. T. A., Foley, J. M., and Schulman, J. L. Effect of mother-child separation and birth order on young children's responses to two potentially stressful experiences. *J. Person. Soc. Psychol. 5*, 162–174 (1967).

15

Maternal Deprivation: Compensatory Stimulation for the Prematurely Born Infant

Anneliese F. Korner, Ph.D.

Without a doubt, the ultimate case of maternal deprivation is that of the infant born prematurely. Such an infant is deprived of all the maternal, physiological regulatory influences which permit him to grow to a stage of maturity which allows him to function as a separate organism. Suddenly and in a state of unreadiness, the infant is forced to cope with temperature regulation, nutritional requirements, the task of oxygenation and the impact of gravity, all of which the maternal organism either regulates, provides, or protects against for the fetus. In addition, the premature infant is deprived of all the sensory experiences which attend life in utero and which one may assume are important for the normal growth and development of the individual.

Great progress has been made over the past 20 years in the medical care of premature infants and in the development of new life-support systems. Attending this progress has been the creation of the highly artificial, technological environment in which the infant grows to term. Until very recently, there has been relatively little concern about the quality of life or of the ecology in which these infants are raised. According to a recent review by Parmelee (1975) which compared the behavioral, neurological and physiological development of infants born at term with that of infants born two to three months prematurely who had grown to term, the development of the premature infants was characterized by a certain unevenness and vulnerability. Contributory factors are apt to be not only the obvious morbidity of this group, but also the highly artificial environment in which these infants are raised, which may hamper the natural unfolding of the infants' maturation.

Given the necessity of the intensive care environment with all its life-support systems, continuous bright lights and its monotonous, white noise, what can be done to provide these infants with sensory experiences which are more naturalistic and which may facilitate the more normal unfolding of their maturation? Intensive-care nurseries have alternately been described as environments of sensory deprivation (e.g., Hasselmeyer, 1964; Neal, 1968; Katz, 1971) and sensory bombardment (e.g., Koronos, 1976; Lucey, 1977). While nothing is known at this time about how preterm infants deal with either sensory deprivation or sensory overload, we know from studies with older individuals that both under- and over-stimulation have a disruptive and disorganizing effect on the physiological and psychological functioning of the organism (e.g., Frankenhaeuser and Johansson, 1974). What the preterm infant in the intensive-care nursery seems to be most lacking is a moderate amount of patterned stimulation which is relevant to the state of his neurophysiological development and that contingently reinforces the developing organization of his own biological rhythms.

A number of recent intervention studies have attempted to provide patterned stimulation to premature infants (see for example the recent review of these studies by Cornell and Gottfried, 1976). The choice of the patterned stimulation given has largely been governed by differing theoretical persuasions. Some investigators have provided visual, auditory and social stimulation to which full-term infants are highly responsive and to which premature infants at various post-conceptual ages begin to respond (Katz, 1971; Williams and Scarr, 1971; Wright, 1971; Scarr-Salapatek and Williams, 1973). Implicitly or explicitly the goal of these interventions is to accelerate the development of premature infants. Other investigators have chosen to impart types of patterned stimulation which are highly prevalent in utero with the explicit intent to compensate for an experiential deficit (Freedman, et al., 1966; Neal, 1967; Barnard, 1972; Korner, et al., 1975; and Korner, 1979). Each of these investigators has used a form of vestibular-proprioceptive or movement stimulation as the main type of patterned stimulation given to premature infants.

My own choice of prividing compensatory vestibular-proprioceptive stimulation to preterm infants was based on a number of theoretical considerations and on a good deal of empirical evidence from our earlier studies with human infants and rat pups which pointed to the fundamental importance of vestibular-proprioceptive stimulation for very early development (Korner and Grobstein, 1966; Korner and Thoman, 1970, 1972; Thoman and Korner, 1971; Gregg et al., 1976). In utero the fetus experiences a great deal of movement stimulation through his continuous flotation in the amniotic fluid, his own movements which are dampened and modulated by his fluid environment, as well as the pattern of his mother's periodic movements. In the incubator, the preterm infant resides on a hard and stationary surface; if he is ill he moves very little and if he is not, his movements are frequently characterized by an overshooting, jerky quality which reflects the immaturity of his inhibitory mechanisms. When moved by others, this occurs mostly at arbitrary and brief intervals when dictated by medical exigencies. The preterm infant is thus deprived of the quantity, the quality, and the rhythmic periodicity of movements he would have experienced in utero.

Evidence from the animal literature strongly suggests that deprivation of movement stimulation may lead to serious developmental deficits. For example, Erway (1975), who works in the area of otolith defects in mice, recently stated that "deficiency of vestibular input either for reasons of congenital defect or lack of motion stimulation may impair the early development and integrating capacities of the brain, especially that of the cerebellum." (p. 20). Mason's work (1968) with nonhuman primates seems to bare out this statement. Mason, like Harlow (1958), isolation-reared infant monkeys on surrogate mothers. Harlow, as a result of these rearing conditions, produced highly abnormal monkeys who engaged in autistic-like, self-mutilating and self-rocking behavior. Mason, by providing isolation-reared monkeys with swinging surrogate mothers, offset the severe developmental deficits and the pathological symptoms typically seen in Harlow's monkeys.

Vestibular-proprioceptive or movement stimulation thus appears to be one of the most important forms of stimulation necessary for the normality of early development. Since the premature birth of a baby deprives the infant of much the movement stimulation he would have experienced in utero, providing him with compensatory vestibular-proprioceptive stimulation may benefit his development. Clearly the goal is not one of accelerating development but to make an attempt at primary prevention of a developmental deficit. The aim then is to facilitate the infant's sensory-motor integration, or to consolidate and optimize the infant's development and, if possible, make it more even. The issue is not whether such intervention can raise developmental quotients measurable months or years after its completion, for we know from many studies that the home environment and the family circumstances over which the investigator has no control exert an overriding influence on developmental outcome (see, for example, Sameroff's review of this topic, 1975). The issue is to produce a child that is clinically and developmentally as intact as possible and who, for that reason, is more capable of coping with whatever home environment he may be entering.

COMPENSATORY VESTIBULAR–PROPRIOCEPTIVE STIMULATION FOR PRETERM INFANTS THROUGH WATERBED FLOTATION

Waterbeds were developed in our laboratory for the purpose of imparting compensatory vestibular-proprioceptive stimulation to preterm infants. It should be stressed, that while the waterbeds create a flotation environment for the premature infant, it was not our aim to simulate intrauterine conditions for this is neither possible nor necessarily desirable. Instead, we merely want impart vestibular-proprioceptive stimulation as naturalistically as possible with some of the formal and temporal characteristics of the movement stimulation which the fetus experiences prenatally. Thus, as will be described below, in addition to providing a flotation environment, we decided to impart movement stimulation which is contingent on the infant's own activity and which, at other times, is superimposed on him in experientially relevant rhythms and intervals.

In developing the waterbeds, we not only had developmental issues in mind, but we also postulated that certain clinical benefits might accrue from their use. For example, we felt that by providing a soft, fluid support to the head we might be able to reduce the incidence of the infants developing asymmetrically shaped, elongated heads which are so frequently seen in premature infants and, perhaps, even the frequency of intracranial hemorrhages. We also thought that the waterbed might help preserve the fragile skin of very small premature infants. Further, we postulated that waterbed flotation might reduce the infants' need to cope prematurely with the full impact of gravity, thus conserving their energy.

Since the levels of vestibular-proprioceptive stimulation which are optimal for development are unknown, we built two versions of the waterbed for use inside the incubator. The basic waterbed provides slight containment for the infant and is highly responsive to each of his movements. The second version is identical in design and consistency, but in addition to the stimulation generated by the infant's own movements, it provides gently rocking oscillations.

Since the studies to be reported were done with the Stanford designed waterbed, a description of these beds is in order. The basic waterbed consists of a high-impact styrene shell, and a vinyl bag covered by a latex membrane in a stainless-steel frame which attaches to the top of the shell. This unit is designed to replace the foam-rubber mattress usually used in incubators. The temperature of the waterbed is entirely maintained by the incubator's heating system. When a waterbed is prepared, the vinyl bag is filled with 2¼ gallons of warm tap water treated with algicide and blue dye. The water temperature chosen is 2° C above the incubator's environmental temperature since thermal tests have shown that the water temperature stabilizes at that level. In more recent years we have begun to use the waterbeds with infants who are cared for on open tables with radiant overhead heaters. Since under these conditions the temperature of the waterbed is not maintained by the incubator heater underneath, we have used a half inch of foam to insulate these critically-ill infants from the waterbed. The blue dye in the water is designed to alert the caregiver in the case of a leak, which over the years has been an extremely rare event. Blue was chosen so as not to be confused with urine, emesis, or blood. Repeated cultures of the water inside the vinyl bag have been negative even after continuous use for more than a month. Between uses, the waterbeds are readily gas autoclaved. The frame of the bed provides anchor points to restrain the infant as needed. When the infant requires elevation or percussion, a styrofoam wedge which sits on the waterbed frame provides a stable surface.

In deciding about the oscillations to be given, I had to address the issues one typically has to confront when setting up an experimental study involving stimulation. I had to decide on the direction, the rise time, the wave form, the frequency, and the amplitude of the oscillations. A decision also needed to be made as to whether to have the oscillations occur continuously or intermittently and at regular or irregular intervals. In making these decisions I tried to avoid arbitrary choices as is done most frequently in experimental studies. Instead, I made every effort to make choices which might have some clinical, biological, or experiential rationale.

Considering this aim, I decided on head-to-foot oscillations. This choice was predicated on the studies by Millen and Davies (1946) and by Lee (1954) which suggest that the direction of this motion may benefit the infant's respiratory effort. Since the infant would be exposed to the oscillations for long periods of time, it was important to make these very gentle. We therefore decided on the amplitude of the oscillations through clinical observations. This was done by exposing several infants to various amplitudes of motion, by ascertaining that the infant had no untoward reactions and by soliciting input from the medical and nursing personnel regarding the feasibility of caring for the infants on different types of oscillating surfaces. As a result of these preliminary studies, a very gentle, barely visible type of oscillation was chosen which measures only 2.4 mm in amplitude at the surface of the bed without an infant in place. In order to make these very small oscillations more perceptible to the infant, a wave with a rise time of only half a second was chosen. This has the effect of producing a very gentle jolt which sets the wave in motion and which is followed by a period of quiescence during which the wave attenuates.

The frequency of the oscillations had to be decided next. Rather than picking an arbitrary frequency from the infinite choice of possibilities, I sought a frequency which might have a biologically and experientially relevant rhythm for the premature infant. In this search I have felt it was safest to provide a maternal rhythm since such a rhythm would probably not interfere with the developing organization of the infant's own biological rhythms, because it would expose the infant to a rhythm to which he would have been exposed had he not been born prematurely. The rhythm of maternal respirations in the third trimester of pregnancy is such an experientially relevant rhythm. Maternal respirations at that stage of gestation are 16 $\pm$ 4 per minute according to Goodlin (1972). The lower rates of this range of frequencies were chosen because I felt intuitively that the lower rates would provide a more peaceful and less restless environment. Twelve to 14 oscillations per minute were thus selected. I also felt that the oscillations should occur at slightly irregular intervals, partly to reduce the chance that the infant would habituate or adapt and therefore tune out the stimulation and partly because irregular pulses would more nearly resemble maternal respirations.

In addition to selecting the frequencies and amplitudes of the oscillations, we had to decide whether to provide continuous or intermittent stimulation. In the first two studies we used continuous oscillations which at the time was an arbitrary decision. It so happened that the continuous pulses were, probably, largely responsible for the unanticipated clinical benefits which will be described below. For developmental purposes, I have since come to appreciate that intermittent stimulation may be far more effective. Intermittent stimulation allows the infant periods of activity and of rest, both of which are probably equally important for the infant's well-being. Intermittent rather than continuous oscillations also provide the infant with the opportunity to activate the waterbed through his own spontaneous movements during periods of nonoscillation, while at the same time insuring that some of the more quiet infants would receive passive movement stimulation, at least part of the day. In deciding on intermittent oscillations, I was also influenced by Denenberg's (1975) review of the animal literature on early stimulation effects from which he concluded that stimulus variation, rather than sensory constancy, is an important, if not indeed necessary condition for adequate development.

Once it was decided to use intermittent oscillations, it was still necessary to choose the kind of intermittency to be used. Rather than using arbitrary intervals of stimulation as is commonly done, I again looked for a maternal rhythm to which the infant would have been exposed had he not been born prematurely and which therefore would not interfere with the developing organization of the infant's own biological rhythms. The basic rest-activity cycle (BRAC) as described by Kleitman (1969) is such a maternal rhythm. In the adult, the average length of this cycle is approximately 90 minutes.

Evidence is accumulating that the manifestations of the BRAC persist throughout the day and express themselves at night through the cycling of REM and NREM sleep (e.g., Kleitman, 1969; Kripke, 1974; Broughton, 1975; and Carskadon and Dement, 1975). From Sternman's research (1967) which points to a strong relationship between maternal sleep stages and intrauterine fetal activity it appears that maternal cycles exert a regulatory influence on fetal behavior. Clearly, the prematurely born infant is deprived of the potentially organizing influences of maternal cycles. The lack of exposure to the maternal cyclicity of physiologic and motor activation may be one of the possible contributing factors to the poor organization of sleep and other behaviors in the premature infant (Dreyfus-Brisac, 1974; and Korner, 1979). We thus concluded that the superimposition of a 90-minute cycle on the infant through oscillating the waterbed for 20 to 40 minutes within each 90-minute period may provide an external aid to the infants' own developing rest-activity cycles. Variable periods of oscillations were chosen because we know from sleep research that REM periods, for example, increase in duration over the night and then decrease (e.g., Aserensky, 1969; and Feinberg, 1974). While the idea of superimposing maternal biological rhythms has never been tried with human premature infants, evidence from the animal literature suggests that this may be beneficial. For example, Hofer (1975a) found that rat pups separated from their mothers showed fragmentation in the organization and rhythmicity of their sleep patterns and a reduced cycle length. In another study (Hofer, 1975b), separation from the mother produced behavioral hyperactivity in young rats which was reduced to the level of nonseparated pups by administering external stimulation over a variety of sensory pathways with a time-patterning similar to the mother's periodic stimulation. Hofer concluded from his research that perhaps the "rhythmicity of maternal behavior acts as a Zeitgeber, a rhythm-giver, for the infant." (Hofer, 1975b, p. 153).

In the studies we have done to date we have as yet not used intermittent oscillations. In the first two studies described in the following pages, we used an Emerson respirator connected to a small inflatable rubber bladder to impart continuous, though irregular oscillations at the rate of 12 to 14 per minute. We later developed a small compact unit built on the same principle which provides the option to use a variety of frequencies and amplitudes of oscillations, if desired. Since then, Narco-Air-Shields, Inc. (a company producing equipment for intensive-care nurseries) has begun to manufacture the waterbed and oscillator for research purposes. This new version of the waterbed is pictured on the following page.

The Air-Shields version of the waterbed has all the stimulus characteristics of the prototypes developed in our laboratory, but the design has been considerably streamlined. The new bed is shallower, permitting more work

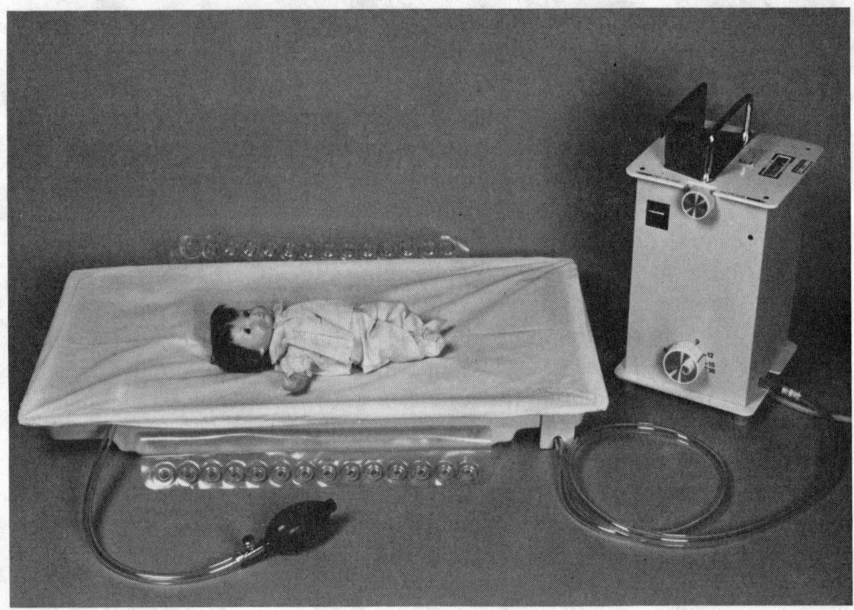

space in the incubator; the latex membrane has been replaced by a loosely fitting sheet. The anchor points for the restraints are now provided through holes in a plastic flap which is attached to the sides of the waterbed. The bulb pictured in front of the bed connects to a pneumatic device which allows the attendant to rigidify and stabilize the waterbed surface for such procedures as lumbar puncture or intubation. We are still experimenting with this feature of the waterbed and we may instead decide to use lightweight styrene boards which can be placed in two seconds over the edges of the waterbed in case of an emergency procedure.

STUDY I

We first undertook at study to determine whether changing the infant's environment on a 24-hour basis by using a waterbed was a safe procedure (Korner, et al., 1975). During 1974, 21 relatively healthy premature infants became available for study in the Stanford Intensive Care Nurseries. This group excluded infants with moderate or severe RDS, small-for-dates infants or babies with congenital anomalies or severe postnatal complications. The sample did include infants with mild RDS, apnea of prematurity, elevated bilirubin, mild hypoglycemia and hypocalcemia.

The 21 subjects were randomly assigned to experimental or control groups.

When a premature baby who met the above criteria became available, consent to use the baby in the study as either a control or an experimental subject was obtained, first from the pediatrician in charge, then from the mother and/or father of the child. Until both consents were obtained, the group to which the baby would be assigned was known to no one (including the person obtaining consent), lest knowledge of the group would influence in any way the decisions made or the treatment the infant would receive.

The infants ranged in gestational age from 27 to 34 weeks and had birthweights ranging from 1050 to 1920 grams. The sample included 10 females and 11 males. The experimental and control groups did not differ significantly from each other in weight or gestational age.

The 10 infants in the experimental group were each placed on a gently oscillating waterbed before the sixth postnatal day where they remained for one week. A comparison of the clinical progress of the two groups during the first nine days of life was made, after which two subjects were transferred back to their referring hospital. The data collected were drawn from the nurses' and the physicians' daily progress notes. To avoid inadvertent bias in recording, the nursing and medical personnel was unaware of the measures of interest to us.

We were greatly reassured to find that the oscillating waterbed in no way affected the babies' vital signs. Respiration, pulse rates and temperature ranges did not differ significantly between the two groups, nor did oxygen requirements or weight changes. Further, the oscillating waterbed did not increase the frequency of emesis.

One very highly significant difference was found between the two groups: the infants in the experimental group had significantly fewer apneas as indicated by the monitor alarms ($P < .01$). The monitor alarms are set to go off in the Stanford Intensive Care Nurseries when the infant's heart rate drops below 100 beats per minute and/or when the infants stops breathing for 20 or more seconds. Figure 1 shows descriptively the pattern of apnea frequency of the two groups.

Figure 1 compares the mean daily frequency of apnea, starting with the baseline average of the first two postnatal days. The differences in the first two days were not significant between the two groups. But as can be seen from Figure 1, after the babies in the experimental group were put on the oscillating waterbed, the incidence of their apneas tended to drop, whereas it continued to increase in the control babies.

STUDY II

Since apnea is thought to be one of the major causes of brain damage, it was important to replicate our finding and to determine whether apnea decreases

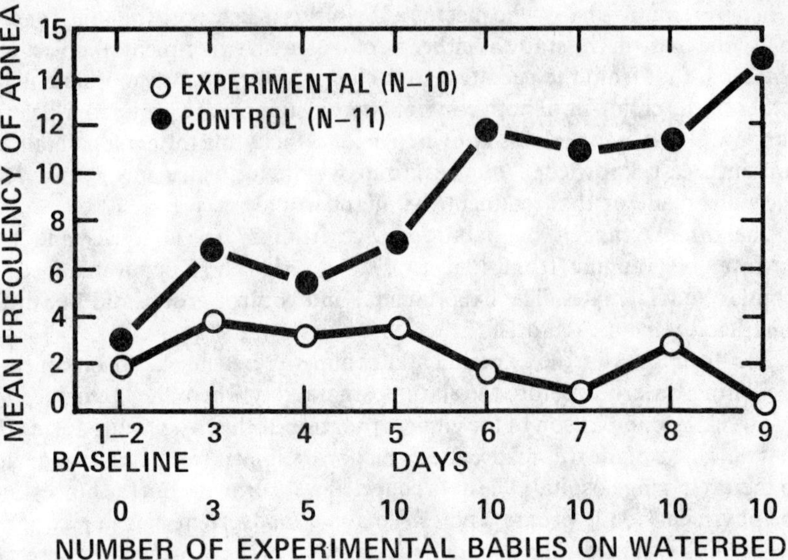

FIG. 1. Comparison between Experimental and Control Groups in the Mean Daily Apnea Incidence. This figure was first published in *Pediatrics*, Vol. *56*, No. 3, September 1975, pp. 361–367.

as a function of waterbed flotation in infants who were pre-selected for having this symptom. We soon had an opportunity to test this question. When Dr. Christian Guilleminault from the Stanford Sleep Disorder Clinic read the results of our first study, he proposed that we do a controlled polygraphic study in which each apneic infant would serve as his own control on and off the oscillating waterbed. This author naturally welcomed this opportunity to have an independent investigator from a separate laboratory using more accurate methods of recording and different ways of appraisal to test the validity of our observation regarding the apnea-reducing potential of the waterbed.

In this new study, the infant's sleep and respiratory patterns were polygraphically recorder over a 24-hour period. Collaborating in this study were Johanna Van den Hoed, M. D., Marianne Souquet and Roger Baldwin, all of whom worked under the direction of Christian Guilleminault, M. D. The 24-hour recordings were divided into four time blocks with the infant being placed on the waterbed during alternate 6-hour periods. To avoid an order effect, half of the infants were placed on the waterbed during the first six hours, half during the second 6-hour block.

The sample consisted of eight apneic preterm infants. We sought to include in the study only infants with true apnea of prematurity by ruling out metabolic, infectious and cardiopulmonary causes of apnea. Seven of the eight subjects were male. Four of the infants were Anglo-Saxon, four were Mexican-American. Gestational ages ranged from 27–32 weeks with a mean of 30 weeks. Birthweights ranged from 1077–1650 g with a mean of 1270 g. On the day of the study the infants' weights were between 1115 and 1600 g with a mean of 1264 g and their postnatal ages ranged from 7–28 days with a mean of 15 days. Three of the infants had been intubated and on assisted ventillation shortly after birth. None were on oxygen within three days of the study. At the time of the study, none received any medication other than antibiotics which were used prophylactically where indicated.

Before the study of each infant began, electrodes were applied. Recordings of each child began within half an hour of noon. They included an electroencephalogram (C_3/A_2 - C_4/A_1), electrooculogram, chin electromyogram, electrocardiogram and respiration which was monitored by two mercury-filled strained gauges (1 abdominal and 1 thoracic) and two thermistors positioned in front of each nostril. Behavioral criteria were systematically checked by an observer and noted on the record during the entire monitoring.

To date, the sleep records have only been partially scored. Thus only the apnea data will be reported here. To compute the results, the data from the two periods on the waterbed and the two periods off the waterbed were combined. Matched paired t tests were used for statistical analysis. For significance levels, two-tailed t tests were used throughout.

The results clearly showed that apneas were significantly reduced while the infants were on the oscillating waterbeds, with the longest apneas and those associated with severe bradycardia being reduced the most. Table 1 shows the number of apneas as indicated by the monitor alarms on and off the

TABLE 1
Number of Apnea Alarms On and Off Oscillating Waterbed

Baby	*Off*	*On*	*Change*	t_7
1	10	8	-20%	
2	16	7	-56%	
3	1	0	to 0	
4	15	9	-40%	3.53*
5	14	13	- 7%	
6	13	10	-23%	
7	5	3	-40%	
8	14	6	-57%	

Matched Pairs t Test, 2 tailed

*$p < .01$.

oscillating waterbeds. Apneas were reduced in each of the infants while they were on the waterbed with apnea reduction being highly significant ($p < .01$).

Stop-breathing episodes as shown from the polygraphic records were classfied as apneas exceeding 10 seconds without bradycardia, apneas exceeding 10 seconds with moderate bradycardia with the heart rate slowing to below 120 beats per minute, and apneas exceeding 10 seconds with severe bradycardia with the heart rate falling below 80 beats per minute.

Apneas exceeding 10 seconds without bradycardia were reduced in seven of the eight subjects while they were on the oscillating waterbed ($t = 2.75$, $df = 7$, $p < .05$, two-tailed). Reductions ranged from 16-50% with a mean reduction of 30%.

Apneas with moderate bradycardia were reduced in the same seven babies out of the eight while they were on the oscillating waterbed ($t = 3.64$, $df = 7$, $p < .01$, two-tailed). Reductions ranged from 16-50% with a mean reduction of 35%.

Apneas with severe bradycardia were reduced the most in the same seven out of eight babies while they were on the oscillating waterbed ($t = 2.26$, $df = 7$, $p < .06$, two-tailed). Reductions ranged from 29-60% with a mean reduction of 46%.

While overall the results point to clear-cut reduction of apneas while the infants were on the oscillating waterbed, they also point to marked individual differences in response. Reductions of apnea varied greatly, with one infant even running counter to the general trend. This infant's response pointed to the importance of an accurate diagnosis of apnea of prematurity at the outset. In retrospect, judging from this infant's apnea history prior to the polygraphic study and his stormy medical course before and after discharge from the hospital, it is likely that this baby's apnea was not purely a function of his prematurity. (For more complete details of this infant's medical history, see Korner, 1979.)

In summary then, the two studies we have done so far which used different research designs and different methods of appraisal both pointed to significant reductions in apnea as a function of the oscillating waterbed. One can only speculate about the underlying mechanism which may bring about this effect. The most plausible explanation appears to be that the continuous irregular oscillations provide afferent input to the respiratory center, thus aborting a number of apneas. Other possible mechanisms of action are currently under investigation. In practical terms, the oscillating waterbed represents a nontoxic, noninvasive method of alleviating a potentially brain-damaging symptom which affects about a third of the preterm infant population. We conclude from our results that clinically it may be wise to give the oscillating waterbed a trial in cases of apnea of prematurity before other, potentially more hazardous modalities of treatment are used.

CLINICAL OBSERVATIONS WITH THE NON–OSCILLATING WATERBED

Over the years, the non-oscillating waterbed has been used extensively at Stanford for a number of clinical purposes. As anticipated, the waterbeds are very helpful in the care of very small premature babies, such as infants weighing between 600 and 1000 g, in that they preserve the infants' fragile skin. The non-oscillating waterbeds have also been found useful in reducing the discomfort of infants with spina bifida, hydrocephalus, disseminated herpes and other skin conditions. In one infant born with blisters all over her body, attending physicians observed that the infant became more quiet and required less sedation when she was placed on the waterbed and from then on, skin breakdown on her back was halted. Further, the non-oscillating waterbeds have been found useful for infants recovering from abdominal surgery or for babies who are on a regimen of parenteral nutrition for emaciation. We have not yet systematically tested our hypothesis that the waterbeds reduce the incidence of asymmetrically shaped, narrow heads which are so frequently seen in premature infants. Our hypothesis was recently confirmed by Kramer and Pierpont (1976) who found that infants placed on waterbeds had more rounded heads. This effect alone has implications for the beginning parent-infant relationship: an aesthetically more pleasing infant should facilitate the bonding process in this relationship.

FURTHER STUDIES

Our current research is going in two major directions: We are further exploring the biomedical and clinical effects of waterbed flotation on premature infants. We also are beginning studies which address the developmental questions which prompted us to develop the waterbeds in the first place.

In the clinical area we are doing yet another replication study of the apnea-reducing effect of the oscillating waterbed. In this study, we are adding a plain non-oscillating waterbed in the comparison to determine whether it is the oscillations or possibly other factors involved in waterbed flotation which create the apnea reducing effect. We also have started a major longitudinal study to determine whether the gentle stimulation and the fluid support provided by the waterbeds will counteract some of the deleterious effects of the prolonged immobilization to which infants on respirators are frequently exposed. In particular, we will be interested to find out whether infants with RDS, with or without apnea, randomly assigned to experimental and control groups, will differ in when they begin to breathe of their own, in their resistance to infections, in the incidence of skin problems and asymmetrically shaped heads, and in the frequency of suspected or confirmed intracranial hemorrhages. Since pressure to the head has recently been implicated in intracranial bleeds (Newton and Gooding, 1975; Pape et al., 1976), the fluid support of the waterbed may diminish this risk. In addition, this study assesses differences in the infants' development of muscle tone, activity level, motor and sensory maturity, alertness and in the capacity to withstand fatigue at the time of hospital discharge and the infants' health status and overall development at ages 1, 2 and 3.

We are also beginning studies which address some of our developmental questions with more normal premature infants in whom major medical complications do not interfere with the developmental process. In particular, we are testing whether the rhythm of the waterbed oscillations given in a temporal pattern similar to the maternal rhythm of rest and activity has a more organizing effect on the infants' sleep organization and motor behavior that does an arbitrary rhythm involving an equal amount of stimulation. We will also study the effects of the intermittently oscillating waterbed on the more long-range motor, neurological and behavioral development of these healthier infants in order to determine whether changing the premature infants' environment through waterbed flotation facilitates in any way the more natural unfolding of the infants' maturation.

ACKNOWLEDGMENTS

Preparation of this chapter was supported by a grant from The Maternal and Child Health Research Division of Clinical Services, PHSDHEW #MC-R-060410-01-0. The research presented here was supported by The William T. Grant Foundation, Public Health Service Grants HD-08339 and HD-03591, the Boys Town Center for Youth Development at Stanford, and Grant RR-81 from the General Clinical Research Centers Program of the Division of Human Resources, National Institutes of Health.

Some of the ideas contained in this chapter were first presented at the Johnson and Johnson sponsored Nantucket Pediatric Round Table on "The Origins of the Infant's Social Responsiveness," Evelyn B. Thoman, ed., to be published by Lawrence Earlbaum Associates, in press.

REFERENCES

Aserinsky, E. The maximal capacity for sleep: Rapid eye movement density as an index of sleep satiety. *Biol. Psychiat. 1*, 147–159 (1969).

Barnard, K. E. *The Effect of Stimulation on the Duration and Amount of Sleep and Wakefulness in the Premature Infant*. University Microfilms: Ann Arbor, Michigan (1972).

Broughton, R. Biorhythmic variations in consciousness and psychological functions. *Can. Psychol. Rev. 16*, No. 4, 217–239 (1975).

Carskadon, M. A. and Dement, W. C. Sleep studies on a 90-minute day. *Electroencephal. Clin. Neurophysiol. 39*, 145–155 (1975).

Cornell, E. H. and Gottfried, A. W. Intervention with premature human infants. *Child Dev. 47*, 32–39 (1976).

Denenberg, V. H. Effects of exposure to stressors in early life upon later behavioural and biological processes. In *Society, Stress, and Disease: Childhood and Adolescence*, L. Levi, ed. Oxford University Press, New York (1975), pp. 269–281.

Dreyfus-Brisac, C. Organization of sleep in prematures: Implications for caretaking. In *The Effect of the Infant on its Caregiver*, M. Lewis and L. A. Rosenblum eds. John Wiley and Sons, New York (1974), pp. 123–140.

Erway, L. C. Otolith formation and trace elements: A theory of schizophrenic behavior. *J. Orthomol. Pschiat. 4*(1), 16–26 (1975).

Feinberg, I. Changes in sleep cycle patterns with age. *J. Psychiat. Res. 10*, 283–306 (1974).

Frankenhaeuser, M., and Johansson, G. On the psychophysiological consequences of under-stimulation and over-stimulation. *Reports from the Psychological Laboratories of the University of Stockholm*. Supplement 25 (1974).

Freedman, D. G., Boverman, H., and Freedman, N. Effects of kinesthetic stimulation on weight gain and on smiling in premature infants. Paper presented at the Annual Meeting of the American Orthopsychiatric Association, San Francisco (1966).

Goodlin, R. C. *Handbook of Obstetrical and Gynecological Data*. Geron-X, Los Altos, California (1972), p. 385.

Gregg, C. L., Haffner, M. E., and Korner, A. F. The relative efficacy of vestibular-proprioceptive stimulation and the upright position in enhancing visual pursuit in neonates. *Child Dev. 47*, 309–314 (1976).

Harlow, H. The nature of love. *Amer. Psychol. 13*, 673–685 (1958).

Hasselmeyer, E. G. The premature neonate's response to handling. *Amer. Nurses Assn. 11*, 15–24 (1964).

Hofer, M. A. Infant separation responses and the maternal role. *Biol. Psychiat. 10*(2), 149–153 (1975a).

Hofer, M. A. Studies on how early maternal separation produces behavioral change in young rats. *Psychosom. Med. 37*(3), 245–264 (1975b).

Katz, V. Auditory stimulation and developmental behavior of the premature infant. *Nurs. Res. 20*, 196–201 (1971).

Kleitman, N. Basic rest-activity cycle in relation to sleep and wakefulness. In *Sleep Physiology and Pathology: A Symposium*, A. Kales, ed. J. B. Lippincott Company, Philadelphia and Toronto (1969), pp. 33–38.

Korner, A. F. Maternal rhythms and waterbeds: A form of intervention with premature infants. In *Origins of the Infant's Responsiveness*, E. B. Thoman, ed. Lawrence Earlbaum Associates, Hillsdale, N.J. (in press, 1979).

Korner, A. F. and Grobstein, R. Visual alertness as related to soothing in neonates: Implications for maternal stimulation and early deprivation. *Child Dev. 37*, 867–876 (1966).

Korner, A. F., Kraemer, H. C., Haffner, M. E., and Thoman, E. B. Effects of waterbed flotation on premature infants: A pilot study. *Pediatrics 56*, 361–367 (1975).

Korner, A. F. and Thoman, E. B. Visual alterness in neonates as evoked by maternal care. *J. Exper. Child Psychol. 10*, 67–78 (1970).

Korner, A. F. and Thoman, E. B. The relative efficacy of contact and vestibular stimulation on soothing neonates. *Child Dev. 43*(2), 443–453 (1972).

Korones, S. B. Disturbance in infant's rest. In *Iatrogenic Problems in Neonatal Intensive Care*. 69th Ross Conference on Pediatric Research (Feb. 1976), pp. 94–97.

Kramer, L. I. and Pierpont, M. E. Rocking waterbeds and auditory stimuli to enhance growth of preterm infants. *J. Pediatr. 88*(2), 297–299 (1976).

Kripke, D. F. Ultradian rhythms in sleep and wakefulness. In *Advances in Sleep Research, Vol. 1*, E. D. Weitzman, ed. Spectrum, New York (1974), pp. 305–325.

Lee, H. F. A rocking bed respirator for use with premature infants in incubators. *J. Pediatr. 44*, 570–573 (1954).

Lucey, J. F. Is intensive care becoming too intensive? *Pediatrics, Neonatology Supplement 59*(2), 1064–1065 (1977).

Mason, W. A. Early social deprivation in the non-human primates: Implications for human behavior in environmental influences. In *Environmental Influences*, D. C. Glass, ed. Rockefeller University Press and Russell Sage Foundation, New York (1968), pp. 70–101.

Millen, R. S. and Davies, J. See-saw resuscitator for the treatment of asphyxia. *Amer. J. Obstet. Gynecol. 52*, 508–509 (1946).

Neal, M. V. *The Relationship Between a Regimen of Vestibular Stimulation and the Developmental Behavior of the Premature Infant*. University Microfilms: Ann Arbor, Michigan (1967).

Newton, T. H. and Gooding, C. A. Compression of superior sagittal sinus by neonatal calvarial molding. *Radiology 115*, 635–640 (June, 1975).

Pape, K. E., Armstrong, D. L., and Fitzhardinge, P. M. Central nervous system pathology associated with mask ventilation in the very low birthweight infant: A new etiology for intracerebellar hemorrhages. *Pediatrics 58*, 473–483 (1976).

Parmelee, A. H. Neurophysiological and behavioral organization of premature infants in the first months of life. *Biol. Psychiat. 10*(5), 501–512 (1975).

Sameroff, A. J. Early influences on development: fact or fancy? *Merrill-Palmer Quart. 21*(4), 267–294 (1975).

Scarr-Salapatek, S. and Williams, M. L. The effects of early stimulation on low-birth-weight infants. *Child Dev. 44*, 94–101 (1973).

Sterman, M. B. Relationship of intrauterine fetal activity to maternal sleep stage. *Exper. Neurol. Supplement 4*, 98–106 (1967).

Thoman, E. B., and Korner, A. F. Effects of vestibular stimulation on the behavior and development of rats. *Dev. Psychol. 5*, 92–98 (1971).

Williams, M. L., and Scarr, S. Effects of short term intervention on performance in low-birth-weight, disadvantaged children. *Pediatrics 47*, 289–298 (1971).

Wright, L. The theoretical and research base for a program of early stimulation, care, and training of premature infants. In *The Exceptional Infant. Vol. 2. Studies in Abnormalities*, J. Hellmuth, ed. Bruner/Mazel, New York (1971), pp. 276–304.

Maternal Influences and Early Behavior

16 Relationships of Human Mothers with Their Infants During the First Year of Life; Effect of Prematurity

Josephine V. Brown
Roger Bakeman

Prematurely born children are in greater danger of being abused than are children born at term. This is the almost uniform report of investigators concerned with the sequelae of prematurity or the etiology of child abuse (Klein and Stern, 1971; Klaus and Fanaroff, 1973; Lubchenco, 1976). But why should this be so? Children are abused for a variety of reasons, at all ages, and often by persons other than their mothers (for a review of child abuse, see Parke and Collmer, 1975). However, we wanted to focus on factors that might help us explain the abuse of young infants by their mothers because this type of abuse represented to us the complete breakdown of mother-infant relationships. We speculated that certain characteristics of newborn infants may contribute to the development of maladaptive mother-infant relationships—relationships that, in the extreme, can result in abuse.

Such a speculation, however, can only be addressed with a prospective study. Yet, prospective studies are unlikely to include even a single case of abuse. First, the fact of being included in a study makes it less likely that a mother would abuse her child, and second, the number of subjects required would be impractically large. However, if we think of mother-infant relationships as lying on a caretaking continuum (Sameroff and Chandler, 1975), one end of which constitutes child abuse, the other optimal care, then a prospective study might include at least a few maladaptive relationships, relationships that do not result in actual abuse but approximate in certain aspects those that do.

During the past few years, we have been studying a group of preterm infants and their mothers and a group of fullterm infants and their mothers, and have observed and recorded both infant characteristics and early mother-infant interactions. Data collection for the first year of life is now complete and the results are described here. Mothers and infants were observed during three feedings: just before being released from the hospital, one month later, and three months later. Because preterm infants are at greater risk of being abused than fullterm infants, we reasoned that an analysis of the early interactions of mothers with preterm infants in comparison with the interactions of mothers with fullterm infants could help us identify patterns that might be implicated in child abuse.

There are good reasons to think that the developing relationships between preterm infants and their mothers might be less than optimal. Preterm infants are different from fullterm infants in several ways that seem likely to affect early mother-infant interactions. For example, preterm infants are more likely to cry and to be irritable (Elmer and Gregg, 1967). In addition, preterm infants are often difficult to feed (Klaus and Fanaroff, 1973), which is one reason why we chose the feeding situation as the context within which to observe mother-infant interactions. We reasoned that because feeding is a very common and important activity, one that is interactive by its very nature, any difficulties between mother and baby would be especially likely to emerge at this time (Brody, 1961). Further, for various medical reasons, preterm infants are typically separated from their mothers for a few weeks after birth, a time that is thought to be particularly important for the development of an attachment between a mother and her baby (Barnett et al., 1970; Leifer et al., 1972).

The mothers who participated in this study gave birth to their babies in an Atlanta hosptial that serves a predominantly indigent, urban population. About 6000 babies are born annually in this hospital and approximately 800 of these are born prematurely. Having access to a large number of preterm infants allowed us to select a reasonable sample of preterms meeting specified criteria. In addition, we were able to select a sample of healthy fullterms whose mothers came from similar social and educational backgrounds as the mothers of the preterms.

In sum, preterm and fullterm infants from a disadvantaged population were examined and their interactions with their mothers were observed three times: just before discharge, one month later, and three months later. We had grounds for supposing that preterm and fullterm infants would be different, but infant examinations were undertaken to document specific ways in which preterm and fullterm infants from this population actually differed, in particular with respect to infant characteristics that could affect mother-infant interactions.

We also expected that the mothers of preterm and fullterm infants and their babies would interact differently soon after birth. Such differences could be interpreted, in the first instance, as reflecting how different infant characteristics elicit different styles of caregiving. But further, as the discussion above suggests, we hoped that the particular ways in which the preterm's interactions would differ from the fullterms' could be interpreted as characteristic of less than optimal interactions, and so would reveal specific interactive features indicative of maladaptive or at least problematic interactions.

Finally, so that we would be able to interpret early differences in the light of later outcome, we collected three kinds of data when the child was about 1 year of age. We used one outcome measure which assessed the quality of the mother-infant relationship directly (the Ainsworth Strange Situation, Ainsworth et al., in press), one which assessed the quantity and quality of stimulation provided by the mother to her baby at home (the HOME Scale, Elardo et al., 1975), and one which assessed the mental and motor developmental status of the infant (the Bayley Scales of Infant Development).

METHOD

Mothers and Infants

Subject Selection

Mothers who were asked to participate in the study had to be in reasonably good health, be 18 years or older, and plan to bottle-feed their babies (at this hospital, less than 6% plan to breast feed). In the interest of sample homogeneity, they also had to be black (at this hospital, less than 20% of the mothers are white). In addition, their infants had to meet the following criteria: if fullterm, be healthy (as judged by the pediatrician and by a 5-minute Apgar rating of 8 or more) and have had an uncomplicated birth; if preterm, weigh between 1000 and 1950 g and have no obvious neurological or physical abnormalities.

Of the mothers who met our criteria, those who had just delivered a preterm infant were significantly more likely to agree to participate in our study than mothers who had just delivered a fullterm infant (73% of the mothers of preterms but only 48% of the mothers of fullterms agreed to participate; chi-square = 4.96, $p < .05$). In most other ways, mothers who declined were not different from mothers who decided to participate. There were no significant differences with respect to the infant's sex, his birth weight, his 1- and 5-minute Apgar scores, and his gestational age (based on the mother's last menses). Furthermore, participating mothers did not differ from decliners with respect to age, parity, previous preterm infant(s), previous abortion(s), education, or income level. Only one bias was detected: Subjects were more likely than decliners to be living alone (29% vs. 18%) or with parents or other relatives (42% vs. 27%) while decliners were more likely to be living with a husband (52% vs. 29%). Indeed a common reason for declining was that the husband did not approve.

Subject Loss

Over the course of the first year, only 7 of the original 56 subjects were lost to the project. One mother of a fullterm infant moved away, three prematurely born infants died, and three mothers of preterm infants did not want to continue for various reasons. All data reported here are based on the 49 mother-infant dyads who remained with the project for the full year (11 preterm and 11 fullterm infants were male, 15 preterm and 12 fullterm infants were female; 9 preterm and 6 fullterm infants were first-born, 17 preterm and 17 fullterm infants were later-born).

Social and Medical Background

Mothers were interviewed with respect to family history, education, current living situation and income, and so forth. In addition, an Obstetric Complications Scale was computed for each mother-infant pair from hospital records (see Parmelee et al., 1976). Selected background characteristics for the 49 mother-infant dyads, given separately for preterm and fullterm infants and their mothers, are detailed in Table 1.

Procedure

Mothers and infants were examined and observed five times in the first 12 months after the infants left the hospital. Since we were primarily interested in the effect of the behavioral characteristics of the prematurely born infants on mother-infant interaction style, we chose our observation and examination times so that the length of time mothers had been responsible for their infants would be about the same for all mothers. Preterm infants were discharged from the hospital approximately one month prior to term but at a chronological age of about one month. As a result, preterms were in fact observed and examined when they were approximately one month younger in

TABLE 1
Background Characteristics for Preterm and Fullterm Infants and Their Mothers

	Preterms (N = 26)	*Fullterms* (N = 23)
Infants		
Gestational age (weeks)*	32.4 (4.4)	39.9 (1.6)
Birthweight (g)	1627 (205)	3269 (379)
5-minute Apgar	7.8 (1.2)	9.5 (0.6)
Obstetric complications (%)†	25.1 (8.7)	13.8 (7.7)
Time in hospital (days)	26.6 (25.6)	3.0 (0)
Conceptional age (weeks)**	37.0 (4.6)	39.9 (1.6)
Mothers		
Age	23.4 (6.5)	22.8 (3.9)
Education (years)	10.6 (2.1)	11.6 (0.9)
Family income ($/month)	378 (224)	400 (279)
Other children	1.6 (2.2)	0.9 (0.8)
Previous pregnancies	2.3 (2.5)	1.3 (0.8)
People in household	6.1 (3.7)	4.9 (2.3)
Living with husband	26.9%	30.4%
Living with parents/relatives	38.5%	39.1%
On welfare	61.5%	69.6%

Note.—Except for the last three rows of percentages, all values are means (standard deviations are given in parentheses). All of the infant, but none of the mother characteristics significantly differentiated between preterm and fullterm dyads ($p < .001$, two-tailed *t*-test).

*Judged by the obstetrician.

†The Obstetric Complication Scale (OCS) is referenced in the text.

**At hospital discharge.

conceptional (gestational age plus age since birth) age but one month older in chronological age than the fullterm infants.

Assessment of Infant Characteristics

The behavioral characteristics of the infants were assessed three times: just prior to hospital discharge, one month later, and three months later. For this purpose we used the Brazelton Neonatal Behavioral Assessment Scale (Brazelton, 1973) in the hospital and one month later, the Prechtl Neurological Examination with Beintema's scoring criteria (Beintema, 1968) prior to discharge, and the Bayley Scales of Infant Development at three months after discharge. Because we are concerned in this report with the effects of newborn characteristics on mother-infant interactions, results of the 3-month examinations will not be reported.

Observation of Mother-Infant Interaction

The interactions of mothers with their infants were recorded during a 30-minute feeding session just prior to hospital discharge and at one and three months after hospital discharge. Prior to discharge, the fullterm infants and mothers were observed in the mothers' rooms, while the preterm infants and their mothers were observed in the preterm nursery. One month and three months later, mothers and infants returned to the hospital where they were observed in a clinic room. Two observers (one observed the mother, the other the infant) encoded the stream of behavior using a code catalog of approximately 120 different predefined behaviors (for example, mother stimulates infant to suck, mother burps infant, mother looks at infant, infant holds nipple in mouth, infant burps, infant has eyes open). Behaviors were recorded with a portable electronic device that records codes and time of entry (Datamyte, DAK-8C). Codes were defined so that data reduction preserved the frequency, the duration, the sequence, and the co-occurrence of all behaviors. Observation procedures were developed in an earlier study (Brown et al., 1975) and are described in several technical reports (Bakeman, Note 1, Note 2; Brown and Bakeman, Note 3). Inter-observer reliability was established before the study began and maintained at levels of 75% (strict criterion, omissions are counted as disagreements) and 90% (loose criterion, omissions are not counted) throughout the study.

Assessment of Outcome at One Year

Nine months after discharge, mothers and infants were visited at home by the social worker on our staff. At that time the quality and quantity of social, emotional, and cognitive support available to the child in the home setting was evaluated with the aid of the HOME Scale (Elardo et al., 1975). The HOME Scale consists of 45 items, each requiring a yes/no answer. About half of the questions are answered in the course of the actual observation of the home environment and the interactions of the mother with her baby (for example, "the child's play environment appears safe and free of hazards," or "mother does not scold, or criticize, or 'run down' the child during visit"). Answers to the remaining items are elicited from the mother during a nonstructured interview conducted by the observer (for example, "someone takes child to grocery store at least once a week," or "mother 'talks' to child while doing her work").

Twelve months after discharge mothers and infants were observed in the "Strange Situation" developed by Ainsworth and Wittig (1969). The Strange Situation was developed as a standardized laboratory procedure during which the infant's attachment behaviors are observed in an unfamiliar environment during a series of eight increasingly stressful episodes, each lasting approximately three minutes. In the course of these episodes, the following behaviors of each infant are recorded: (a) his exploratory behavior both in the mother's presence and in her absence; (b) his response to mother's absence, when alone and when left with a stranger; (c) his response to mother's return after her absence in comparison to his response to the stranger after her absence. The quality of the mother-infant relationship is then judged on the basis of these responses during the Strange Situation. Several studies indicate that the relationship of the mother and infant during the Strange Situation is related to specific earlier patterns of interactions experienced by the infant with his caregiver (Ainsworth, et al., in press). During the Strange Situation, the actual behaviors of the mothers, the infants, and the stranger were recorded with a procedure that was very similar to the one used to record behaviors during the feeding (Bakeman et al., 1976).

During that same visit, but prior to the observation in the Strange Situation, the Bayley Scales of Infant Development were again administered to each infant.

HOW DID PRETERM AND FULLTERM DYADS DIFFER DURING THE FIRST THREE MONTHS?

Differences in Infant Characteristics

Preterm and fullterm infants were examined in the hospital and one month after discharge. The purpose of these examinations was to document how the two groups of infants differed with respect to the kinds of behaviors that could affect early mother-infant interaction styles. Differences in the examination scores of preterm and fullterm infants were analyzed with two-tailed t-tests. Developmental differences between scores obtained in the hospital and one month later were analyzed with one-tailed sign tests. Unless otherwise noted, only differences at the .05 level of significance will be discussed. (The infant examination data are discussed in greater detail in Brown et al., Note 4.)

The results of our analyses indicate that the behavior of the two groups of infants was quite distinct in the hospital and one month later. Further, a comparison of the developmental trends of the two groups of infants during this period revealed some additional interesting differences. All our findings suggest that the preterm infants were more difficult to care for, less satisfying to feed, and less responsive than the fullterm infants. Specific differences are documented below.

In the hospital, preterms were less active, exhibited weaker motor movements, had poorer head control, poorer hand-to-mouth control, and less well developed rooting and sucking responses. They also exhibited fewer startles, cried less and with lower intensities and for shorter durations, and were less irritable. In addition, the preterms smiled more and were more tremulous than the fullterm infants. Contrary to our expectations, however, the preterm infants did not differ from the fullterms in their ability to orient to auditory and visual stimuli.

One month after hospital discharge, the preterm infants were significantly less alert and less responsive to auditory and visual stimuli and were more difficult to console than fullterm infants. Furthermore, they still exhibited poorer rooting and sucking responses.

The ways in which preterm and fullterm infants changed during that first month are also different and may have implications for how mothers of preterms viewed their babies. Preterm infants became more active and more irritable but did not improve in their ability to orient to auditory and visual stimuli, while fullterm infants became much more alert and better able to orient to auditory and visual stimuli. No wonder that several mothers of preterm infants remarked to us that their babies did not seem to like being at home. In the hospital their babies had been quiet and undemanding but now, one month later, these same babies were irritable and active, but still sucked poorly and still responded poorly to auditory or visual stimuli.

Differences in Mother-Infant Interaction

In the previous section we described how preterm and fullterm infants differed when examined by us; in this section we will describe how those infants interacted with their mothers during a feeding. First we will describe how preterm and fullterm dyads differed with respect to frequency and duration of specfic interactive behaviors. And second, we will view the interaction more abstractly—as a "behavioral dialogue"—and again describe group differences, but with respect to interaction style.

Interactive Behaviors

Conclusions based on the frequencies and durations of specific behaviors and behavior categories recorded during the feeding observation are in general agreement with those derived from the infant examination data: In comparison with fullterms, preterm infants were more difficult and less satisfying to feed and seemed less fun to interact with. However, differences during the feeding sessions were most apparent prior to hospital discharge and one month later; three months later most of the preterm/fullterm differences—at least with respect to the specific behaviors discussed here—had disappeared. Specific differences are described below. (Again, only significant differences are discussed. Data for selected summary behavior categories are given in Table 2, which gives some feeling for how mothers and infants spent their time during the feeding session. In most cases, summary categories were formed by aggregating specific behaviors, for example,

TABLE 2
Summary Scores for Selected Behaviors by Type of Infant and Time of Observation

	Hospital		*1 Month*		*3 Months*	
	Prem	*Full*	*Prem*	*Full*	*Prem*	*Full*
Infant						
gross motor	6.7	6.6	17.4	26.4	25.0	25.1
fine motor	15.2	18.1	17.1	16.6	16.3	16.5
touching/grasping	9.7	12.7	6.8	4.7	6.1	7.7
eyes open	28.8	40.5	60.7	72.8	80.3	71.6
looking at mother	(4)	(14)	12.3	15.2	12.4	10.3
looking at surround	(2)	(2)	7.7	29.6	56.5	50.7
vocalizing	1.9	1.2	9.3	10.3	13.7	15.5
Mother						
looking at infant	92.3	91.7	94.3	94.4	95.8	84.0
vocalizing to infant	13.6	8.1	17.8	15.1	25.7	15.8
tactile stimulation	26.7	20.0	16.2	15.3	13.4	10.7
vestibular stimulation	19.3	9.8	17.9	11.5	13.4	7.9
bottle feeding infant	20.4	33.1	27.7	28.4	16.3	20.3
spoon feeding infant	(0)	(0)	10.9	11.3	14.9	14.0

Note.—Summary scores are mean durations, based on 26 preterm and 23 fullterm dyads and expressed as percentages of the half-hour observation sessions. If at a given observation time less than half of either preterm or fullterm dyads engaged in a particular behavior then the number of such dyads is noted in parentheses and no mean duration is given.

"infant vocalizes" includes infant whimpers, cries, babbles, etc. These data are discussed in greater detail in Bakeman and Brown, Note 5.)

Preterms fed less vigorously than fullterms, at least during the hospital observation. They were less likely to signal their readiness to feed by opening their mouths and by rooting. Their mothers expended more effort throughout the hospital interaction. They issued more directive commands, and thumped, poked, pinched, and rocked their infants more. All these efforts, however, were rewarded with less success. The infants fed less and there were fewer of the usual signs to indicate that feeding was progressing smoothly: Preterm infants burped less and their mothers wiped their mouths less frequently.

In addition to the fact that preterm infants were initially more difficult to feed, they were also less social. They looked less at their mothers (in the hospital and at one month) and less at the environment (at one month). And, although preterms and fullterms did not differ in the total amount of time they vocalized, the vocalizations of the preterms in the hospital consisted primarily of gasping inhalation sounds, while fullterms tended to make more sucking noises. By three months, the fullterms babbled and cooed more than the preterms, while the preterms continued their earlier gasps and sighs.

Behavioral Dialogues

A particular concern of ours has been to develop indices of interaction that could be derived from concretely defined behaviors and yet would characterize the structure of the interaction independent of those particular behaviors. For this purpose, we view mother-infant interaction, not as a sequence of particular behaviors, but instead as a "dialogue" or "conversation," the elements of which are not just vocalizations but a broader class of communicative behaviors. (This approach is discussed in more detail in Bakeman and Brown, 1977.) In a sense, a class of interactive behaviors or "communicative acts" are equated to the phrases and sentences of adult conversation, and the entire interaction is reduced to sequences of mother "talks" (mother acts), infant "talks" (infant acts), both "talk" (mother and infant co-act), or neither "talks" (both quiescent).

Specifically, 42 behaviors from the code catalog were designated "mother communcative acts" and 30 were designated "infant communicative acts." These included such behaviors as mother rocks, rubs, pats, pokes, vocalizes, shifts position, offers bottle, etc., and infant cries, whines, babbles, burps, looks to mother, smiles, wiggles, waves arms, rejects nipple. Then each ½-hour session was segmented into 360 5-second intervals, and each interval was categorized: as quiescent (Q) if none of the mother and none of the infant communicative acts occurred within it; as infant-alone (I) if one or more infant communicative acts but no mother communicative acts occurred; as mother-alone (M) if one or more mother but no infant communicative acts occurred; and as co-acting (C) if one or more infant and one or more mother communicative acts occurred.

In summary, observation sessions were reduced to sequences of the four dyadic states defined here. (A segment of an interaction might look like this: QQQQMMMCCMMMCMMQQQIIIQQ....) A advantage of viewing mother-infant interaction simply as sequences of these four "dyadic states" is that certain characteristics of the interaction can easily be quantified (e.g., the proportion of time spent in the various dyadic states and the probability with which various states follow each other). We regard these scores as relatively "content-free" indices of interaction, as indices of "interaction style" that let us describe the structure of the interaction in a relatively abstract way. It was our hope that analyses of these indices would reveal preterm/fullterm differences that were not readily apparent from the analyses of specific behaviors.

The rates of most specific infant behaviors increased with time and so it is not surprising that the overall rate of infant activity (p(I + C), the probability of the infant acting alone pus the probability of co-action) also increased with time (see Figure 1). The mother's rate of activity (p(M + C)), however, was

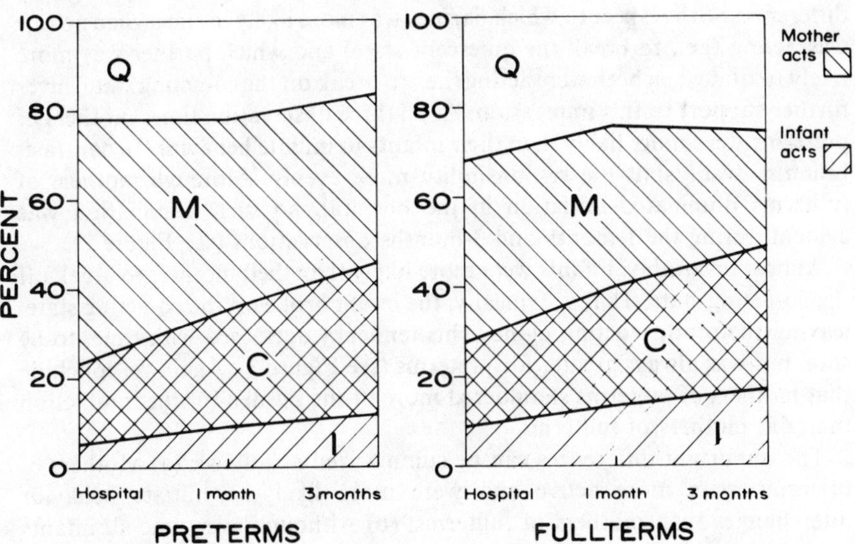

FIG. 1. Mean dyadic state probabilities by type of infant and time of observation.

quite stable. As a result of increased infant activity and stable mother activity, the probability of co-action (p(C)) increased and the probability that the mother would be acting alone (p(M)) decreased. And so with time, as the infant engaged in more communicative acts, the interactions became characterized by more concurrent activity and less mother-acting-alone time. This was generally so both for preterm and fullterm dyads.

While the rates for specific behaviors distinguished preterm and fullterm dyads primarily in the hospital, the values of the dyadic state probabilities distinguished the two groups of mothers and infants consistently at all three observation times. Mainly, mothers of preterms were considerably more active than mothers of fullterms, while the preterm infants were somewhat less active than the fullterms. Since the rate of concurrent activity was similar for both groups of dyads, the mothers of preterms were more often acting alone, while their infants were less often acting alone, than were the mothers of fullterms and their infants. It almost seems as though the mothers had a notion of an "appropriate" amount of concurrent activity and strove to meet that quota. Because preterm infants were less active, their mothers exerted considerably more effort in reaching the quota, while mothers of fullterms, who reached their quota with considerably less effort, were then free to let their infants act alone.

These findings suggest that mothers of preterms bore an unequal share of the responsibility for the flow of the interaction. An examination of group differences with respect to which partner was more likely to start when no one was acting (i.e., to break the quiescent state) and which partner was more likely to quit when both were acting (i.e., to break off the co-acting state) gives further support to this impression. At all three observation times mothers of preterms were more likely than their infants to initiate behavior. In contrast, fullterm dyads split the responsibility more evenly. Although mothers of fullterms dominated initiation in the hospital, no such domination was evident during the 1-month and 3-months observations (see Figure 2).

Almost invariably, infants were more likely than their mothers to break off the co-acting state. That is, typically, the infant broke off the co-acting state, leaving the mother acting alone. This tendency decreased with time, to be sure, but was always greater for preterms (see Figure 3). Again we conclude that mothers of preterms shouldered more of the burden for the interaction than did mothers of fullterms.

The important differences can be summarized as follows: (a) Mothers of preterms were more active and were more likely to initiate behavior interchanges than mothers of fullterms; (b) Although over time all infants became more likely to initiate behavior interchanges so that the mother-infant dialogues became more balanced, this tendency was less for the

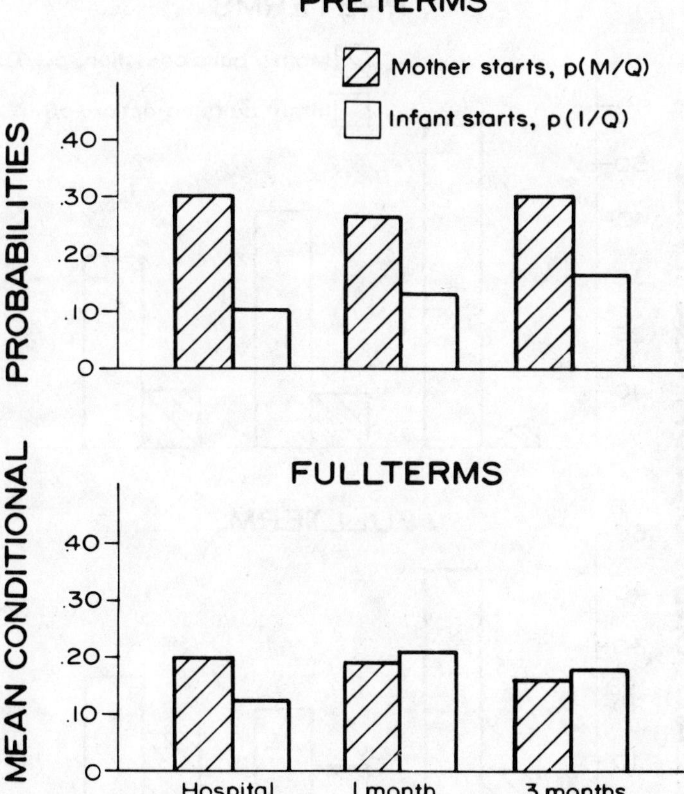

FIG. 2. The probability of breaking the quiescent state, for mothers and infants, by type of infant and time of observation. The figure depicts mean values for 26 preterm and 23 fullterm dyads. Considering individual dyads, "mother starts" was greater than "infants starts" for most preterm dyads at all three observation times (for 23, 21, and 20 out of 26, $p < .001$, .01, and .01 by sign test), but for fullterm dyads only at the hospital observation (for 18, 10, and 8 out of 23, $p < .05$, NS, and NS).

preterm than for the fullterm infants; (c) Although the rates of *specific behaviors* changed over the first three months and preterm and fullterm mother-infant dyads became more similar in terms of their specific behaviors, the differences in interaction style during this time period remained stable. (For additional detail see Bakeman and Brown, Note 5.)

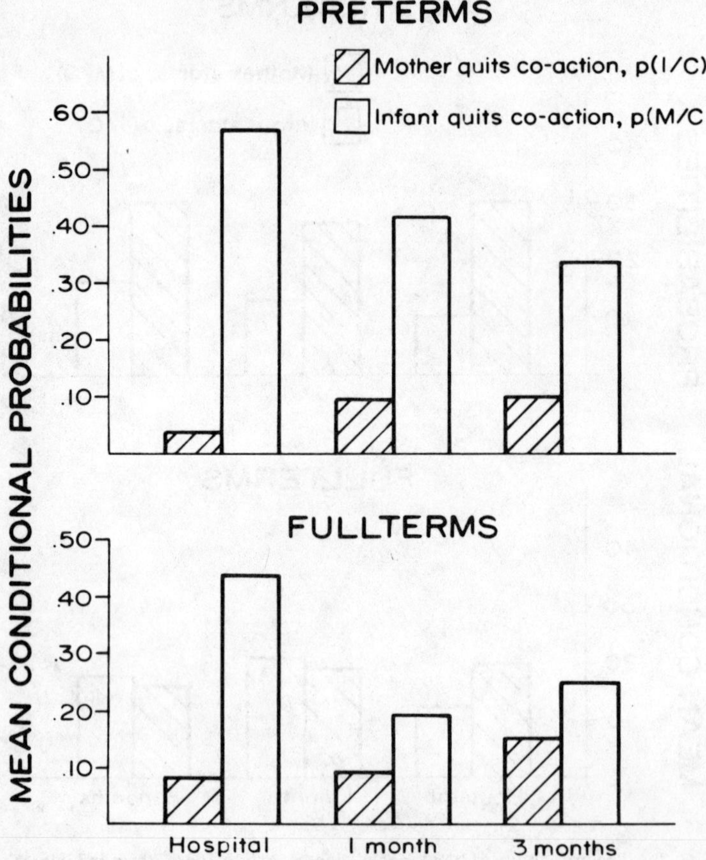

FIG. 3. The probability of breaking off the co-acting state, for mothers and infants, by type of infant and time of observation. The figure depicts mean values for 26 preterm and 23 fullterm dyads. Considering individual dyads, "mother quits" was almost invariably greater than "infants quits" for all dyads at all observation times (for 26, 24, and 23 of the 26 preterm and for 23, 21, and 21 of the 23 fullterm dyads, $p < .001$ for all).

HOW DID PRETERM AND FULLTERM DYADS DIFFER AFTER ONE YEAR?

So far we have demonstrated that the behavior of the preterm and fullterm infants during their first three months at home was very different, that their mothers responded to these behavioral differences, and that, as a result, the interaction styles of the two groups of mothers and infants also differed. If these group differences are related to later differences in either infant characteristics or quality of mother-infant relationships, we would expect that our outcome measures would also signficantly differentiate the two groups of mothers and infants. But they did not. Below follows a brief description of these results.

The Quality of Stimulation in the Home

Mothers were interviewed and observed with their babies at home nine months after the babies had been discharged from the hospital. The social worker visited the mothers at a time that was convenient for them, while their babies were awake, and administered the HOME Scale.

Although there were no group differences in the total HOME scores, the overall scores were low (i.e., 29 for mothers of preterms and 32 for mothers of fullterms). The scores were, in fact, similar to those reported by Caldwell for her original standardization sample and reflect the underpriviledged background of the mothers in our sample.

Although the mothers in general scored very high in the area of "emotional and verbal responsivity," they lost points in all other areas. A majority of infants in our sample were reared in an environment that was not free of hazards, had no toys that would permit hand-eye coordination (e.g., blocks), were without access to books or music, and had no special place where their possessions were kept. The mothers typically did not teach their infants names of things, play or look at picture books with them, and, at the same time, they restricted their infants' physical movements and used physical punishment to control their behavior. Fathers typically did not share in the caregiving of the child (mainly because most fathers were not present in the home).

The Baby's Mental Development

Twelve months after hospital discharge, the Bayley Scales of Infant Development were administered to all infants. When corrected for prematurity, the scores of the preterm and fullterm infants were within normal limits and did not differ from each other. The corrected Mental Development Indices were 111 and 109 and the corrected Psychomotor Development Indices were 110 and 113 for preterms and fullterms, respectively. The uncorrected indices of the preterm infants, however, were significantly below those of the fullterm infants (MDI = 92 and PDI = 96).

Preterm infants functioned at a mental age of 12.8 months and at a motor age of 13 months, while the mental and motor ages of the fullterms were 13.6 and 14 months, respectively. Hence, when the preterm infants went home from the hospital, their mean conceptional age was one month younger than that of the fullterms, and 12 months later they still functioned at a maturity level that was approximately one month below that of the fullterms. An analysis of the kinds of items failed by preterms but passed by fullterms revealed that the preterms lagged in gross and fine motor development and in language-related social skills. For instance, significantly fewer preterms walked alone, were able to put three cubes in a cup, repeated a performance when laughed at, jabbered expressively, or used gestures to make wants known.

The Quality of the Mother-Infant Relationship

After the observers had coded the behaviors of the infant, the mother, and the stranger during the Strange Situation, all codes were merged on the basis of time of entry and the record of each observation was transcribed. All infants were subsequently classified as either A, B, or C babies on the basis of these transcripts by two independent judges who were unaware of the birth status of the child.

An infant was classified as "avoidant" (A baby) if he avoided his mother in the reunion episodes, cried little, and explored whether his mother was present or not. He was designated as "normal" (B baby) if he explored in the presence of his mother, but less so in his mother's absence, and if he showed other clear signs of preferring his mother over the stranger. Finally, if a baby would not let his mother out of his reach during the first reunion episode, explored little and cried much whether his mother was present or not, yet could not be easily comforted by his mother, he was classified as "ambivalent" (C baby).

The judges initially assigned each infant to one of eight subcategories (for details, see Ainsworth, et al., in press): A1, A2, B1, B2, B3, B4, and C1, C2. We felt that the initial use of these finer distinctions would result in classifications that were ultimately more reliable. If one regards these eight categories as lying on an ordinal scale, then the initial agreement can be described as follows: There was perfect agreement in 24 cases; in 15 cases the judges disagreed by 1 scale point; and in 10 cases the judges disagreed by 2 scale points. The final classification was arrived at by arguing to consensus.

Although slightly more preterm than fullterm infants were classified as either ambivalent or avoidant, these differences were not statistically significant. Of the 26 preterm infants, 13 were classified as normal, 7 as avoidant, and 6 as ambivalent. Of the 23 fullterm infants, 17 were classified as normal, 2 as avoidant, and 4 as ambivalent.

SUMMARY AND CONCLUSIONS

The data described here are derived from an ongoing study concerned with the effects of early infant characteristics and mother-infant interactions on subsequent development. In this chapter we reported data that were collected during the infants' first year of life. Our strategy has been to compare a group of preterm infants with a group of fullterm infants, first with respect to newborn characteristics, then with respect to early mother-infant interaction styles, and finally with respect to the quality of the mother-infant relationships and the infants' developmental status at the end of the first year.

We had hoped that this comparison would help us understand why the rate of abuse of prematurely born babies is higher than that for babies born at term. Specifically, we had speculated that certain characteristics of the newborn may elicit the kind of maternal interaction styles that contribute to the development of maladaptive mother-infant relationships and that these characteristics may be more prevalent among prematurely born infants. If this were so, then an examination of the early interaction style of a group of mothers with preterm infants in comparison with that of a group of mothers with fullterm infants would help us identify interaction patterns that might be implicated in the etiology of child abuse.

But the interpretation of earlier group differences, with respect to both infant characteristics and interaction styles, depends on outcome. For example, if the preterms had scored lower as a group than the fullterms with respect to our outcome measures, we would have argued that the modal interaction style of mothers with their preterm infants was maladaptive. As it is, the outcome measures did not distinguish the two groups, and so, at this time, we are not justified in regarding one group's style as any more or less adaptive than the other's.

The findings described here can be summarized as follows: (a) Preterm infants differed from fullterm infants in a variety of ways that suggest that prematurely born infants are less rewarding and more difficult to care for. (b) The ways in which mothers interacted with preterm and with fullterm infants were quite different from the beginning and remained different during the infant's first three months at home. Preterms contributed less to the interactive flow than fullterms and the burden of maintaining that flow fell disproportionately on the mothers of preterms. (c) In spite of these earlier group differences, no differences between preterm and fullterm dyads were detected with respect to the quality of the mother-infant relationship or the infant's developmental status at one year.

What can we concude from these findings? First, it seems likey that mothers of preterms adapted to the characteristics of their infants and established an interaction style which, in the absence of later differences in outcome, presumably was appropriate to the infant. Still, interaction style demonstrated a degree of "functional autonomy" because differences in interaction styles of both groups of mothers and infants persisted over the first three months, while differences in frequencies and durations of specific interactive behaviors largely disappeared. We conclude that early mother-infant interaction style is influenced greatly by infant characteristics, results from the maternal adaptation to the infant, and may or may not have further consequences. In any case, from the evidence presented here, we have no reason to assume that the modal interactive style of the preterm dyads was any more or less adaptive than that of the fullterm dyads.

How can we explain the lack of group differences in the outcome measures used in this study? Perhaps our measures were not sufficiently sensitive, even though all had been used effectively in several studies. Or, perhaps we simply did not wait long enough, and differences will emerge at age 2 or 3 when the cognitive and social demands made of the infants are more complex (for a similar argument, see Scarr-Salapatek, 1976). On the other hand, it is possible that no group differences will ever emerge. The preterms in our sample were relatively healthy and it has been shown that the prognosis of preterms with few neonatal complications is good (Caputo and Mandell, 1970). Finally, it may be that the preterms and their mothers benefited more from being in the study than the fullterms and their mothers so that potential differences were obliterated. It is true that mothers of preterms asked the social worker on our staff for help significantly more often than mothers of fullterms and it may be that greater support provided by our social worker to the mothers of preterms enabled them to focus more attention on their infants. This explanation is supported by the work of Garbarino (1976), who reported that New York State counties with more adequate parental support systems had lower child abuse rates.

But the fact remains that we did not find differences in group outcome, at least at 1 year. We began with the fact that prematurely born infants are more likely to be abused (Klein and Stern, 1971; Lubchenco, 1976) and thought that we could link earlier differences between preterms and fullterms to later maladaptive relationships and even child abuse. At this time, our data do not support, but do not necessarily preclude, the notion of such a linkage. However, there are still other interesting questions we can ask. One such question is whether there are any relationships between our early measures and outcome at 1 year. To answer such a question we should regard the preterm and fullterm dyads as one sample (albeit a rather small one) and focus on individual rather than group differences. Analyses along these lines suggest that obstetrical complications and infant characteristics, rather than indices of mother-infant interactions, predict infant developmental status and quality of mother-infant relationship at 1 year. These are tentative results, and before exploring them further we prefer to wait for additional later outcome measures. However, the results of these preliminary analyses do suggest that the most effective means for preventing poor infant development and problematic mother-infant relationships at 1 year might well be improvement of social and economic conditions that are associated with perinatal problems. (Richards, 1977, makes a similar argument.)

Finally, these results underscore the flexibility of the relationship between the human mother and her infant. Even under quite unfavorable environmental circumstances, the mothers in our study compensated for the condition of their infants and cared for them appropriately. Perhaps this result should not surprise us. After all, investigators working with nonhuman primates (e.g., Berkson, 1975), who have studied the development of infants with handicaps more severe than those of the preterms in our study, have demonstrated the compensatory power of the primate mother-infant relationship.

ACKNOWLEDGMENTS

This research project was supported by Grant MH26131 awarded by the Center for the Study of Crime and Delinquency, National Institute of Mental Health, DHEW. The authors want to thank Dr. Susan Essock-Vitale and Dr. George Etlinger for their helpful comments on an earlier version of this chapter.

REFERENCE NOTES

1. Bakeman, R. Data editing procedures (Tech. Rep. 1). Atlanta: Georgia State University, Infancy Laboratory, January 1975.
2. Bakeman, R. Data analyzing procedures (Tech. Rep. 2). Atlanta: Georgia State University, Infancy Laboratory, January 1975.
3. Brown, J. V., and Bakeman, R. Mother-infant behavior codes, birth through three months (Tech. Rep. 3). Atlanta: Georgia State University, Infancy Laboratory, June 1975.
4. Brown, J. V., Aylward, G. P., and Bakeman, R. The development of a group of preterm and fullterm inner-city black infants during the first year of life (Tech. Rep. 7). Atlanta: Georgia State University, Infancy Laboratory, 1978.
5. Bakeman, R., and Brown, J. V. Mother-infant interaction during the first months of life: Differences between preterm and fullterm infant-mother dyads from a low income population (Tech. Rep. 5). Atlanta: Georgia State University, Infancy Laboratory, December 1977.

REFERENCES

Ainsworth, M. D. S., Blehar, M., Waters, E. and Wall, F. *Patterns of attachment: Observations in the Strange Situation and at home.* Earlbaum, Hillsdale, New Jersey (in press).

Ainsworth, M. D. S. and Wittig, B. A. Attachment and exploratory behaviors in one-year-olds in a strange situation. In *Determinants of Human Behavior IV*, B. M. Foss, ed. Methuen & Co., London (1969).

Bakeman, R. and Brown, J. V. Behavioral dialogues: An approach to the assessment of mother-infant interaction. *Child Dev. 48*, 195–203, (1977).

Bakeman, R., Wolkin, J. R., Karger, R. H., and Brown, J. V. A behavior code catalog for the Ainsworth Strange Situation. *JSAS Catalog of Selected Documents in Psychology 6*, 105, (1976).

Barnett, C. R., Leiderman, P. H., Grobstein, R., and Klaus, M. Neonatal separation: The maternal side of interactional deprivation. *Pediatrics 45*, 197–205 (1970).

Beintema, D. J. *A neurological study of newborn infants.* Clinics in Developmental Medicine No. 28. Heinemann, London (1968).

Berkson, G. Social responses to blind infant monkeys. In *Aberrant Development in Infancy: Human and Animal Studies*, N. R. Ellis, ed. Earlbaum, Hillsdale, New Jersey (1975).

Brazelton, T. B. *Neonatal behavioral assessment scale.* Clinics in Developmental Medicine No. 50. Heinemann, London, (1973).

Brody, S. Preventive intervention in current problems of early childhood. In *Prevention of Mental Disorders in Children*, G. Caplan, ed. Basic Books, New York (1961).

Brown, J. V., Bakeman, R., Snyder, P. A., Frederickson, W. T., Morgan, S. T., and Hepler, R. Interactions of black inner-city mothers with their newborn infants. *Child Dev. 46*, 677–686 (1975).

Caputo, D. V. and Mandell, W. Consequences of low birth weight. *Dev. Psychol. 3*, 363–383 (1970).

Elardo, R., Bradley, R., and Caldwell, B. M. The relation of infants' home environments to mental test performance from six to thirty-six months: A longitudinal analysis. *Child Dev. 46*, 71–76 (1975).

Elmer, E. and Gregg, G. S. Developmental characteristics of abused children. *Pediatrics, 40*, 596–602 (1967).

Garbarino, J. A preliminary study of some ecological correlates of child abuse: The impact of socioeconomic stress on mothers. *Child Dev. 47*, 178–185 (1976).

Klaus, M. H. and Fanaroff, A. A. *Care of the High-Risk Neonate*. W. B. Saunders Co., Philadelphia (1973).

Klein, M. and Stern, L. Low birthweight and the battered child syndrome. *Am. J. Dis. Child. 122*, 15–18 (1971).

Leifer, A. D., Leiderman, P. H., Barnett, C. R., and Williams, J. A. Effects of mother-infant separation on maternal attachment behavior. *Child Dev. 43*, 1203–1218 (1972).

Lubchenco, L. O. *The High Risk Infant*. W. B. Saunders Co., Philadelphia (1976).

Parke, R. D. and Collmer, C. W. Child abuse; An interdisciplinary analysis. In *Review of Child Development Research*. Vol. 5, E. M. Hetherington, ed. University of Chicago Press, Chicago, (1975).

Parmelee, A. H., Kopp, C. B., and Sigman, M. Selection of developmental assessment techniques for infants at risk. *Merrill-Palmer Quarterly, 22*, 177–199 (1976).

Richards, M. P. M. An ecological study of infant development in an urban setting in Britain. In *Culture and Infancy: Variations in the Human Experience*, P. H. Leiderman, S. R. Tulkin, and A. Rosenfeld, eds. Academic Press, New York (1977).

Sameroff, A. J. and Chandler, M. J. Reproductive risk and the continuum of caretaking casualty. In *Review of Child Development Research*, Vol. 4, F. D. Horowitz, ed. University of Chicago Press, Chicago (1975).

Scarr-Salapatek, S. An evolutionary perspective on infant intelligence: Species patterns and individual variations. In *Origins of Intelligence*, M. Lewis, ed. Plenum Press, New York (1976).

Maternal Influences and Early Behavior

17

A Model for the Study of Early Mother-Infant Communication

Evelyn B. Thoman
Margaret P. Freese

Through the evolutionary process the newborn infant's capabilities are designed to permit adaptation to its environment and survival. As the mother typically constitutes the major environment for the infant, the meshing of her behaviors and those of the infant is a significant determinant of the infant's survival and early development. A great deal of sophisticated research has identified the infant's potential for adapting to the environment in terms of sensory discrimination abilities, response repertoire, and modifiability of stimulus-response relations. In view of the sensitivity of these response capabilities, it is generally agreed that from the time of birth the infant is an active, not a passive, participant in interaction. However, the actual functioning of these capabilities in the communicative process between mother and infant has only begun to be explored.

The purpose of our research is to observe infants in their natural habitats and to describe some of the important behavioral characteristics of infants and mothers, and the ways in which their behaviors fit together. The general viewpoint of this research is that mothers and infants are in continuous communication from the early weeks of life. The general framework for the research is general systems theory. Our procedural approach is that of longitudinal study with intensive—and extensive—observations made under circumstances which are as natural as possible.

In the first part of the paper, we will present a framework for viewing the ealry interactive system of mothers and infants, and an argument that the communication during the early weeks of life is not only extremely significant, but is uniquely different from communication at a later age. In the sections that follow, we will present a rationale for the procedures we use to study the communication system, the behaviors that are recorded, and examples of data analyses that derive from the application of a systems view of the early mother-infant adaptation process.

MOTHER-INFANT INTERACTION AS COMMUNICATION

Linguistic Models Are Not Applicable to Early Communication

A major assumption for our model of mother and infant interaction is that it constitutes a communication system from the time of birth. Obviously, communication with a newborn baby is not linguistic in nature. Furthermore, linguistic models are not applicable in any attempt to understand the early communication.

Because of great interest in the emergence of language, linguistic models have been an inspiration for many studies of early interaction. The prelinguistic period is generally viewed as a precursor to the development of language. The mother-infant interaction during this period is viewed as a training stage on which the mother plays the role of modeler, shaper, and otherwise director of the infant with the objective of helping her infant to become socially competent, i.e., language speaking. Bruner (1975) espoused this view when he said that the infant's success in achieving joint action virtually leads into language. That is, through the mother's responsiveness, the rules for regulating her behavior become apparent to the baby. The infant's effectiveness in "achieving ends" provides the infant with the concepts regarding agents, actions, objects, and recipients that are the basis for language. Thus, the mother-infant situation is one in which fundamental cognitive schemata necessary for language are acquired.

This linguistic pespective has had some major consequences for theoretical views of early mother-infant interaction. One consequence is that attention has been paid primarily to the second half year of life when the baby is demonstrably acquiring concepts or schemata which will later be integrated and expressed linguistically. Such studies have been designed to identify ways in which the infant accumulates information about the world from the social environment. Because of this emphasis on concept-acquisition, too little attention has been paid to the first six months of life. The first half year of life is viewed more as a precursor of the prelinguistic period, a time when the infant's potential for information acquisition is developing, but one which has little direct relevance to language acquisition and therefore is of little interest.

A second consequence of this perspective is that the linguistic model is seen as most appropriate for exploring the nature of nonlinguistic communication. However, the linguistic-cognitive models would argue that early communication is relatively simple, and that cognitive differentiation leads to greater complexity in communication with time. There is growing evidence that this notion may be untrue, or at least greatly exaggerated with respect to the simplicity of the early interactions. An unexpected subtlety begins to be apparent in evidence for the newborn's immediate imitation of an adult's movements (Meltzoff and Moore, 1977; Trevarthen, 1977), Condon and Sander's (1974) demonstration that an infant's motor movements may be synchronized with an adult's speech, and studies of mother-infant interchanges which reflect maternal responses to cues given by the infant which are not directly apparent to an observer (Thoman et al., 1970; Thoman et al., 1972; Sander et al., 1979).

The communicative capabilities of infants during the early weeks of life have only begun to be explored, and their complexity has probably been vastly underestimated. This complexity is emphasized by Thorpe (1967), who stated that "the selective pressures that led to the emergence of language must have been social, and among the more likely specific possibilities is the prolongation of social dependence which brought with it the need for more subtle social adjustments and more elaborate forms of cooperation" (p. 12).

The complexities of communication in the first six months of life may not be analogous to those seen in later linguistic communication. Although the early interaction certainly includes vocalization, its characteristics are very different from later verbal patterns. Mothers talk to their babies, but without an expectation of their words being comprehended. In fact, some mothers even respond, with change of intonation, for their babies—and thus carry on a "conversation" with themselves. Babies may grunt, vocalize, fuss or cry; but their mothers must make inferences if they are to relate the vocalizations to the baby's status of hunger, pain, discomfort, or even boredom.

The totality of mutual involvement in this early communication has no analogy in linguistic exchange. For example, if the mother picks the baby up and holds it close to her, she may feel the infant's soft skin against her cheek, the baby's motor movements, and its molding to her body. She may smell the infant's skin odor, or feces. She may watch the infant's visual gaze, grimacing, and various limb or body movements. Simultaneously, the infant may be moved about in space, may have the visual image of the mother's mobile face, may perceive auditory stimulation from the mother's vocalization; the infant may also have tactile, kinesthetic, and proprioceptive stimulation from her movements; and the infant may feel her body warmth. All systems are involved as mother and infant communicate with their entire bodies and all sensory and response modalities.

In the study of this very complex communication, the simultaneity of behaviors defies sequential analysis—although many of us have tried this approach. The simultaneity of behaviors also has no parallel in linguistic exchange. If two partners attempt to speak simultaneously, in fact, communication "breaks down" and the interaction becomes disorganized. Thus, it is not appropriate to conceptualize the early mother-infant interaction as being a simpler form of communication which is analogous to linguistic communication at a later age.

Early Communication Is Affective in Nature

Another unique aspect of the earliest communication system which has only begun to receive attention is the pervasiveness of affect. Clearly, "information" in the traditional sense is not being transmitted between mother and infant, whether communication takes the form of vocalization, of gesture, or of body movement. Research with older infants generally emphasizes the importance of pleasurable sensations only as a mechanism for reinforcing the learning of important messages being communicated by the environment. Thus, emotional factors act as an indirect influence on the ongoing process of acquisition of bits of information that will be put together to form cognitive schemata. For example, during play the mother performs an act repetitively and to the extent that the repetition occurs when the infant is in a pleasurable state, the repeated act may have a higher probability of being remembered. Additionally, nonrepetitive acts of the mother become salient because they elicit pleasure—or displeasure. By contrast, rather than the *indirect* involvement of affect as a source of reinforcement during interactive events, study of the early mother-infant interaction must be concerned with the *direct* involvement of affect as the very essence of the interaction.

The affective nature of the interaction is an inherent quality of the early communication. It expresses itself in behaviors by both partners simultaneously, so that the flow of their behaviors or communication is very closely integrated and may be expressed with great subtlety. A variety of research techniques may be needed to thread out the related patterns and their changes over age. A number of researchers have been engaged in fruitful research in this area (Brown et al., 1975; Dunn and Richards, 1977; Beckwith et al., 1976).

A very molecular approach has been taken by Tronick et al. (1975),

Condon and Sander (1974), and Stern (1971, 1974a,b). Using time lapse photography and frame-by-frame analysis of the films, they have demonstrated temporal relations between the behaviors of mothers and infants. In these analyses, behaviors are found to occur either simultaneously (i.e., in the same time-frame) or so close together sequentially that it is impossible to view the behaviors in an initiator-responder framework. Their research emphasizes again the importance of observing the behaviors of both members of the system simultaneously if the behavior of either member of the pair is to make any sense. This evidence for a much more complicated communication network between mother and infant than has previously been expected opens new vistas in the area of empirical study of the infant as a social and feeling being.

Almost certainly the principles involved in the early affective communication between mother and infant differ from those involved in later linguistic communication. We are not the first to maintain that the principles applied to the study of language are not applicable to early communication. Chomsky (1967) has taken a very strong stand on this issue, contending that the nonlinguistic communication of animals and infants has no continuity with the nature of language. Without limiting ourselves to Chomsky's formal linguistic framework, we should heed his warning that very different principles may apply to linguistic and prelinguistic communication. This may also be the case for nonlinguistic communication in the older child, which may develop concurrently with the acquisition of specialized, conventional verbal forms of communication but according to very different principles.

MOTHER–INFANT COMMUNICATION AS A SYSTEM

The guiding theoretical model for our research is that of general systems theory. Thoman, Denenberg, and their collaborators (Thoman et al., 1978; Thoman et al., 1979) have presented extensive arguments for the applicability of systems theory notions to the development of mother-infant interaction. We have profited greatly by the writings of Sander (1964, 1974, 1979; Sander et al., 1970), who has been working with this theoretical framework for a number of years. In this paper, we will focus primarily on the implications of such a framework for the study of early communication.

It should be noted that for many years, researchers have talked about the mother and infant as a "system," meaning that the mother and infant mutually influence one another. By searching for the source of influence, their research reflects a causal model which cannot take into account the ongoing feedback process that actually occurs. Bunge (1968) has pointed out that whenever there is feedback in a system, the notion of causal relations is inapplicable. This does not mean to preclude other noncausal forms of determinism. To take the systems notion seriously, the mother-infant relationship must be viewed very differently than it has been from the causal perspective.

The distinction between causal and noncausal forms of determinism is more than a semantic one. It is obvious that any behavior on the part of mother or infant may be determined by all of their interactive experiences prior to that point, but to focus on any one sequence or class of events as being causal for either the infant's or the mother's behavior may be trivial. (Extreme and catastrophic events are not a part of this consideration.) The research orientation for developmental study has traditionally been analytic, whereas the developmental process is essentially integrative, a process of synthesis of highly complex determinants (Sander et al., 1979). As Denenberg (1979) has pointed out, causal concepts enable us to do refined and sophisticated research in the laboratory. However, the developmental process as it occurs in the real world may not reveal itself in the laboratory.

If we are deprived of the search for causes, what is left? An answer is the study of the processes by which behaviors are integrated and by which the form and organization of behaviors change with age. Patterning of mother-infant behaviors has to be studied over successive time periods. A major problem is the identification of the behaviors that may reflect the process. This is the issue of units of measure. From a biological perspective, there is some agreement as to the unit at each level of organization from the single cell to groups of cells, body tissue, and the total central nervous system. From a behavioral perspective, and particularly at the social systems level, the units are not so readily apparent. The individual mother and infant are clearly the subsystem units of the dyadic system and their behaviors compose the system elements. There are also emergent properties of any system as a whole which are not apparent in the behaviors of any subsystem units. The system has an integration of its own and the laws that describe systems have to be obtained by studying it as a complete entity, rather than by studying the component parts (Denenberg, 1979).

An implication of this systems model is that just as there are characteristics of the integration process for various levels of organization with an individual organism, there are undoubtedly characteristics of the integration process for a mother-infant system. These are yet to be defined. Clearly they will have to be derived from the study of patterning of behaviors.

Golani (1976) has provided very dramatic evidence for the importance of relating multiple behaviors in the identification of patterns. He has examined in great detail the motor movement patterns in a variety of species, and has found that measures of a single behavior may not reveal regularity, whereas the patterning of combinations of movements may reveal regularities of behavior which are characteristic of an organism, animal or human. He has referred to this patterning as the "orchestration" of behavior. Golani's work provides a working model for the search for adaptive behaviors of infants and for the orchestration of adaptive behaviors of mothers and infants. A major objective for the researcher is to identify the complexes of behaviors of mothers and infants that constitute units which may reveal regularities in their patterning—and thus provide information on the interactive process.

A related issue is the temporal interval within which behavior patterns may emerge or be meaningful. Several investigators (Condon and Sander, 1974; Tronick et al., 1975; and Papousek and Papousek, 1977) have used behaviors that occur in successive fractions of a second. At the other extreme, our research includes descriptions of patterns of behaviors of mothers and infants over a total day's observation or even over several weeks. The purpose of the system is to maintain its own integrity by coping with instabilities that occur both within the system and from the vicissitudes imposed on the system externally. Oscillations or variations of patterns may have a wide range of temporal rhythms. Iberall and McCulloch (1969) have pointed out that some kinds of behaviors have very brief momentary variation, while others vary over greater periods. They call the mother-infant relationship a mother-child "symbiotic oscillator system." This notion emphasizes the wide variation in temporal characteristics of the dynamic action modes of the mother-infant system.

ONE APPROACH TO THE STUDY OF THE MOTHER—INFANT SYSTEM

Our approach to study the mother-infant system is an apparently simple one. It begins with an intent to study the system in action under conditions that are as natural as possible. Observations are made in the hospital on the day after delivery, and they are made in the subjects' homes thereafter. Ethological study has provided the guidelines for our procedures, and this will become more apparent as we describe each aspect of the study.

We have selected behaviors to record which require minimal subjective judgment. They are identifiable by common descriptive terms such as: the mother is patting, caressing, moving, looking at, talking to her infant; or the infant is alert, sucking, moving, fussing or crying. Actually, as anyone knows who has tried to record objectively such "simple" behaviors, they are not discretely on-or-off characteristics, as this description might make it sound. One must continually struggle to maintain reliability on even so small a distinction as that between a "pat" and a "caress." Reliability in such studies must be assessed in an ongoing manner. During every observation we make, there is an "overlap" period when two observers record simultaneously for subsequent reliability assessment.

Another major facet of our research is that we record as many behaviors as we can and still maintain relatively high reliability. Approximately 75 codes are used, but they are typically not used singly even when referring to a specific behavior. That is, the code system is viewed as a language, with "nouns," "verbs," and "modifiers," because the codes can be combined in various ways to describe any one behavior. The code system has been devised to be applicable from birth through one year of age. Some simple examples from codes that are appropriate for the older baby will remove some of the mystery from this brief description:

| Baby is in upright position—standing alone;
|o Baby is standing upright, holding on for support; with *o* in mother's position: baby is standing upright with mother's support;
L Baby is upright and walking;
Lo Baby is upright and walking, holding on for support.

Similar elaboration and combinations of symbols are used for the younger infants, but examples would have been more complicated to present. Reliability in recording these kinds of codes must be calculated for the specific complex code used for any analysis. Analyses are also made on mother and infant behavior-combinations, and these combination-variables must also be assessed for their reliability.

Only by recording a large number of behaviors is it possible to derive those combinations of behaviors that are meaningfully clustered for any one mother-infant pairs (Thoman et al., 1978; Thoman et al., 1979). An example emphasizes the importance of the search for relatedness among multiple behaviors that may occur in a seemingly random fashion when observed in isolation.

Another reason for recording a large number of mother and infant behaviors is that the results of our studies have indicated that the same behaviors may not be components of meaningful behavior patterns in all mother-infant pairs (Thoman et al., 1977; Thoman et al., 1978). An example of this point is the case of one mother and infant relationship in which the infant's open-eyed REM during active sleep became a cue for the mother to breast-feed the baby. The relationship between these behaviors was a highly systematic one. Such a combination of behaviors would not be expected to form a meaningful pattern for many, if any, other mother-infant pairs. Few infants have the large amount of open-eyed REM characteristic of this particular infant. Additionally, very few mothers would interpret the behavior as a signal for feeding. However, this mother and infant pair may have commonalities with other pairs when the organization of their behaviors is examined at a higher level of generality. There are many babies that give potent cues, although the cues may not be open-eyed REM, and there are certainly many other mothers that respond extremely readily to perceived behavioral cues from their infants. Thus, uniqueness at one level in their hierarchically organized behaviors does not preclude the identification of patterns of interaction that are common to other dyads at a different level of organization. The identification of a group of mother-infant pairs with commonality at any level of organization may be the basis for generality and may have greater implications for process analysis than any overall description of a randomly-selected group of mothers and infants. This principle will be illustrated in the data analyses described in the following sections.

BEHAVIORS RECORDED

Very generally the kinds of behaviors we record in the home are designed to give information on the infant's behavioral states throughout any observation; the infant's sleep states, state-related behaviors, and respiration during periods of time in the crib; maternal behaviors that describe her location with respect to the infant, the position in which she holds or places the infant, stimulation given to the infant including tactile, movement, vocal, gestural, and visual attention; and the nature of her activities during periods of caretaking interaction including feeding, changing, or bathing the baby.

It should be noted that all behaviors recorded are regarded as characteristics of the mother-infant system, even though it is necessary to record some as mother behaviors and some as infant behaviors. The activities of each member of the dyad are considered to be a function of the total interactive system. Even when the infant is asleep, as indicated above, there may be an exchange between the partners. And characteristics of the sleep states may reflect the immediately previous interaction during the infant's wake period, as well as the ongoing rhythmicity attained in the relationship. The variables that are selected for analysis may thus include single or combined infant and/or mother behaviors. The frequency or rate of occurrence of a behavior may be expressed with the total observation as the background period, or some other variable may be chosen for background. For example, we may choose to examine the proportion of the total observation a mother looks at her infant, or we may choose to examine the proportion of those epochs in which she holds her infant that she looks.

DESIGN OF THE STUDY

The general format for the major project from which the data are reported can be described very briefly, as the complete details of the procedure are described elsewhere (Freese, 1975; Thoman et al., 1978; and Thoman et al., 1979). The infant's sleep-wake states and respiration are observed at 2 days of age while the mother and infant are still in the hospital, and on the same day, two mother-infant feeding periods are observed. Four weekly observations are made in the home on weeks 2, 3, 4, and 5. These latter observations last for a seven-hour period on each day, with the day divided equally between two observers (and an overlap observation time of 15 minutes). The recording procedure includes code recording the occurrence of any of the 75 mother and infant behaviors during each successive 10-second period throughout the observation. Thus, there are 2520 epochs of recorded behaviors from each home observation. The results described below illustrate analyses we have done with the objective of describing early interactive or communicative processes in the mother-infant system.

INDICES OF IRRITABILITY AS A SYSTEMS MEASURE

Some characteristics of the social interactions of mothers and infants are examined in conjunction with variations in the crying behaviors of infants (Freese, 1975). Infant crying has received a great deal of attention as an elicitor of maternal behaviors (e.g., Thoman et al., 1974; Bernal, 1972) or as an antecedent to later behaviors (e.g., Bell and Ainsworth, 1972; Moss, 1974). However, most studies have focused on crying as an exclusively infant behavior, and the identification of linear causal relations between crying and other variables has been the typical objective. However, there are various circumstances, or background conditions, which may serve as qualifiers for obtaining meaningful measures of infant crying. For example, some infants cry primarily when alone and in their cribs but soothe readily when held; other infants cry under both circumstances. Not only do infants vary with respect to their crying under various conditions, but the extent to which these qualifying conditions occur may vary in different mother-infant relationships. For instance, mothers vary with respect to the amount of time they hold their infants and engage in caretaking activities. The relating processes may be obscured if we assume those processes to be the same in all relationships and rely on group analyses exclusively in exploring relationship data for patterns.

For the purposes of a systems analysis, infants were selected who cried a great deal throughout the observations and who were not readily soothable when the mothers interacted with them. In this way, 3 babies were identified as irritable from a group of 11 by criteria including both mother and infant behaviors. Other characteristics of the mother-infant relationships were examined to identify commonalities in interactive patterns that differentiated the subgroup of three pairs from the remaining eight in the sample. Then individual infants within the entire group were described to demonstrate that the remaining subgroup of eight displayed variations of interactions that must be examined further if the process of interaction, or communication, is to be the focus of study.

INTERACTION PATTERNS IN MOTHER—INFANT SYSTEMS CHARACTERIZED BY IRRITABILITY

From an initial group of 11 infants, four particularly fussy infants were identified on the basis of the total number of 10-second epochs they fussed or cried during the four successive 7-hour home observations. The crying of one of these infants was concentrated in long periods when the mother was not interacting with the infant, and the infant did not seem to be particularly fussy during interactions. That infant will be discussed separately. The remaining three infants seemed to be generally difficult for their mothers to soothe and will be discussed as a group. Figure 1 shows the number of minutes of fussing or crying for these three infants and the other eight infants during the observations for weeks 2-5, along with the standard errors of the means. An analysis of variance with repeated measures confirmed that the three infants fussed and cried more than the other eight infants ($F = 12.28$; $df = 1,9$; $p < .01$).

Since mothers frequently respond to infants' cries by holding their infants, it seemed reasonable to determine the amount of time mothers held fussy infants compared to other infants. These data are presented in Figure 2. The mothers in the three systems characterized by irritability held their infants for an average of 171 minutes of each home observation, while the mothers of the other eight infants held their infants an average of 87 minutes. This difference is significant ($F = 20.02$; $df = 1,9$; $p < .01$). Presumably there are other differences between these two subgroups related to the three mothers' attempts to soothe their infants while they held them. At some later date, it will be helpful to evaluate differences in the amounts and forms of stimulation provided by these mothers and other mothers during holding.

Since the three mothers in systems characterized by irritability held their infants more than the other mothers did, the question arises whether that behavior effectively decreased the rate at which their infants cried relative to the other group of infants. An appropriate measure of this is the amount of

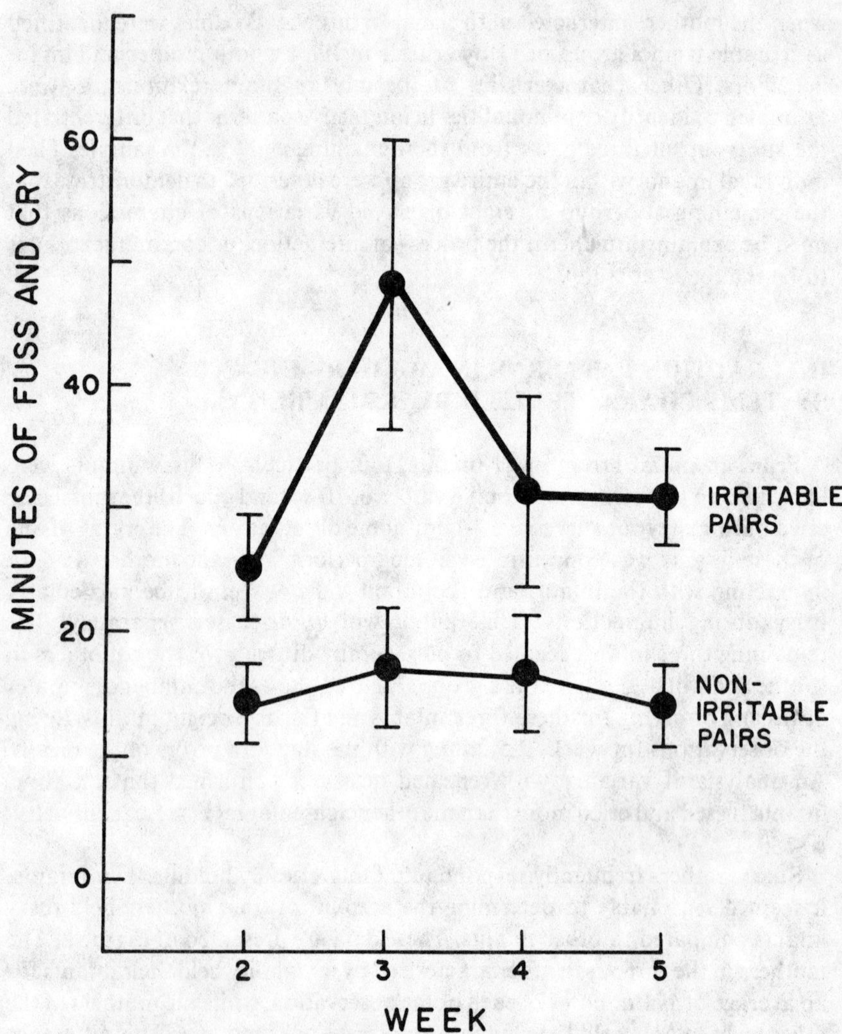

FIG. 1. Mean amount of Fuss or Cry for the group of 3 Irritable Pairs and the 8 Nonirritable Pairs. (Mean ± SEM).

crying the two subgroups of infants did during social interaction, which is defined here as holding that does not occur in the context of the caretaking interactions including feeding, bathing, and changing. The amount of fussing or crying during social interaction was calculated separately for the two subgroups of mother-infant pairs, and the results of this analysis are presented in Figure 3. For the subgroup of eight mother-infant pairs, an

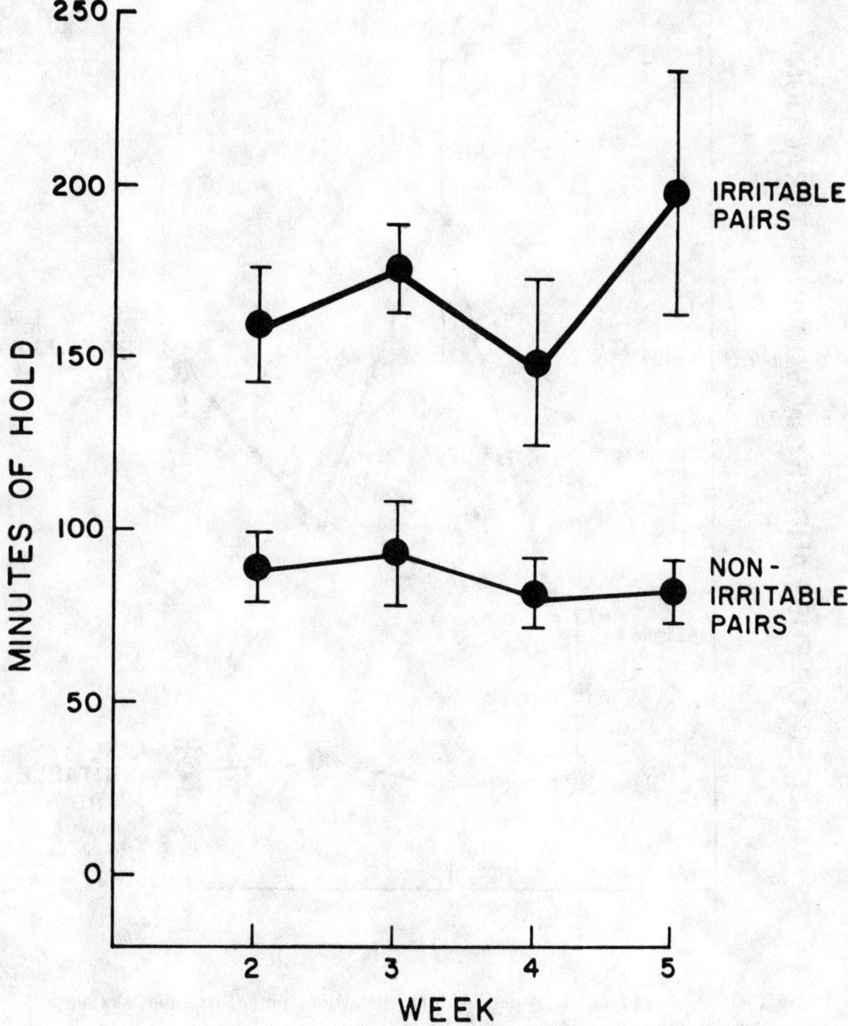

FIG. 2. Mean amount of Hold for the 3 Irritable Pairs and the 8 Nonirritable Pairs. (Mean ± SEM).

average of two minutes of fussing or crying during social interaction occurred for each 7-hour observation. For the subgroup characterized by irritability, the amount of crying that occurred in social interaction was much more variable, but averaged 16 minutes per observation, significantly more than for the other mother-infant pairs ($F = 45.96$; $df = 1,9$; $p < .01$).

Another difference in systems behaviors associated with irritability was

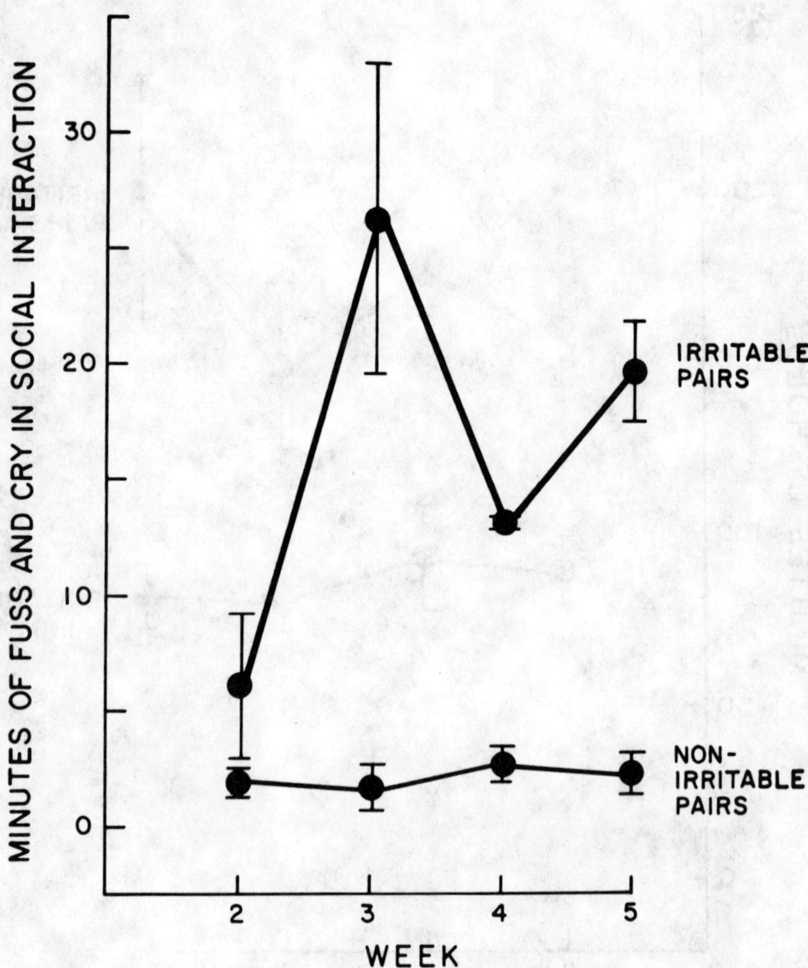

FIG. 3. Mean Fuss or Cry during Social Interactions for the 3 Irritable Pairs and 8 Nonirritable Pairs. (Mean ± SEM).

mothers' visual contact with their infants during social interaction. To be scored as looking at their infants during social interactions, mothers were required to look at their infants for more than half of any given 10-second epoch. The mothers of this subgroup of three infants looked at their infants for a significantly smaller proportion of their social interaction than did mothers of other infants ($F = 5.18$; $df = 1,9$; $p < .05$). These results are presented in Figure 4. The mothers in systems characterized by irritability looked at their infants for an average of 61 minutes of their 171 minutes of

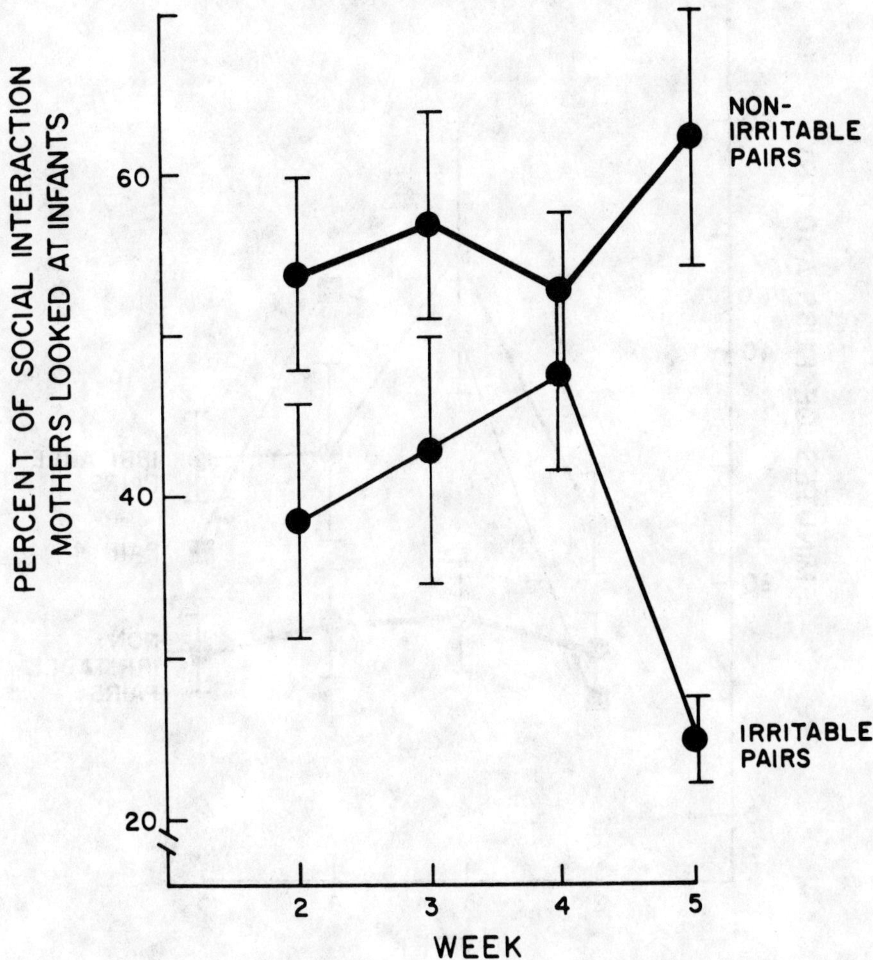

FIG. 4. Mothers' Looking during Social Interactions for 3 Irritable Pairs and 8 Nonirritable Pairs. (Mean ± SEM).

social interaction, while the other mothers looked at their infants for an average of 48 minutes of the 87 minutes they were engaged in social interaction with their infants. At least in terms of looking behavior, the mothers of the irritable infants were not making use of the additional interaction time they spent with their infants. This may reflect their frustration at the lack of success of their soothing efforts or the unreceptiveness of their infants to visual attention.

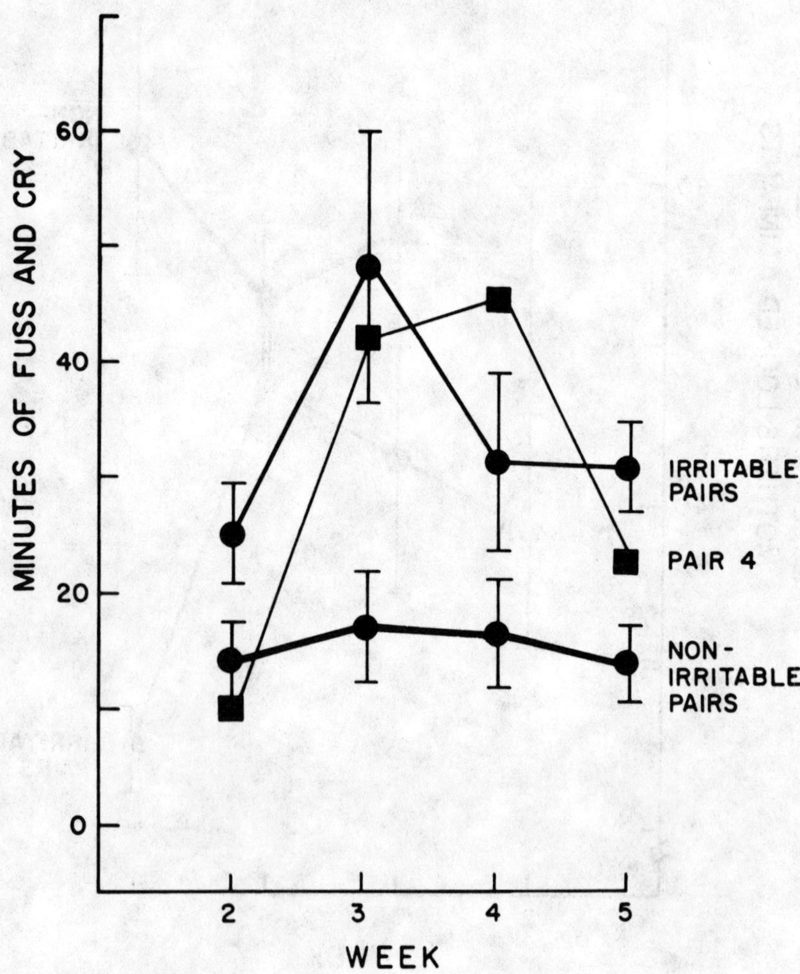

FIG. 5. Mean amount of Fuss or Cry for Pair 4 compared to Irritable and Nonirritable groups. (Mean ± SEM).

RESPONSE LATENCY TO CRYING AND INTERACTIONAL SYNCHRONY

Let us return now to the fourth infant, who was identified as fussy in the initial screening on the basis of total amounts of fussing or crying, but whose pattern of fussing was different from the patterns in the other three mother-infant pairs in which there was considerable fussing or crying. Figure 5 shows

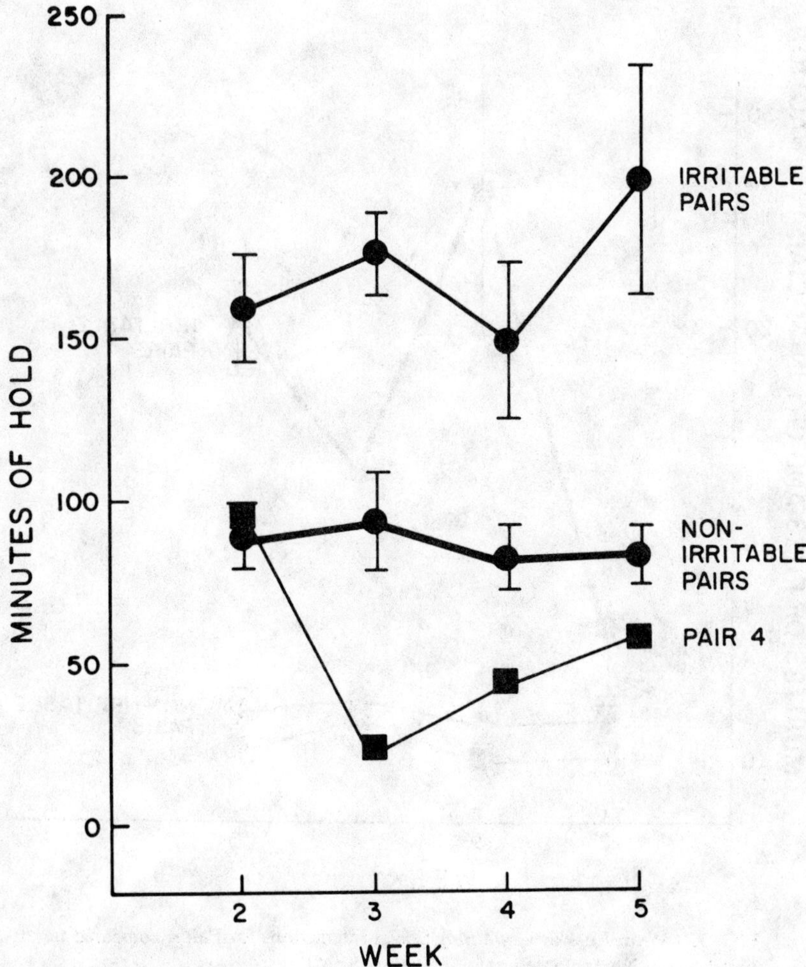

FIG. 6. Mean amount of Hold for Pair 4 compared to Irritable and Nonirritable groups. (Mean ± SEM).

that in terms of the total amount of time this infant fussed and cried, he was indistinguishable from the subgroup of three infants. However, as illustrated in Figure 6, Infant 4 was held even less than the mean for the subgroup of eight pairs in which little crying occurred. Additionally, as seen in Figure 7, this infant cried very little during social interaction. This characteristic clearly differentiates Mother-Infant Pair 4 from the three mother-infant systems previously discussed.

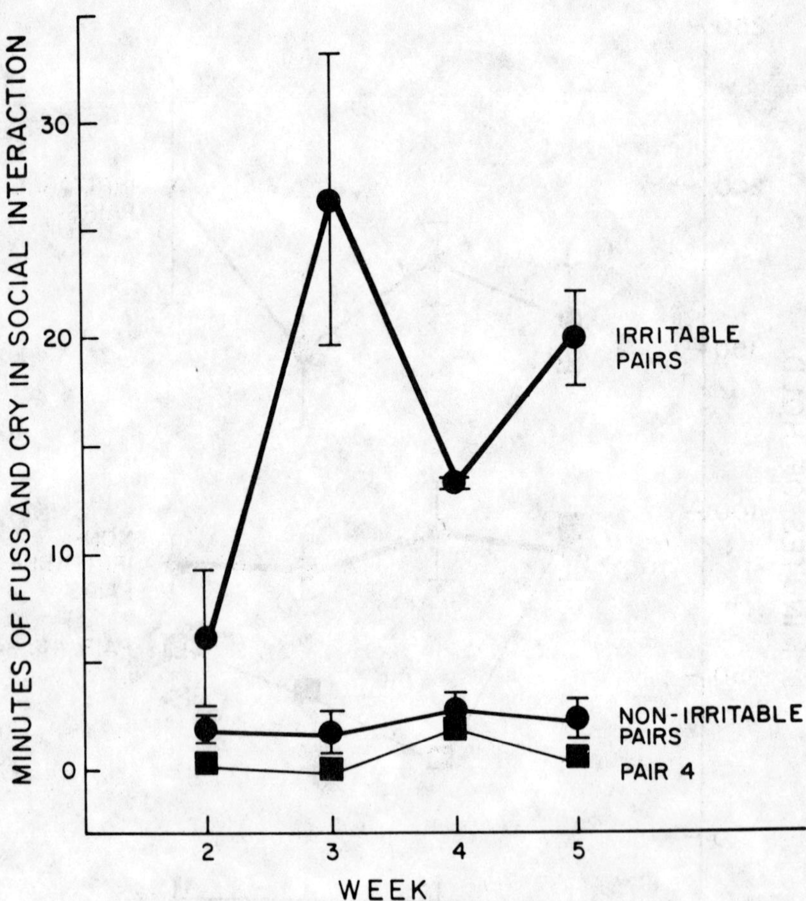

FIG. 7. Mean Fuss or Cry during Social Interactions for Pair 4 compared to Irritable and Nonirritable groups. (Mean ± SEM).

Thoman, Denenberg, Becker, Gaulin-Kremer, Poindexter and Shaw (1974) have examined the effects of varying latencies of responses to infant vocalizations. In their study, they noted that infants who were picked up within 90 seconds of the initiation of fussing or crying almost invariably soothed within 10 seconds. Infants who were allowed to cry for longer than 90 seconds took on average almost one minute to soothe. These data suggest that a mother's response latency to her infant's cries is an important measure of response synchrony in the system.

To explore changes in this facet of mother-infant synchrony for Mother-Infant Pair 4, the number of cry episodes that continued for 90 seconds or

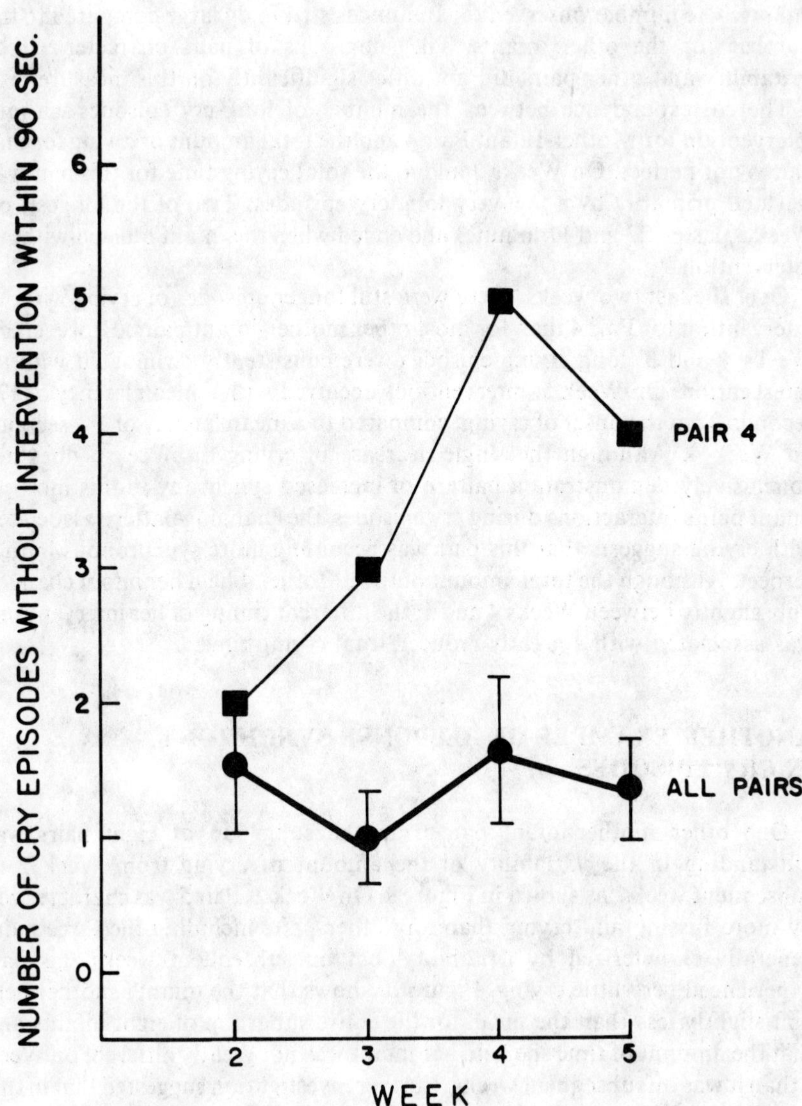

FIG. 8. Number of Long Cry Episodes for Pair 4 compared to the mean of all pairs.

longer without intervention was tabulated for each home observation. Figure 8 shows these episodes plotted by weeks for Infant 4 and the entire group of 11 infants. The number observed for Infant 4 is strikingly large compared to the number for the other infants. The subgroups of pairs characterized by irritability and other pairs did not differ significantly on this measure.

The correspondence between the number of long cry episodes without intervention for Mother-Infant Pair 4 and the total amount of crying for that pair is not perfect. On Weeks 3 and 4, the total crying time for this pair was elevated primarily by a few very long cry episodes. Two of the longest, on Week 3, lasted 27 and 11 minutes and ended when the infant quieted without intervention.

Over the last two weeks, there were still longer episodes of crying without intervention for Pair 4 than for most other mother-infant pairs. However, on Weeks 4 and 5, long crying episodes were consistently terminated with an intervention. On Week 5, interventions occurred with a mean latency of 170 seconds from the onset of crying, compared to a mean latency of 284 seconds on Week 4. Although the single decrease in crying on Week 5 does not conclusively demonstrate a pattern of increased synchrony in this mother-infant pair's interactions during cry episodes, the changing pattern associated with crying suggests that this pair was becoming more synchronous in that respect. Although the total amount of time Mother 4 held her infant changed only slightly between Weeks 4 and 5, the different timing of her interventions was associated with a greatly reduced total crying time.

ANOTHER EXAMPLE OF RESPONSE SYNCHRONY IN CRY EPISODES

One other mother-infant pair from the subgroup of eight pairs was outstanding in the variability of the amount of crying from Week 2 to subsequent weeks, as shown in Figure 9. On Week 2, Pair 5 was characterized by more fussing and crying than any other pair, including the three pairs generally chracterized by irritability, but on subsequent weeks this pair experienced very little crying. Figure 10 shows that the infant's mother held him slightly less than the mean for the entire subgroup of eight infants and that the amount of time she held her infant was not greatly different on Week 2 than it was on subsequent weeks. Further investigation suggested that in this mother-infant pair, synchrony with respect to a rapid response to crying developed very rapidly. In Figure 11 the number of cry episodes for Pair 5 that continued for at least 90 seconds before intervention are presented by weeks, along with the means for the entire group of 11 infants. Although there were five instances of long response latencies to crying on Week 2 for Pair 5, on

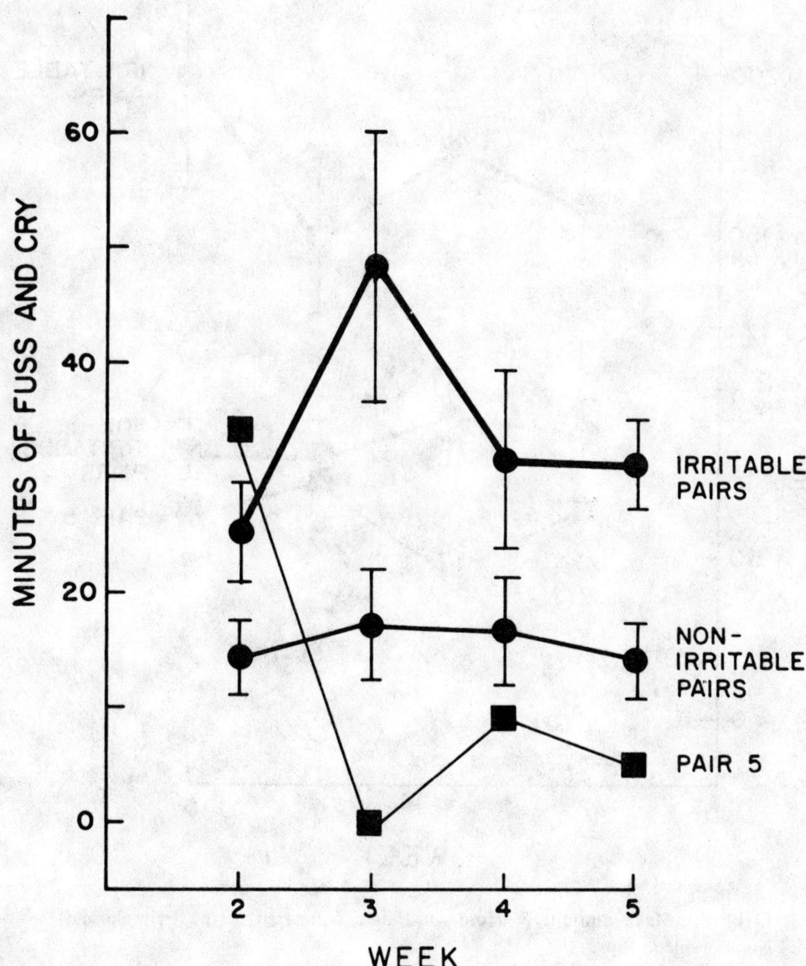

FIG. 9. Mean amount of Fuss or Cry for Pair 5 compared to the Irritable and Nonirritable groups. (Mean ± SEM).

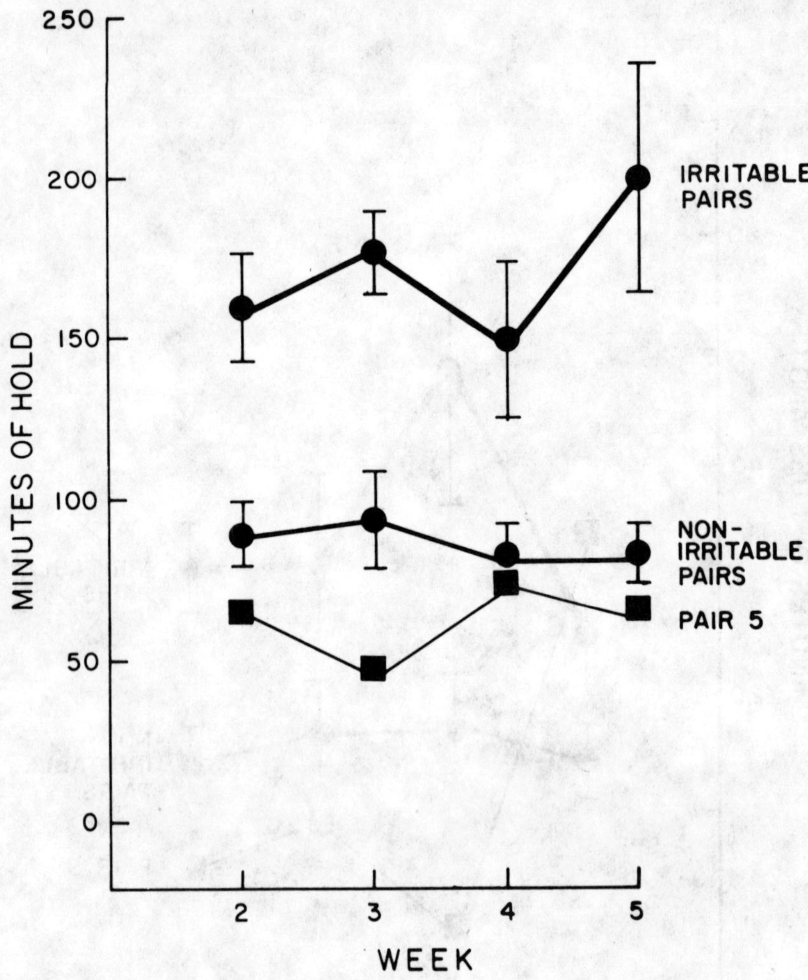

FIG. 10. Mean amount of Hold for Pair 5 compared to the Irritable and Nonirritable groups.

Weeks 3, 4, and 5 there were no such instances. This synchronous pattern was associated with very little crying for Pair 5 during Weeks 3-5.

DISCUSSION

From the data described for two of the subjects, it would appear that the timing of the mother's intervention with respect to her infant's crying had a

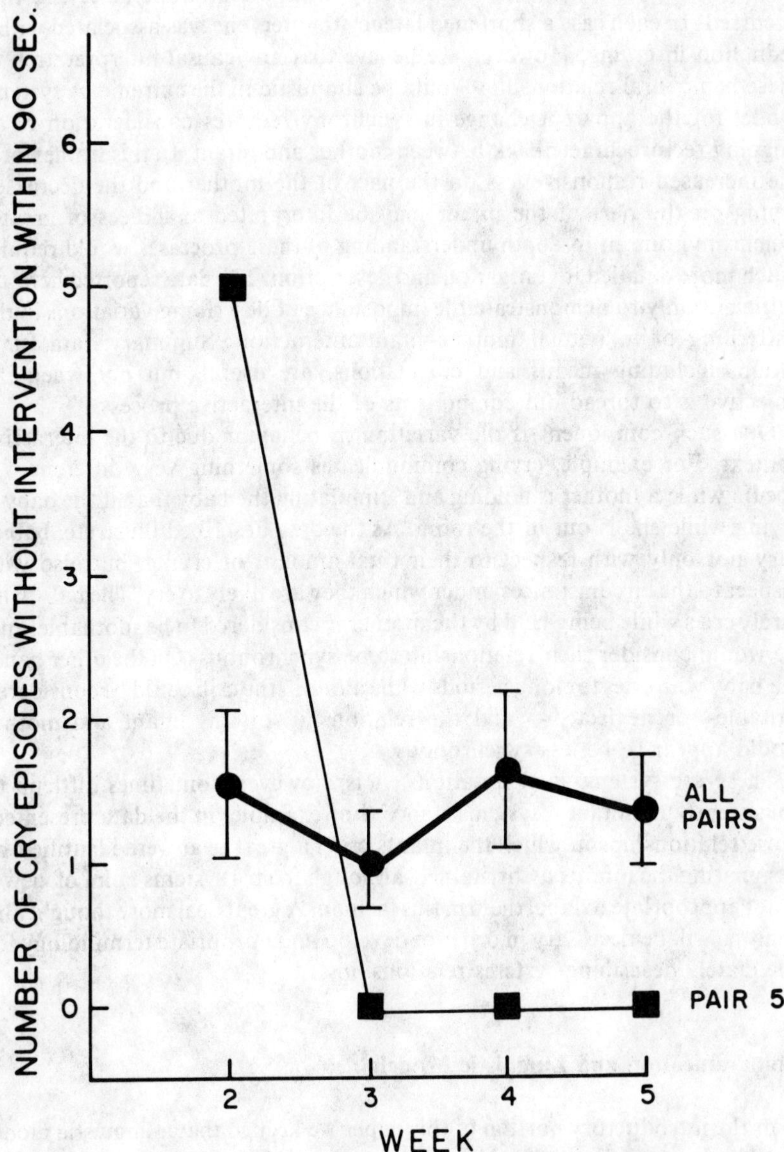

FIG. 11. Number of Long Cry Episodes for Pair 5 compared to the mean for all pairs.

direct, and possibly causal, relationship with the amount of crying that occurred. In each case a shortened latency to intervene was associated with a reduction in crying. However, we believe that any causal interpretation of these behavioral relationships would be simplistic in the extreme. A systems model for the apparent change in synchrony requires consideration of an ongoing reciprocal feedback between mother and infant. In this framework, the increased responsiveness on the part of the mother and the decreased crying on the part of the infant may be interpreted as indices of greater synchrony, but an in-depth understanding of these processes would require much more detailed investigation and description. The data reported here are sufficient only to demonstrate the importance of describing variations in the patterning of individual mother-infant interaction. Summary data for a group, including means and correlations, are useful, but not when the objective is to thread out components of the interactive process.

One such component is the variation in behavior due to the interactive context. For example, crying communicates something very different if it occurs while a mother is holding and stimulating the baby than if the baby is crying while she is out of the room. As the data described illustrate, babies vary not only with respect to their total amount of crying, but also with respect to the circumstances under which they are likely to cry. The baby who rarely cries while being held by the mother is considered to be soothable, and we would consider their relationship to be synchronous. On the other hand, the baby who cries for long periods while alone in the crib could be considered irritable—or neglected— and the relationship of this infant and mother would appear to be less synchronous.

These are systems interpretations. It is, however, sometimes difficult to consistently maintain a systems stance. For example, in the data presented, those relationships in which the infants cried a great deal were identified by designating the infants as "irritable," although from a systems point of view it is not appropriate to label them in this fashion. A great deal more thought and analysis will be necessary in order to develop an appropriate terminology for adequately describing systems relationships.

Communication and Linguistic Models

In the introductory portion of this paper we argued that a linguistic model would not be applicable to the earliest mother-infant communication. Early nonlinguistic communication was described as uniquely different, involving multimodal, ongoing and simultaneous exchanges by both members of the dyad. Communication of this nature can not be analyzed using a model based on the sequential exchange of verbal messages. To illustrate from the data described, the infant may cry while the mother is holding him, while she is looking at and talking to him. The scene can as readily be depicted with the mother as the subject: the mother is holding the infant, looking at and talking to him, while the infant cries. In neither case is the action unimodal, static, nor sequential. The other unique chracteristic of early communication, the pervasiveness of affect, is also implicit in this particular scene.

However, in due time, some portion of the communication begins to occur in a turn-taking manner. Likewise the infant comes to use certain exchanges, particularly during play periods, as intended messages. In mutual imitation of words, sounds, or gestures we see the activity which is so eloquently described by Bruner (1975) as a precursor to language acquisition. There is also increasing evidence for the many ways in which the mother functions as a model for learning conventional signals. With the onset of verbal skills, communication becomes more specialized in nature. Nonverbal communication continues, but as the child grows older attention from both parents and researchers is focused more and more on the spoken word, and models for this very specialized form of communication are in the province of linguistics.

Some consideration must be given to the function of early communication as a prelude to the development of linguistic competence. However, so little is known about language development, and especially about early language reception, that any statements about the linkage between nonlinguistic communication and subsequent linguistic capabilities must be primarily speculative.

A variety of complex maturational and learning processes prepare the infant for language acquisition. The nature of neural development, the nature of the learning that occurs during the early months, and the relationships between these levels of development are largely unexplored. We do not propose to deal with these complexities other than to suggest ways in which species-typical experiences serve to prepare the infant for later language acquisition.

A major contribution of the early communication period is not only the development of the potential for language acquisition, but also the development of the expectation of an ongoing exchange. Bell and Ainsworth (1972) have speculated that the mother's response to an infant's cry does not reinforce the crying behavior, but on the contrary strengthens the infant's expectation of being able to communicate and to interact effectively with the environment. We suggest that the synchronous relationship may be one in which such communication is more fully developed, and the infant is thereby better prepared for the specialized form of communication required for language learning. The possibility that effective early communication facilitates later language acquisition is a testable hypothesis; but in order to investigate this question, intensive longitudinal research of the type we have described would be required.

Our approach to this research question is consistent with recent work coming from linguistics. Naremore (1978), in reviewing language research on young children, emphasizes the value of examining individual subject data as a way of explicating group data. She notes that our search for "universal" trends leads us to obscure the important information which can be derived from careful description of what *each individual* child does with language. Thus, the models for linguistic and nonlinguistic behaviors may differ, but the developing research approaches are consistent.

A final speculation with respect to the function of early interaction, or communication, comes from a recent symposium on the Neurological Bases of Language Disorders in Children (1978).* During the discussions, Dr. Norman Gerschwind suggested that the major achievement during the early months of life is the development of attentional processes, and that appropriate experience is of primary importance while specific brain centers are developing. The mother-infant relationship presumably provides the opportunity for the infant to acquire the most relevant experiences under the most optimal conditions. A major component of these experiences would be the affect prevailing during interactions with the environment, particularly with the mother. The infant begins to attend to the mother, her characteristics and her actions very early, and mutual attention to other aspects of the environment soon follows. It may be that a successful communication system between mother and infant facilitates both the broadening and sharpening of the infant's attentional capabilities. These and other questions can only be explored by developmental, that is, longitudinal study of individual mother-infant pairs.

ACKNOWLEDGMENTS

The research described in this paper was supported by The William T. Grant Foundation, NICHD Grant HD-08195-01A2, and NIMH Predoctoral Fellowship 5268-81-13645.

REFERENCES

Beckwith, L., Cohen, S. E., Kopp, C. B., Parmalee, A. H. and Marcy, T. G. Caregiver-infant interaction and early cognitive development in preterm infants. *Child Dev. 47*, 579–587 (1976).

---

*Symposium on The Neurological Bases of Language Disorders in Children: Methods and Directions for Research. National Institutes of Health, Washington, D. C., 1978.

Bell, S. M. and Ainsworth, M. D. S. Infant crying and maternal responsiveness. *Child Dev. 43*, 1171–1190 (1972).

Bernal, J. Crying during the first 10 days of life and maternal responses. *Dev. Med. Child Neurol. 14*, 362–372 (1972).

Brown, J., Bakeman, R., Snyder, P., Frederickson, W., Morgan, S., and Hepler, R. Interactions of black inner city mothers with their newborn infants. *Child. Dev. 46*, 677–686 (1975).

Bruner, J. S. The ontogenesis of speech activities. *J. Child Lang. 2*, 1–19 (1975).

Bunge, M. Conjunction, succession, determination, and causation. *Int. J. Theoret. Phys. 1*, 299–315 (1968).

Chomsky, N. The general properties of language. In *Brain Mechanisms, Speech and Language*, F. L. Darley, ed., Grune & Stratton, New York (1967), pp. 73–80.

Condon, W. S. and Sander, L. W. Synchrony demonstrated between movements of the neonate and adult speech. *Child Dev. 45*, 456–462 (1974).

Denenberg, V. H. Paradigms and paradoxes in the study of behavioral development.In *The Origins of the Infant's Social Responsiveness*, E. B. Thoman and S. Trotter, eds. Erlbaum, Hillsdale, New Jersey (1979), in press.

Dunn, J. B. and Richards, M. P. M. Observations on the developing relationship between mother and baby in the neonatal period. In *Studies in Mother-Infant Interaction*, H. R. Schaffer, ed. Academic Press, New York (1977).

Freese, M. P. Assessment of maternal attitudes and analyses of their role in early mother-infant interaction. Unpublished doctoral dissertation, Purdue University, 1975.

Golani, I. Homeostatic motor processes in mammalian interactions—a choreography of display. In *Perspectives in Ethology*, Vol. 2., P. P. G. Bateson and P. H. Klopfer, eds. Plenum Press, New York (1976), pp. 69–134.

Iberall, A. S. and McCulloch, W. S. The organizing principle of complex living systems. *J. Basic Engineering*, June, 290–294 (1969).

Meltzoff, A. N. and Moore, M. K. Imitation of facial and manual gestures by human neonates. *Science, 198*, 75–78 (1977).

Moss, H. A. Communication in mother-infant interaction. In *Nonverbal Communication*, L. Kramer, P. Pliner and T. Alloway, eds. Plenum Publishing Corp., New York (1974).

Naremore, R. Symposium on the Neurological Bases of Language Disorders in Children: Methods and Direction for Research. National Institutes of Health, Washington, D. C. (1978).

Papousek, H. and Papousek, M. Mothering and the cognitive head-start: Psychobiological considerations. In *Studies in Mother-Infant Interaction*, H. R. Schaffer, ed. Academic Press, New York (1977).

Sander, L. Adaptive relationships in early mother-child interaction. *J. Amer. Acad. Child Psychiat. 3*, 231–264 (1964).

Sander, L. Infant and caretaking environment: Investigation and conceptualization of adaptive behavior in a system of increasing complexity. In *Child Psychiatrist as Investigator*, E. J. Anthony, ed. Plenum Publishing Corp., New York (1974).

Sander, L., Stechler, G., Burns, P. and Julia, H. Early mother-infant interaction and 24-hour patterns of activity and sleep. *J. Amer. Acad. Child Psychiat. 9*, 103–123 (1970).

Sander, L. W., Stechler, G., Burns, P., and Lees, A. Change in infant and caregiver variables over the first two months of life: Integration of action in early development. In *Origins of the Infant's Social Responsiveness*, E. B. Thoman and S. Trotter, eds. Lawrence Erlbaum Associates, Inc., Hillsdale, New Jersey (1979), in press.

Stern, D. N. A microanalysis of mother-infant interaction: Behavior regulation social contact between a mother and her 3½-month-old twins. *J. Amer. Acad. Child Psychiat. 10*, 501–517 (1971).

Stern, D. N. Mother and infant at play. In *The Effect of the Infant on Its Caregiver*, M. Lewis and L. Rosenblum, eds. Wiley, New York (1974a).

Stern, D. N. The goal and structure of mother-infant play. *J. Amer. Acad. Child Psychiat. 13*, 402–421 (1974b).

Thoman, E. B., Acebo, C., Dreyer, C. A., Becker, P. T. and Freese, M. P. Individuality in the interactive process. In *The Origins of The Infant's Social Responsiveness*, E. B. Thoman and S. Trotter, eds. Erlbaum, Hillsdale, New Jersey (1979), in press.

Thoman, E. B., Becker, P. T. and Freese, M. P. Individual patterns of mother-infant interaction. In *Observing Behavior*, Vol. 1, G. Sackett, ed. University Park Press, Baltimore (1978).

Thoman, E. B., Denenberg, V. H., Becker, P. T., Gaulin-Kremer, E. Poindexter, M. M. and Shaw, J. L. Analysis of mother-infant interaction sequences: A model for relating mother-infant interaction to the infant's development of behavioral states. In *Maternal-Infant Life Conferences*. Wisconsin Perinatal Center (1974).

Thoman, E. B., Leiderman, P. H. and Olson, J. P. Neonate-mother interaction during breast-feeding. *Dev. Psychol. 6*, 110–118 (1972).

Thoman, E. B., Turner, A. M., Leiderman, P. H., Barnett, C. R. Neonate-mother interaction: Effects of parity on feeding behavior. *Child Dev. 41*, 1103–1111 (1970).

Thorpe, W. H. Animal vocalization and communication. In *Brain Mechanisms Underlying Speech and Language*, F. L. Darley, ed. Grune & Stratton, New York (1967).

Trevarthen, C. Descriptive analyses of infant communicative behaviour. In *Studies in Mother-Infant Interaction*, H. R. Schaffer, ed. Academic Press, New York (1977).

Tronick, E., Adamson, L., Wise, S., Als, H. and Brazelton, T. B. The infant's response to entrapment between contradictory messages in face to face interaction. Paper presented at meetings of the Society for Research in Child Development, Denver (1975).

Maternal Influences and Early Behavior

18

Individual vs. Multiple Mothering in Mammals

John C. Gurski
J. P. Scott

In a recent *Science* editorial, Etzioni (1977) addressed himself to the future of the family. He noted that 1) the number of nuclear family groups has decreased in the last 11 years, 2) there are several theories that attempt to account for both the causes and ultimate effects of this decrease, some decrying and some heralding the demise of the nuclear family, and 3) the evidence necesary to adequately assess the benefits and disadvantages of alternative family styles (communal families, contractual marriages) is not yet available on a grand enough scale to permit an adequate assessment of the situation. Although this may be so, data are being gathered on the social patterns of many species, including data on the caregiver-offspring relations, both in laboratory and natural settings. These data provide comparisons upon which to judge whether for species that organize themselves in certain ways we may expect to find typical caregiving patterns.

In this chapter we review the caregiving behavior of most of the members of the mammalian class in which such behaviors have been investigated. We will concentrate on social aspects of the caregiving patterns and examine the organization of those patterns along lines that are either predominantly individual (usually by the mother or both parents) or cooperative (caregiving by nonrelated and related members of the group in addition to and without interference from the biological parents). While this review may not fully answer Etzioni's criticism, it will allow consideration of whether for mammalian caregiving there are any particular factors that are typical and how these factors might be more or less adaptive in certain situations, either for human or infrahuman groups.

Parental behavior—that cluster of behavior patterns which has as its ultimate goal the survival of the species—is undoubtedly one of the most important from an evolutionary point of view. In any species that cares for the next generation in some systematic way, responsbility for that generation can be said to belong to the caregivers until the young have progressed to a point where they can operate satisfactorily on their own. In species that deposit fertilized eggs, physiological maternal care begins at conception and extends at least to the point of egg-laying. In numerous other species epimeletic behavior (Scott, 1968) itself begins at birth, whether that birth process takes the form of hatching from the egg or some form of parturition. In species that provide postpartum care for the young, this care takes two basic forms: provisioning and sheltering. These two aspects of caregiving are found in physiologically primitive invertebrate organisms, e.g., social insects (Wilson, 1971), as well as in the physiologically complex species, e.g., *Homo sapiens*. Thus, provisioning and sheltering appear to be of central importance in the rearing of the young.

We (*H. sapiens*) belong to the class Mammalia, in which initial provisioning is provided by the mother or her surrogate through delivery of milk from the mammary glands. Females have of course evolved the mechanisms of both birth and provisioning in all members of this class. Sheltering can range from protection from the elements or from predators by shielding with the body to the construction of permanent nests or houses, depending on both the species involved and important ecological factors. Responsibility for sheltering may be assumed by different sex-and-class members of the group. Regardless of the form they take, provisioning and sheltering appear in all species in our class. However, the different forms these behaviors take should give some indication of the psychology of each species.

In the following sections of this chapter we will review studies that are representative of the caregiving patterns of several species. The orders considered are arranged in typical taxonomic hierarchies. Each order is represented by several studies of representative species that display patterns of single or multiple mothering. The chapter concludes with a discussion of the relationship of attachment formation to dependence.

MULTIPLE MOTHERING IN RODENTS

Myomorphs

Deermouse

Although most research with rodent species in this area has been with *Mus musculus*, one of the earliest reports of shared care of the young was not with this genus. King (1963), in discussing maternal behavior in *Peromyscus*, writes that wild *P. maniculatus bairdii* have been observed in their nests with more than one family, in a "nursery aggregation." He stated that exchange of the young between the females occurs and that the young suckle the mother and adopted mother indiscriminately. About 3% of the total number discovered (6/185) were multiply mothering the offspring in this way. One pair was composed of mother and daughter; two others were found with their own litters and one or two males. It is possible for the litters to be of different ages with no detrimental effects. King comments that this sort of living situation gives rise to considerable variation in the social environment of the developing young.

House Mouse

In the wild house mouse (*Mus musculus*) kept in semi-natural observation areas, Crowcroft and Rowe (1963) reported that when two females became pregnant at the same time, they were observed to make communal nests which they continued to share with their litters, and later with the litters of their daughters. On occasion, when only one female in a nest became pregnant, she would expel a female which had been sharing her nest. Southwick (1969) has also reported communal nesting in wild house mice in a semi-natural setting. He observed two females to share both nest and pups frequently and with a good survival rate: he observed three females communally nesting without incident, but there was a decrease in survival rate as the number occupying a nest increased beyond this number. The young were abandoned as density increased to the point where as many as eight or nine litters were in attendance by only two mothers.

Laboratory study of this phenomenon began with Sayer and Salmon (1969; 1971). They noted that the growth rates of mouse pups are enhanced by the presence of more than one mother even though the pup-to-mother ratio remains the same. This appears to be due to the tendency for the mouse mother's milk supply to increase as the total size of the litter which she is caring for or sharing increases. Other possible factors such as social facilitation by mothers, more efficient thermal regulation, and increased quality of milk supply were given no support.

Sayer and Salmon (1971) speculate on the selective value of communal nursing, including defense against predators, more efficient early warning of danger, and an increase in the probability of the litter's surviving in the event of loss of one of the females during the lactation period.

Care of the young by virgin females under communal condition has also been observed (Gandelman et al., 1970). The virgin females were housed with lactating mothers and their litters. These virgin mice aided in the care of the young and sometimes in their delivery. Male mice on the other hand only exhibited caretaking behavior when housed individually with the litter. Gandelman et al. (1970) reported that the nest was moved frequently during the 10-day observation period. In some instances the virgin females were more solicitous of the pups than were the lactating mothers. The behavior of these virgin females was presumably in response to the stimuli associated with pups rather than to any particular hormonal influences associated with the maternal condition.

Finally, communal nursing has been observed to occur when mothers of different inbred strains are placed together (Werboff, et al., 1970). Both A/J and C57BL/6J pups showed enhanced growth rates as the result of communal nursing. Whereas Sayer and Salmon (1971) reported no difference in the activity level of their subjects (BALB/c), Werboff et al. (1970) reported that the A/J young showed higher activity levels especially when multiply mothered by both A/J and C57BL/6J mothers. They also reported that the C57 young in the mixed-strain multiple mother condition showed the heaviest weight. These strain-specific effects indicate that the behavior shows genetic variation. It also indicated, as in cross-fostering experiments (e.g., Reading, 1966), that there is a possibility that deficiencies in one strain are offset by qualities of the other strain. These deficiencies are presumed to have occurred through generations of inbreeding.

In a recent study, one of us (Gurski) investigated the results of a rigorous form of multiple mothering. Female mice from three inbred strains (C57BL/6J, DBA/2J, and C3H/FeJ) were communally housed until their estrus cycles synchronized; they were then placed into a cage with a male of their own strain and allowed to mate. Females that successfully gave birth to a litter of at least four pups formed the population from which the samples were chosen for the study. With the exception of the control group the female with litter formed part of a triad of dams with pups from either (1) the two other strains or (2) her own strain. All the pups in any triad also had to meet the criterion of having been born within three days of each other as this restriction greatly improved the survival rates of the younger litters. In this way four experimental groups were formed by combining the factor of between-and-within-strain triads together with the daily rotation of either the mother or the litter to a different nest belonging to one of the family groups in the triad (see Table 1). The daily rotation of either the litters (E_1 and E_3) or the mothers (E_2 and E_4) continued from Day 1 to weaning day (Day 21); the biological mother was reunited with her own litter in this manner every third day and with one of the other two litters every third day as well. The Control group (C) dam reared her own offspring during the same period and the family group was not rotated. The pups of this group had no experience with other adult females of their own or other strains prior to weaning.

TABLE 1
General Experimental Design (Gurski, 1977)

Name of Group	*Unit Rotated*	*Strains of Foster-Mothers or Offspring*	*No. of Mother-Litter Units from each Strain*	*Mothers*	*Pups*
C	(not rotated)	(not fostered)	4	12	48
E_1	Litter	3 (incl. own)	4	12	48
E_2	Mother	3 (incl. own)	4	12	48
E_3	Litter	1 (own strain)	4	12	48
E_4	Mother	1 (own strain)	3	9	36
		Totals	18	54	216

Inbred Strains: C57/BL6; C3H/FeJ; DBA/2j

Results of the study showed that mothers having a litter rotated into their nest box (E_1 and E_3) retrieved that litter within five minutes after coming into contact with them, with most retrieving them to the nest immediately (see Figure 1). Litter weights of these groups were not significantly different from Group C pups of the same strain at any time during the study. On the other hand, mothers that were rotated daily (E_2 and E_4) to another nest showed a different pattern: they did not readily retrieve the foster young nor their own young when rotated back to them; rather they spent many minutes exploring the nest box and the young. In all cases, however, the young had been adopted within several minutes after the mother had been rotated to the nest box, either by the mother's retrieving them to the strange nest or by her carrying nesting material from the nest site to the site where the litter had been deposited, normally being the corner on a diagonal opposite the nest site, and rebuilding the nest around the litter. Daily weighing of these litters also revealed only the usual strain differences; compared to the controls there was neither a positive nor a negative effect of rotation upon litter weights.

On weaning day the mothers and litters were separated; the pups in each litter were housed together in a strange cage and the mother stayed in her cage. An open-field test was run on each pup: no significant group differences were observed on the pups' ambulatory behaviors in a novel environment, again indicating that the experimental pups did not undergo changes in normal developmental history as a result of multiple mothering. On Day 22 a test of attachment was run. Each pup was placed into the open-field enclosure where there were now four adult female mice. The experimental groups' (E_1 - E_4) females were the pup's biological mother, the two foster mothers, and a stranger from the pup's own strain; the control group pups were each tested with their biological mother and with a strange female from each of the three

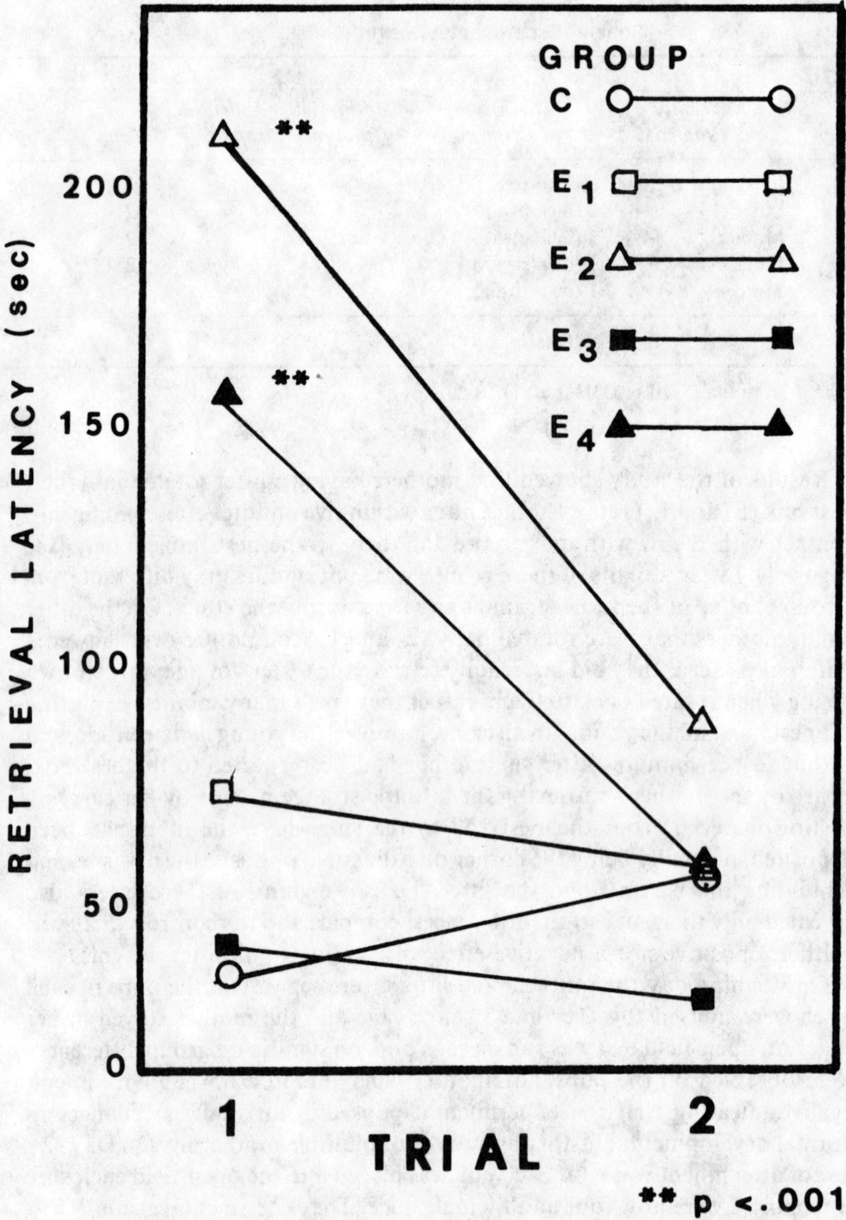

FIG. 1. Mean Retrieval Latency Scores of Mothers in each Group at Trial 1 and Trial 2 of the 24-Hour Test. (Asterisks indicate that the scores were different from all others at that Trial for the *p*-value listed.) Gurski (1977).

strains. The number of seconds the pup was within one tail-length of the female and which female that was, were both recorded. Results of this test indicated that pups from the experimental litters differentially distributed their preferences for females that they had been reared by, compared to the control group which preferred the biological mother. In total scores the groups in which mothers were rotated (E_2 and E_4) were not different from controls, whereas pups from rotated litters gave lower scores indicating a somewhat weaker attachment to all mothers including their biological mother.

Summary. Summarizing this study, multiple mothering affected retrieval latencies of rotated mothers while it did not affect the latencies of those mothers that had pups rotated into their nest boxes; pup development measured by weight gain proceeded normally, unaffected by multiple mothering; multiply mothered pups scored equally with mothers and surrogate mothers in post weaning tests of proximity and following, and differently from control pups, which chose the biological mother most often. The study extended the conditions under which the mouse can multiply mother its offspring and, if the attachment test is regarded as valid, points to an environmental factor in the acqusition of maternal attachment in the mouse based upon significant contacts of dependence at the early developmental ages.

Laboratory Rat

There is no study in the literature of communal nursing in the rat in either a natural or laboratory setting. There are several experimental studies which indicate that the rat mother will adopt a strange litter of her own or of a different species (Denenberg et al., 1962; Ottinger et al., 1963). These studies attempted to use the rat as an animal analog of the effects of maternal emotionality in a situation where she was rotated every 24 hours between her own and a foster litter. While these studies were designed to explore the maladaptive aspects of the rotational situation, and in fact may have precipitated these negative effects by the design (e.g., shocking of mother before depositing her in the pup's cage) the majority of pups survived under these rigorous conditions, although their body weights were somewhat reduced when compared to controls. Another way of interpreting these results is that, even under conditions which stressed the maternal-infant system beyond any parameters it could have been selected to endure, the system proved quite durable in that the "next generation" was produced and survived to weaning.

A novel aspect of experimental multiple mothering, between-species care, has been explored thoroughly by Denenberg and his associates (Denenberg et al., 1964; Rosenberg et al., 1970; Denenberg et al., 1973). They placed rat "aunts" with a lactating mouse mother and her litter and assessed the effects under a number of situations. Weanling mice were observed to show lowered open-field activity, decreased fighting when paired with another mouse, and lowered corticosterone levels in a novel environment. The pups showed a decreased survival rate, however. Apparently the effects were due to the increased handling rather than to any particular nutritive effects, since the Rosenberg et al. (1970) study used thelectomized (mammary glands removed) rat "aunts" with the same overall results as in the other studies in this series.

Hamster

Whereas the female mouse (including nulliparae) shows reponsiveness to pups not her own under a variety of conditions, and the rat somewhat less so but still relatively responsive, the female hamster will adopt only under very limited conditions. Rowell (1960) reported that even normal mothers occasionally attacked and ate their own young, and although they were usually good foster mothers, they sometimes attacked strange pups which were consigned to them. She points out (Rowell, 1961) that hamsters and mice are differently organized socially, the hamster being a more solitary animal and the mouse more capable of living in social groups.

In the 1961 study Rowell presented a strange pup to each of 33 females: 20 females first encountered the pup on the cage floor and immediately cannibalized it; the other 13 females found the pup in the nest—and 8 of these 13 ate the pup at once; 4 pups were eaten after being licked and the last pup was licked until it fell out of the nest whereupon it was eaten. Although Rowell did not indicate which females did what, 15 of the 33 were pregnant during the test and 13 were mothers at some time previous to the test. This study taken by itself seems to obviate any multiple mothering in nonlactating female hamsters. But younger hamsters are observed to tolerate pups when not with their mother even after they became sexually mature, a finding which suggests the presence of a developmental or critical period factor, since when with the mother the young female hamster attacks pups before the onset of sexual maturity.

Richards (1967) in a review paper cites his own research which implicates other variables than a simple aversion of the hamster to foster pups other than its own. Instead of a single pup, he offered virgins, nulliparous pregnant, and primiparous lactating females three pups each. The last two groups were tested within 24 hours of parturition. While the virgins ate or at least killed all the pups, the nulliparous females usually attacked one and mothered the rest while but one of all the primiparous females fostered the pups.

It appears then that multiple mothering is possible in the hamster only in limited situations and that the solitary social life of the species is a critical factor limiting this possibility.

Hystricomorphs

Guinea Pig

Little information is available for the guinea pig (*Cavia porcellus*) in the present context. King (1956) states that some natural fostering probably occurs since the young tend to attach themselves to females other than their natural mother. Kunkel and Kunkel (1964) report that in small groups some mothers would nurse infants other than their own; however casual adoption was not found. Morris (1965) states that other mothers feed the abandoned litter if a mother is killed while she is still nursing.

Fullerton et al. (1974) studied mother-infant interactions in laboratory guinea pig subjects. They concluded that although the system shows some specificity it is a loose type of organization, as evidenced by the young organism's greater amount of time spent with females other than its mother.

Recently, Pettijohn (1977) studied the reactions of adult guinea pig parents, male and female, to a recording of neutral or distress vocalizations of infant guinea pigs, or white noise. His results indicate that the age of the stimulus infant was a critical variable in the parent's response to the distress signal, with most mothers scoring high in Week 1 and decreasing thereafter to chance level by Week 5. The results of the study lead Pettijohn to conclude that paternal reactions to distress vocalizations are nonexistent and that after the first weeks of life the maternal reaction also extinguishes.

Summarizing the data on these four separate genera, they show a spectrum of behavior ranging from complete acceptance to almost complete rejection of young other than their own. The pups seem to benefit by multiple mothering where it occurs (King, 1963; Morris, 1965; Werboff et al., 1970; Sayer and Salmon, 1971). Attachments of young to mother or her surrogates are conditioned by the early rearing pattern to which the young are exposed (Gurski, 1977). The social organization of each genus seems to be critical in the ultimate acceptance or rejection of nonrelated offspring. Synchrony of estrus facilitates multiple mothering, although this is not a necessary factor.

MULTIPLE MOTHERING IN CARNIVORES

Felines

Members of the cat family are typically solitary mammals. The exception to this rule is the lion (*Panthera leo*) which is quite social. Lions form a social group which is called a pride. The permanent nucleus of a pride is a group of related females with a range of ages (Bertram, 1975). Schaller's observations on the Serengeti lion (1972) include a description of the communal rearing of the young. Sometimes two or three lionesses in a pride have cubs at the same time. They become companions and care for the cubs jointly. The lionesses do not attempt to separate their young from the rest of the pride. When the litters are about 8 weeks old the lionesses usually combine their litters. Schaller describes this occurrence: five lionesses having a total of 13 cubs between them, ages 6 weeks to 4 months, combined their litters and cared for them communally. Schaller states that he personally had difficulty in assigning cubs to mothers, the integration was so complete.

There are advantages to this arrangement: it is quite adaptive when the mother has a large litter and either has 1) less milk or 2) is "dried up," incapable of delivering milk, whether her litter is large or small. Schaller states that disadvantages are also evident when the cubs become quarrelsome while suckling; the system favors the larger cubs, and the smaller cubs usually are less able to nurse.

Rudnai (1973) provides other information on lion epimeletic behavior: the lioness leaves the pride prior to parturition and gives birth in a secluded shelter. For six to eight weeks postpartum she divides her time between the pride and her cubs. Rudnai observed that a litter over 4 months old that is already in the pride may cause the lioness to leave the pride with her new and younger litter when they are old enough to travel. However if they are no more than two months apart, all the cubs are reared together. Communal rearing does not destroy any bond between the mother and own young according to Rudnai, as a frightening situation usually send the cubs to their biological mother's side even though they may have been sitting with another mother.

In a recent article (Bertram (1975) provides some data on the social system of lions, which may give some clues as to the function of multiple mothering in the ecology of this species. He states that males are unlikely to be genetically related to females in the pride but are closely related to one another. This combination of closely related males with closely related (to themselves) females contributes to their unique social structure, and points to kinship factors as important to the practice of multiple mothering in this group.

Lionesses do not have a regular estrus cycle in the wild, but are often in heat synchronously—a phenomenon observed in the mouse also—although mice do have regular estrus cycles. In the lion synchronously-produced litters have a better survival rate than solitary litters, because communal suckling and rearing is possible; it results in a more regular food supply and more regular attention to the young. Bertram (1975) speculates that communal hunting by mothers could make for more successful hunting and a larger and more plentiful food supply.

Canines

The literature on canine social behavior is not complete nor even what could be called adequate yet. However, it is growing. The work of Scott and his colleagues (Scott and Fuller, 1965) and Fox (1975) have provided much needed laboratory and field data on various Canids, including the domesticated dog.

Information that is available on both wild and captive wolves and the African cape hunting dog gives rise to the conclusion that multiple mothering is an integral part of the social system of many members of this family. In his classic study of the wild wolf, Murie (1944) observed that a female not related to the pups by parenthood spent much time with the pups which were developing in the pack at the time. The bitch was very attentive to them and played with them. Murie observed that females with litters do not den together but do den near each other when having their own litters. Both males and females in the pack brought food to all the young.

These observations have been generalized to the captive wolf pack. Wolves at the Brookfield Zoo in Chicago have been observed to cooperate in the rearing of the young of a single mother (Rabb et al., 1967). An additional observation helps to explain why mothers do not normally den together: Rabb et al. (1967) observed that two mothers, giving birth to separate litters, brought them to a common shelter. Amicable relations lasted one night. The following night all pups were killed, most having been pulled in half by the two mothers, each attempting to possess all the pups herself. In spite of this, Rabb et al. (1967) see the attention of the adults to all the young as adaptive.

> "Ritualized group activities, altruism shown in the care and raising of the young by non-parents, and low levels of reproductive activity in some male leaders suggest that wolves have evolved their social structure with some selective pressure for traits of value to the group, and not just the individual." (p. 310).

Wolves hunt in packs. This is also an integral part of their social behavior. Communal feeding occurs in the pack hunter as well as in jackals and coyotes

(Kleiman, 1967). It has evolved in its most ritualized form in the Cape hunting dog.

The Cape hunting dog (*Lycaon pictus lupinus*) has been studied by Kuehme (1965). He observed a pack of eight adults (six males and two females) and 15 pups (4 pups with one female and 11 pups with the other female). At the beginning of his observation they were, respectively, 1 and 3 weeks old old. Each of the females nursed all the young and "tried to steal them from the other" (p. 443), a phenomenon already noted in the wolf.

During a hunt, dogs tore open the belly of their living quarry, bolted down hand-sized chunks of meat and skin without chewing, returned to the burrow within five minutes, and disgorged the meat in front of the begging pups and their guards. The "guards" are the females and certain males who share this duty. The females would digest portions of this food and store it for later, at which time they disgorged it. Kuehme (1965) speculates that this guard system is similar to what prehumans may have used, i.e., guarding of the young by some, hunting by some, and the hunters sharing the kill with the young and their guards. The cape hunting dog also has a high adult death rate (Bekoff, 1975); multiple mothering would have a presumed selective advantage here in providing alternate caretakers in the event of death to the biological parents. It should also improve the survival rate of the pups.

It is not uncommon for group-oriented mammals to share in the care of the young. It is somewhat more surprising when solitary species practice multiple mothering: although most solitary Canids do not, Bekoff (1975) reports that sharing of care occurs in the Golden Jackal (*C. aureus*) and Gier (1975) reports similar behavior in the coyote (*C. latrans*). In the former multiple caregiving is kinship related, with the female offspring remaining with the parents to help with care of the next litter. Coyote maternal bitches have been recovered from dens where two litters were located; the relationship can be kinship found (mother-sister; sister-sister) or both bitches might have been sired by the same male. An adoption appears to be a likely possibility on those occasions where one bitch has been found with litters of pups too dissimilar in age for her to have carried both. Under wild circumstances, however, the mothers' share in caring for young housed communally is not yet determined.

The caregiving systems of the Canids of India is similar to that of African Canids. Davidar (1975) reports that a single Dhole or Indian wild dog (*Cuon alphinus*) bitch or pair may bring up the young in a cave or earth on their own. Communal nurseries are also common, made up of several separate earths or in a common cave where bitches give birth to and bring up their young. Davidar also observed whelping bitches fed by members of the pack, which regurgitate food for them. Groups of 10–12 pups have been found with one bitch; they may have been litters of more than one dam.

Summary

Summarizing the literature presented here on Canids, multiple mothering occurs in several species and contributes to the survival of the young where it occurs. Males and females participate in the feeding of the young; where nursing pups are present, two or more mothers who both have litters allow nursing by all pups, as occurs in wolves. Denning together by two or more wolves may not occur in natural settings because the mothers compete in attempting to adopt the helpless young, resulting in the deaths of these pups. This was demonstrated in the behavior of captive wolf mothers. Although the research in the domesticated dog remains to be done, the literature on wolves suggests that multiple mothering would occur naturally if dogs were still socially pack-oriented, rather than being socialized to a human owner. Fox (1975) also urges, along lines originally developed by Crook (1970) for infrahuman primates, that as social organization advances cooperative practices such as care of the young by many members of the group is enhanced and may become a selective factor: the pack in Canidae social organization is the ideal situation for selection of group-oriented behaviors.

MULTIPLE MOTHERING IN ARTIODACTYLS

Caprines

The review of communal epimeletic behavior in rodents and carnivores has demonstrated that in these orders the practice is evident in several species and that it is related to social structure. The epimeletic behavior of the herd animals is an exception to this trend. These mammals, concerned with survival in a flock which is moving and grazing constantly, allow adoption and communal rearing under only the most rigorous experimental conditions.

Hersher et al. (1963) and Smith (1965) discuss the phenomenon of lamb theft in sheep, a phenomenon which is different from that observed in wolves, where mothers attempted to rear young which were born to other females. In sheep it is preparturient mothers who steal the young of other dams. These preparturient mothers often drive the natural mother from the lamb when she tries to care for it (Hersher et al., 1963). As soon as she gives birth to a lamb of her own this behavior disappears.

The caretaking behavior of sheep is precisely timed. Although a ewe will mother any young immediately before or after giving birth, she will reject all young if not allowed access to them soon after parturition. Hersher et al. (1963) have used several techniques to test the parameters of this virtually closed system of behavior. They allowed mother goats 5–10 minutes contact with the young at birth, then separated the pair at two or three months for about 6–10 hours. Following this period they placed the mother with her own and two other kids in an observation room. The mothers either nursed both their own and the other kids, or refused to nurse any kids, even their own. The ewes were divided 50:50 as to tendency to adopt.

Hersher et al. (1963) also separated sheep and goat mothers from within 12 hours after birth and then harnessed the mother so that she would not be able to butt the youngster. Results indicated that she would accept a youngster whose age varied from a few hours to several days old but it took a while for this to occur. Cross-species acceptance was also possible with does-accepting lambs and ewes-accepting kids after the "critical period" had been passed if they were prevented from butting them for a time. The difficulty with which adoption takes place would seem to indicate a poor prognosis for the health of the young, but Hersher et al. (1963) reported that kids reared by sheep and lambs reared by goats grew faster, gained weight more rapidly, and appeared healthier than controls reared by same-species females.

Smith et al. (1966) looked at the critical period in attachment between lambs and ewes in some detail. Certain important points should be considered. First the young are precocial, as are birds who have short critical periods of imprinting, strong attachment, and no multiple mothering. The young of the other species discussed up to now are altricial, born both blind and helpless. Second, ewes will accept the first lamb (or two, possibly three) presented to them, even if these lambs are unrelated, provided there is no contact with other lambs in the interim between birth and adoption. Third, acceptance of an unrelated kid appears quite easy and spontaneous if, after a period of separation from her own young, both her own young and the unrelated kid are simultaneously presented to her. Smith et al. (1966) tried this with 21 ewes and 37 lambs. The body weights of control and experimental lambs showed no significant differences; the experimental lambs, if anything, were slightly heavier. The results indicated that this type of short-term separation did not affect their health or development. Smith hypothesized that the postparturient ewe will become attached to and distinguish any newly-born lamb which she licks in the anogenital region for 1/3 to 1/2 hour postpartum.

Several researchers have extended Smith's hypothesis. Lindsay and Fletcher (1968) separated lambs of 2–22 days of age for three hours and found that eyesight was important to recognition but that even when a correct choice was made by sight the mothers nuzzled the lamb's anogenital region and refused to allow an alien to suckle.

Most research has been done with domestic sheep and goats; Shillito and Hoyland (1971) observed Soay sheep which are reported by them to be the most primitive of domestic sheep of an "unimproved" type in Europe (i.e., they are somewhat closer to a wild genetic stock). These researchers observed some ewes making maternal responses to all new lambs even though they already had lambs of their own. Attachment appeared to be dependent on mutual recognition. Parturient and pregnant ewes who were within a few days of lambing approached newborn or day-old lambs, licking and calling, following until their mothers butted them away. The ewes appeared to be responding to specific stimuli presented by lambs. That these stimuli were typically olfactory was explored further by Baldwin and Shillito (1974). They ablated the olfactory bulbs of eight pregnant Soay ewes, which resulted in anosmia. Four of the ewes were observed not to lick the lambs properly after birth; six ewes fed lambs with no attempt to butt them away. Olfaction was concluded to be concerned with the identification of the lamb at close quarters and in forming the typically strong ewe-lamb relationships.

Cervines

Altmann's (1956) long-range study of the elk or wapiti (*Cervus canadensis nelsoni*) of the Jackson Hole, Wyoming, herd gives information about cooperative caregiving in this family. She reports that cooperative protection of the young calves was observed, and named the groups where this took place "calf pools." She states: "One or two cows serve as guardians and stay with the young while the others graze and return at intervals for nursing and licking their calves" (Altmann, 1956, p. 66). After about 3 weeks of age the calf leaves the pool and is able to follow the herd. Thus it appears that the calf pool functions as a short-term protective system which the young leave as soon as they are able to join the herd's daily activities.

Summary

Summarizing this section, the appearance of multiple mothering in these herd mammals occurs chiefly under experimental conditions and, with the exception of the elk, might often be considered aberrant when it occurs in nonexperimental animals. These herd animals live in large, highly mobile groups, a factor that could endanger the young if multiple mothering occurred. If the young could nurse indiscriminately, some young would be overfed and some would be underfed; some mothers would nurse many young while others would not nurse any young.

The strong attachment system appears to be quite adaptive and as close to "instinctive," in Bowlby's (1969) sense, as is any social behavior which has cohesiveness as its goal. However, the attachment is limited by the mother and not the young. That the separations and subsequent within and between-species adoption did not prove maladaptive to the lamb is an interesting finding, and possibly contrary to any general theory of attachment.

MULTIPLE MOTHERING IN MARINE MAMMALS

Since work with marine mammals is not as advanced as that with land mammals, much of what will follow in this section is necessarily anecdotal.

Pinnipeds

Considering the mammals of the order *Pinnipedia*, no cooperative feeding has been observed in the sea otter (*Enhydra lutris*), seal (*Callorhinus ursinus*), sea lion (*Zalophus californicus*), or harbor seal (*Phoca vitulina*) (Evans and Bastian, 1969). These animals are characterized by loose social organization, strongest bonds between mother and pup, with adults forming aggregations only during breeding season.

Cetaceans

The herd marine mammals of the order *Cetacea* are much different from the pinnipeds. Their behavior is also an interesting contrast to those land mammals (e.g., sheep and goats) which move in herds and also have precocial young. The following incidents are reported by McBride and Kritzler (1951). A male bottlenose dolphin (*Tursiops truncatus*) was found on the beach. It was 2 weeks old and its mother had probably died or abandoned it. When the infant was put into the living tank, two captive pregnant females already in the tank cared for it, allowing it to "nurse." The male chose one of the females for its foster parent. The infant died even though given care, because the females did not yet have milk. (They were two months prepartum; milk is not available until four days prepartum.) Another female, placed in a tank with a younger female who was not yet weaned, was ready to give birth. The younger female immediately went to her and attempted to nurse. The female, who was ready to deliver, allowed the nursing. The younger female continued her attempts at nursing throughout the delivery period. Finally, McBride and Kritzler reported that two females swam with an infant between them for the first few days after birth: this probably facilitates survival. Solicitude for the safety of the young, which is shown by nonmaternal females, persists for several weeks after the birth of an infant. When an emergency occurs the rest of the group encircles the trio until the emergency is over.

Tavolga (1966) also reports that a nonparous dolphin may show certain types of maternal behavior. An example was the following: one year before giving birth a nonparous female spent much time in the company of three young dolphins. This female escorted the young dolphins without interference from the mothers; mothers would usually interfere when the young attempted to swim with other dolphins, thus facilitating attachment to her. This nonparous female kept the young dolphins with her on the far side of their living tank during periods of public entertainment. Both of these activities are ordinarily seen only in a mother dolphin with a young calf.

Caldwell and Caldwell (1966) report that there is also parental cooperation among females. Mothers of young infants sometimes take charge of and direct other infants, thereby allowing the other mother to feed. The mother who has fed then "relieves" the first escort who can then use the time to feed. This care-sharing behavior has also been reported for a male but it is considered unusual. There may be an experimental factor here since elsewhere they (Caldwell and Caldwell, 1968) report that primiparous mothers attempt to reclaim their young earlier than do multiparous mothers.

Information on the whale is even more anecdotal, coming mainly from historical reports. Caldwell et al. (1966) speculate (based upon other reports) that the existence of whale "aunts" is possible in the sperm whale; this "aunt" would be another female of the herd or group that aids the mother in rearing the young.[1]

Although the information in this section is anecdotal and somewhat idiosyncratic, it can be said that the evidence is reliable, since these independent sources agree, and it suggests what is possible in these groups without experimental manipulation. From the observations of Caldwell and Caldwell (1966) it would seem that herding per se in mammals does not preclude multiple mothering if the survival of the young of the species is improved by it.

MULTIPLE MOTHERING IN PRIMATES

Infrahuman Examples

Because of their relationship to us by common ancestry, the social behavior of apes and monkeys has been much studied as a source of possible

[1]They state that this occurs in the elephant *Loxodonta africana* and *Elephas maximus* but do not cite their source.

information regarding the evolutionary roots of human behaviors. In fact, Bowlby (1969) cites several primate sources as support for his theory of attachment. However, the variations found in primate behavior tell us, if anything, that there is some degree of latitude in the way social behavior may be expressed.

It was the Harlows (Harlow et al., 1963) who drew attention to the need for studying epimeletic behavior in the primate in the context of a system, drawing attention to the ways in which each member changed and the effects of that change on the other member or members of the system.

Hinde (1969) followed this with a detailed analysis of the maternal filial dyad in the rhesus monkey. He reported that the balance between acceptance and rejection, which is controlled by the mother in the early weeks, is critical in promoting independence in the young. The rhesus macaque mother responds to the social context, however; she is much more rejecting when experimentally isolated from conspecifics than when in the group-living situation: she is protective of the young when the possibility of harm arises, and experimental isolation from conspecifics removes the possibilty of outside danger. The attachment of mother to infant can be more clearly seen in the group context: when separated from her infant for a period of time it is she who encourages a weaker attachment upon reunion, by rejection, and the infant who attempts to strengthen it, by maintaining contact. The changes that occur within the dyad are always potentially influenced by the reciprocal interactions between the partners.

In an early paper, Jay (1963) described maternal care in the Hanuman langur (*Presbytis entellus*). She observed multiple mothering from the infant's first day of life: the youngster clings to and is nursed by a number of females, who may take the infant some distance from the mother without incident. She comments that langur male adult relations appeared more "relaxed" than do those of male baboons. DeVore (1963) reports that the infant is a center of attention for the baboon troop but the youngster is not shared by passing it around. The infant is guarded by them: this allows the mother to care for the infant in safety. The primarily terrestrial existence of the baboon, distinguished from the partially arboreal existence of the langur, may play a role in the more guarded nature of baboon social relations: baboons would be more vulnerable to predators without warning.

Poirer (1972) has also noted that north Indian (Hanuman) and Nilgiri langurs practice multiple mothering while south Indian langurs do not. He has contrasted the langur and baboon society also. He notes that the langur society is almost matriarchal whereas baboon society is not. The langur female has the primary responsibility for protection of the young whereas in the baboon society the male participates by protecting the troop along with other males.

Among vervet monkeys, mothers are "relaxed" about approach by females but do not pass their young around as does the Hanuman langur (Lancaster, 1972). Females juveniles show interest and will touch, cuddle, carry, and groom infants whenever they have an opportunity to do so. Vervets have separate dominance hierarchies by sex; some females do display dominance over some males, however. Males do not figure importantly in infant care, at least until after the infant is 3 months old.

Quite the opposite system is seen in the *Macaca sylvana* of Gibraltar. Here the leader males may take the infant from the mother as early as 1 day of age. For the infant's first two weeks, the male is the major influence. According to Burton (1972) this encourages biological maturation. The male, who is the putative biological father, orients the infant away from himself, the mother, and other adults, and towards subadult males. Through these subadult males the infant makes juvenile and age-mate contact. Females are not usually permitted to hold the infant until the infant is able to walk, around day 10. The obvious exception is the nursing mother. The subadult males, towards whom the head male directs the infant, care for and "sit" with it. Socially, subadult females are an isolated group, while adult females are more involved in the socialization of juveniles and subadults.

While the observation of complex primate social behavior is possible in the wild or in natural settings, it is analyzable more easily and in greater detail when the group is in captivity. Emerson (1973) studied infant-sharing in captive *Colobus* monkeys in the Los Angeles Zoo. These primates use a complex method of initiating a subadult female into their caretaking system. In the wild it is reported that there is one dominant male and three or four adult females, one or two subadult females and one infant in a typical group. Sometimes a second male is observed. In the groups studied the female subadult was 2–3 years old: the male and the infant's mother spent time with the subadult female until she could share the infant without injuring or frightening it. After the sharing had been done successfully the 3-week-old infant was seen to be moving back-and-forth between the mother and subadult at different intervals. Emerson speculates that the lack of predation pressure in the wild in this arboreal species may contribute to the evolution of infant-sharing as the need for quick retreats is obviated.

The question naturally arises as to whether the behaviors observed in captivity arise primarily because predator pressure is gone or whether it has evolved in at least a potential form during the history of the species. Brueggeman (1973) studied the most common laboratory primate, the rhesus monkey (*Macaca mulatta*) in a seminatural setting, on Cayo Santiago, Puerto Rico. She reports that care is given by all age classes of males and females to infants and yearlings of both sexes. She also comments that it is adaptive and promotes survival, probably through the process of social learning. The late stage-one infancy period is the point at which multiple caretaking begins. There is no complete loss of the bond between the mother and infant since the infant is periodically brought back to the mother, an indication of her relationship to and "ownership" of the infant. This ubiquitous caregiving behavior is also reported by Lindburg (1973), with special emphasis on the care given by the adolescent female.

In the laboratory most research has concentrated on deprivation of maternal care, in the hope that its lack would increase our knowledge of its function when compared with controls. This approach, while possibly answering questions about severe or extreme deprivation, seems inadequate when used to understand a system of interaction between living organisms. The deprived infant is losing more than its mother in most situations: it is also losing all contact with any substitute caretakers. A more fruitful approach seems to be that of Griffin (1966) who conducted a multiple mothering experiment with rhesus mother-infant pairs. At a mean age of 2 weeks the infants were separated from their mother for 2.5 hours after which they were united with one of the mothers who had been separated from her infant. This was done every two weeks for 32 weeks so that, among the four mother-infant pairs, each infant was with each mother, including its biological mother, four times. Griffin reported that all mother-infant pairs accepted each other within a few hours. While the variance of interactions was greater for this group compared with nonseparated controls, he judged the mother-infant system "relatively insensitive to radical changes in the relationship" (p. 31). This condition did not produce lasting effects or deficits in the social behaviors of either mothers or young.

An equally fruitful approach has been that of Kaufman and Rosenblum with two species of macaque monkey, the pigtail (*Macaca nemestrina*) and bonnet (*M. radiata*) (Kaufman and Rosenblum, 1969; Rosenblum, 1971, 1973; Kaufman, 1973). They report that the ecologies of the two species are not different, but a genetic difference must exist as evidenced by the characteristic responses to separation of infant and mother. Even though in a social group, pigtail infants show the responses typically defined as the depressive reaction so intimately related to Bowlby's attachment theory (Kaufman, 1973). The infant withdraws completely from the group for about three days. Activity does not approach the pre-separation baseline for about four weeks. During the severe depressive period no adult female attempted to comfort or adopt the infant. By contrast, the bonnet infant when subjected to the same manipulation experienced no severe deprivation. Adoption by the other animals in the group was immediate; this presumably obviates a depressive reaction. The infant, accustomed to close social contact with all members of the group, immediately sought care and received it from the other mothers, and sometimes from the males. There was no difference in the pre-

and post-separation activities of the infant. When reunited with their mothers the pigtail infants became intense and clinging while the bonnet resumed normal relations without what might be considered by some to be "anxious" attachment.

These two species are developmentally different in a number of ways. The pigtail infant's exploration is restrained by its mother, the family unit is more isolated and weaning is a severe ordeal. The bonnet infant undergoes less restraint, has more positive interactions with related and unrelated adults, participates in more social play during the first year, and endures less intense punishment for transgressions. Rosenblum (1973) also emphasizes the difference in intraspecific aggressive encounters and maternal vigilance when the infant becomes mobile, both behaviors being more intense in the pigtail.

Another species studied by Kaufman and Rosenblum is the squirrel monkey (*Saimiri sciureus*). Squirrel monkeys form close and relatively enduring relationships with one or more other female members of the group in addition to the mother. Females act maternally toward young which are not their own; this is allowed by the mother. The squirrel monkey "aunt" is usually an associate of the mother (Rosenblum, 1973) although this is not always the case. There have been maladaptive results in this multiple mothering system not observed in bonnets: some young have died of malnutrition (Rosenblum, 1971). Whether this is something that occurs more in captivity than in the wild is not clear. It is fairly well-established that the mother and the "aunt" do not compete with each other for the infant (Rosenblum, 1971).

One other area should be mentioned—the paternal role in caregiving. Except for the above-cited report of *M. sylvana*'s active control of the infant, most males range from tolerance to ambivalence. Pigtail males are tolerant but aloof, for instance, while bonnet males do not engage in interaction until the infant is ready to play. However, adoption by the male has been reported for baboons (*Papio hamadryis* and *P. anubis*) and rhesus (*M. mulatta*) (Mitchell and Brandt, 1972).

There are various systems of mothering in primates (Jolly, 1972). When all species are considered the precocial vs. nonprecocial dichotomy becomes more of a continuum and so becomes somewhat less important in determining the way in which members organize themselves. Early care of the young is still no less related to the species' ecology, although similar ecologies can produce entirely different systems of mothering. In addition, similar genera may produce quite varied species differences. For example, Jolly has also described the quite dramatic differences between north Indian and south Indian langur infant care. Among all primates it seems usual for females to take an interest in each other's young. "Aunts" which help rear the young are not always blood relatives (Jolly, 1972; Rosenblum, 1973).

The subject of "aunting" in primates has recently been reviewed in detail by Hrdy (1976), who concludes that such behavior can provide protection for the young when imminent emergencies arise, as well as a possibility of subsequent exploitation of those young by surrogate parents who have previously cared for them. The former is by far the more common situation for many of the species cited in the present paper, e.g., Hanuman and Nilgiri langurs, baboons, and squirrel and colobus monkeys. In several species sitting with the infant and adoption by both male and female nonrelated adults has been observed. When infants are "exploited" by male anubis baboons, Nilgiri langurs, vervets, Barbary macaques, Japanese macaques, and Hamadryas baboons, it is for protection of the adult from agonistic encounters with other males. Referred to by Dean and Crook (1971) as "agonistic buffering," attacks by the more powerful male are inhibited when the subordinate one is carrying the infant.

Incidents of aggression toward infants are observed more often in males than in females: Hanuman langurs from male troops have been observed to invade troops and kill infants sired by other males, a practice that may enhance their reproductive success. It is interesting that the species also has a ubiquitous multiple mothering practice, that of passing around of the infant from female to female soon after birth (Jay, 1963; Poirer, 1972). The possible selective advantage to the infant is that, in the case where the mother is attacked or is defending herself, another female may be sufficiently attached to the infant to protect and care for it 1) until the mother can resume her responsibility or 2) in case of her death. Since the sexes do not mingle unless females are in estrus, the responsibility for protection of infants devolves upon the females: multiple mothering in this species may have evolved as a survival mechanism against attacks by male invaders.

Hrdy (1976) also reviews studies that indicate how the infant's age may condition the onset of aunting: the criterion of possible harm to the infant (as judged by the mother) conditions her permissiveness in allowing other females access to it. Early vulnerability would inhibit early aunting. In those species that practice it, three benefits are conferred: 1) foraging freedom for the mother, 2) socialization of the infant, and 3) potential help in the case of other contingencies. An additional benefit is possible: "play mothering" (Lancaster, 1971) by the immature female provides her with skills needed when she becomes sexually mature and produces an infant of her own. She in turn is assumed to be bonded strongly enough to the nonrelated infant to provide protection and relief for the mother, and possible adoption in the event of the mother's death.

Summarizing this section, the diversity of infrahuman primate social behavior extends to the care of the young. Even as the langur shares the young in an almost completely unrestricted manner, the pigtail macaque mother is extremely singular and protective, at least in those maternal-filial dyads observed in captivity. Where multiple mothering occurs it sometimes includes both sexes and sometimes just the female or the male (multiple fathering), depending upon group composition and social dominance structure. Multiple mothering in infrahuman primates appears to provide a selective advantage to the group by providing a greater number of significant social contacts between adults and young at the early stages of development and to the individual young by increasing the number of experienced caretakers that can offer it protection in emergencies.

Human Examples

In this section, four general examples of multiple mothering will be reviewed. The most well-known and well-researched experiment in communal childrearing, the Israeli kibbutz, will be considered first. Following this, the communal movement in American, the day-care approach of the West Berlin New Left, and, finally, the practices of the Peoples' Republic of China will each be described.

Kibbutzim

The first kibbutz, Deganya, was established in Palestine in 1909 with 12 members (Hazan, 1973). Presently it is reported that there are 226 kibbutzim with a total population of about 90,000 including about 31,400 children and youths. From a small movement conceived in Europe and begun in Palestine it has become today a "communal agroindustrial entity" (Hazan, 1973, p. 3). The following description of the childrearing practices of the kibbutz is drawn from a combination of sources (Spiro, 1958; Rabin, 1965; Bettelheim, 1969; Katz and Lewin, 1973).

From the first day of his life the infant is a child of the kibbutz. He lives in a communal nursery, is reared by a metapelet (nurse), and later by a nursery teacher and teacher. He is housed with about 15 other peers of both sexes. This cohabitation continues throughout his childhod and adolescence. At the age of 1 year he is moved to a Toddler House, where the adult-child ratio decreases to 1:8. At age 4–5 two Toddler groups are merged, thus reestablishing the ratio at 1:16. This is the unit in which he stays until entering high school at the age of 12. All social activities are engaged in together, whether this be eating, sleeping, showering, school, or recreation.

The metapelet is always a female who volunteers for the position. Parents and educators make choices from among the volunteers based on the criteria of congeniality, compatibility, training, and personality. The metapelet is the basic transmitter of the kibbutz culture, and since her personality can become either a catalyst or catastrophe in the parent-child-nurse triad of interaction, great care is taken in choosing nurses who will prove to be catalysts. The metapelet role was an organic development from the strongly egalitarian political principles on which the kibbutz was founded. The women refused to be left out of the work of the original group. Communal ownership, abolition of money within the kibbutz, and male-female equality set the stage for group ownership and rearing of the children.

Although the nurse has primary responsibility for care and nurturing of the child, the parents are still among the most important people in the child's life. In infancy the child is visited at least once a day by the father and several times a day by the mother. The mother will breast feed the child on these occasions unless she cannot produce milk: in that case the infant is bottle-fed cooperatively by either its nurse or its mother.

At six-months of age the infant may be taken to the parents' room for an hour per day; this period increases to two hours when he is moved to the Toddler's House and to three hours when at kindergarten age. These periods are spent in close interaction, which the various sources agree is free from normal tensions which arise when parents have a role of authority to play as well. Following this free period the parents return the child to his home and put him to bed.

Parents are intensely attached and devoted to their children. The child's independence of the parents, presumably suggestive of a looser attachment towards them, at times forces the parents to overreact, leading to conflicts between them and the children. This can also happen with nurses who may be somewhat insecure and need the children's love more than they need hers.

The modern kibbutz is an extended family, sometimes with three or four generations still in the kibbutz together. The primary centers of the child's life are his parents' and his own home; the secondary centers are his grandparents' homes. The father's authority is internal, emanating from his image as perceived by the child and not from his external paternal role. Boys are more often attached to the father than the mother in this context. This is very different from what Cohen and Campos (1974) have shown with children in the American family, where the mother is significantly more often chosen by the child in a two-choice situation.

What is the effect of this kibbutzim society on the child? Every child in the community is exposed to the lack of opportunity to develop a close relationship to the mother figure during the first three years, maternal deprivation for limited periods, and inconstancy of mothering figures, three dicta which Bettelheim states are contraindicated by Bowlby (Bettelheim, 1969). The answers are not complete but they are sufficient enough to give some idea of the child's early personality: the kibbutz child reaches his second birthday somewhat inferior in both social maturity and general development. Rabin (1965) hypothesizes that multiple mothering at this age causes frustration and anxiety leading to withdrawal. Withdrawal in turn leads to reduced identification; in addition, a high child-adult ratio reduces changes for social-learning from the caretaker. By 10 years of age this early disadvantage is corrected to a degree; the I. Q. and ego strength are higher in the kibbutz-reared child, and he is superior to the nonkibbutz child in both positive attitudes towards his family and in the expression of altruistic goals. He still expresses more anxiety and guilt when compared to the nonkibbutz youngster at this age, however.

By 17 years, the kibbutz adolescent is superior in I.Q., adjustment, and personal growth. He shows less conflict with his family and less ambition in the sense of a personal career apart from the kibbutz. Rabin concludes that "Multiple mothering... has no long-range deleterious effects upon personality development and character structure" (p. 210). Jay and Birney (1973), using many of the same measures as Rabin, generally confirm` Rabin's findings. Shapiro and Madsen (1974) tested 8- to 11-year old kibbutz and nonkibbutz children in groups of four on a cooperation board game in which the players represented themselves in one condition and the group in the other condition. Kibbutz children scored higher in cooperative tasks and were more influenced by the group-representative condition than the nonkibbutz youngsters, even when it was economically nonadaptive to the player. The kibbutz children were competitively motivated but it was channeled into between-group and not between-player competition. Considering the principles and goals of the kibbutz founders it appears that the method of multiple mothering produces a child who is socialized to become a functioning member of the society in generally the way it was desired. The kibbutz raised Israeli is concluded to be

> "nonpathological, effective, shows only moderate but positive attachment to others, and shows a reduction in intimate rivalry and ambivalence (Beit-Hallahmi and Rabin, 1977, p. 536)."

In spite of the success of the kibbutz movement, and partially as a result of this success, communal rearing patterns are giving way to nuclear family arrangements: children more often sleep at home and mothers more often assume maternal and domestic duties than in the earlier revolutionary years. As economic improvements continue the equality of function among the sexes has decreased as males continue in the production-oriented roles and employ outside help and females assume a nuclear family sex-typical role (Beit-Fallahmi and Rabin, 1977).

American Communal Movement

Compared to the kibbutz and its smoothly running social machine, the American communal movement appears to have been not completely built before it was put into service. Although communal experiments began in the seventeenth century, the only consistent enduring commune in America has been that of the Hutterite sect (Levine, et al., 1973). The most common characteristic of the modern commune is dissent with the mainstream of society (Eiduson et al., 1973): this dissent may be due to religious or economic idealism on the part of its members; political movements of the 1960's and women's consciousness-raising practices of the 1970's have contributed strongly. Communes emphasize sharing of materials, housing, food, and childrearing. Most members are of middle class origins; in spite of the general rejection of the conventional (expressed by experiments with minor and major hallucinogens) traditional marriage and sex relationships seem to prevail.

In general, children are communally reared to minimize favoritism. Problems arise when the parents differ as to how this practice should be implemented, and this has led to members leaving communes because they could not agree on how much or how little care children should receive and parents should give. It was Bettelheim (1969) who made the point that multiple mothering is made far easier for the child when one strong central value system is held in common by the mother-figures. As much for this fact as for any other, Eiduson et al. (1973) state that the impact of multiple mothering on the child is difficult to answer yet, for the modern American commune. Recent research indicates that couples in commune societies experience pressures from their peers to share and relate on an equal social footing. Parents relinquish absolute control in the socialization of their children and an increased amount of feedback regarding their childrearing patterns. Children aged 5–11 years are on the receiving end of more social structuring by a greater number of authority figures who may not always agree with each others' approaches (Kanter et al., 1975).

Day-Care Movement in West Berlin

It was also political dissent that gave rise to the day-care movement in West Berlin (Sedoun et al., 1973). Women who were excluded from political activism due to lack of day-care facilities started centers which represented the first alternative to childrearing practices available at that time (1968) in West Germany. The guiding principle was that of "nonauthoritarian education," based upon the belief that the child's helplessness in the family was the basis of the authoritarian personality characterized by emotional and psychological rigidity in the face of authority. They attempted to correct this rigidity by using a synthesis of principles from Vera Schmidt's Child Care Laboratory of Moscow and A. S. Neill's Summerhill School. The centers were structured around unrestricted free play, meals according to the child's needs, and freedom of self-expression. Each center was a child collective where external order was based on principles of sharing responsibilities and pleasures.

Early successes were later overturned when the West German government withdrew its economic support. The members began to disagree as to their goals, some believing in the original mission of teaching the children the collective political objectives of their parents and socializing them to carry these on; others felt that the extension of day-care service to the working class was more important than maintaining the student-centered movement.

Although not generalizable to the West Berlin Storefront Day-Care Centers, research on day-care centers in the United States and United Kingdom has argued for the principle of day care as a satisfactory substitute for working parents. Caldwell et al. (1970) found no difference in attachment to parents between home-reared and day care children at 30 months of age. Tizard and Tizard (1971) found no gross disturbances in London residential nurseries in 2-year-old children when compared with working class home-reared children, although the nursery children showed less willingness to approach strangers and somewhat more social immaturity. This appears to be what Rabin (1965) discovered in the young kibbutz child. Schwarz et al. (1973) matched children at three to four years of age who had attended day care centers from infancy with those who had just started. Both groups were beginning at a new center. They found that the early experience with centers resulted in a significantly greater positive response to the new center, suggesting that a change of caretaker did not depress the experienced children where it did depress the children leaving home for the first time.

Multiple Mothering in the Peoples' Republic of China

Concern with the worker has shown its most positive effect in the multiple mothering of the Peoples' Republic of China. Although information is anecdotal and not plentiful enough for any final judgment, Sidel (1974) writes of two factories in which the care center is located on-site. Women workers can bring their newborn babies to the factory's nursing room when they work. The caretaker-child ratio is from 1:4 to 1:7 on the average. The children called the caretakers "Auntie." Aunties are chosen from among workers for "responsibility and patience." They are not given any special training, however.

The Peoples' Republic has a strong central value system that includes sexual equality. These should contribute to the success and satisfaction with the system of multiple mothering practiced there. The infant can thrive physically and emotionally if the mother-substitutes are constant, warm and giving (Sidel, 1974). Multiple mothering, there as in the Israeli kibbutz, is part of the "new human being the Chinese are trying to fashion" (p. 105). This satisfaction reportedly extends to the 24-hour nurseries that are also in operation. The parents are away from the children for 24 hours a day, and as much as six days of the week. The children are reported to adapt in less than three months while the parent-child relationship remains close. The child goes to these nurseries at 1-½ years and may live there until 7 years of age. The move back to the house is usually without incident, especially when the parents and child remain in touch with each other during his stay in the nursery.

Summarizing the material in this section, multiple mothering in humans is usually prompted by a social motivation. Its relationship is less to the biological and more to the social-ecological environment. This is not surprising in view of the position taken by modern anthropologists that the nuclear family unit evolved as a response to political and economic, and not to biological pressures (Campbell, 1974). The weight of evidence does not support predictions of gross pathology; rather, it supports statements that caretaking can be safely distributed among several individuals.

ATTACHMENT, DEPENDENCE, AND MULTIPLE MOTHERING

Attachment

Several theorists have written on the topic of maternal-filial attachment. Their positions range from an ecological-instinctivist approach (Bowlby, 1969) that precludes multiple attachments to an associationist learning approach (Cairns, 1966; Gewirtz, 1972) that allows for multiple attachments to occur. We take the position that attachment is a multiprocess-developmental phenomenon which is inevitable as to its appearance in the mammalian offspring but is not fixed as to how it must be expressed nor as to the number of individuals to which it must be directed. Attachment is an affectional bond representing a special relationship to an individual or individuals; it is not necessarily conditioned by dependence on food, shelter, etc. needs, but is not necessarily completely independent of those needs either.

Many theorists have written of the offspring's attachment to the mother; few have written of the caregiver's attachment to the infant. Even so, it must be assumed that caregiving behavior is at least partly conditioned by the caregiver's bond to the infant, whether or not the infant recognizes this bond or prefers the caregiver over other individuals. Therefore under most circumstances the caregiver will form an attachment to the infant or infants cared for; this attachment serves to keep the caregiver in proximity to the dependent infant during that period of time that it is the caregiver's responsibility. We would predict that a close affectional bond between caregiver and infant would be positively correlated with the kinds of variables that are considered indicators of better quality care. In infrahuman mammals these are sufficient food and shelter, and in humans they also include lively social interaction and response to the youngster's signals and approaches (Bowlby, 1969).

Multiple Mothering, Dependence, and Attachment

The possibility exists that a child can form attachments towards more than one important figure. Since the strength of attachment of the principal caregiver to the infant could reduce significant contact with others (Kaufman and Rosenblum, 1968) the principal caregiver must be in part responsible for the number of attachments the offspring will make. On the other hand, even if attachments to many figures are not possible, most of the species reviewed here are at least partially cooperative in the rearing of the young and some ubiquitously so (Sayer and Salmon, 1969, 1971; Jay, 1963). Since genetic as well as environmental factors must account for these behaviors there must be an adaptive benefit to multiple mothering in those species that practice it. We agree with those theorists (e.g., Gewirtz, 1972) who see dependence relationships as important ones. Our position is that multiple mothering increases the number of possible caregivers who are 1) attached to the young and will help in emergency situations as well as in providing food and shelter when the biological mother is not available to do so, and 2) possible recipients of the attachment behaviors of the young. While the advantages of emergency and survival aid are obvious, especially in those cases cited above where socialization, relief for the mother and protection from harm in emergencies were discussed (see also Hrdy, 1976), the advantages of having alternative attachment figures are seen as equally as important and as closely related to the presence of multiple mothering as is the advantage of emergency aid. In the species where multiple mothering is practiced not only does the young organism receive significant input from at least one other source; it also interacts significantly with caregivers other than the principal one. This gives it an opportunity to learn about them. In the case of death or of abandonment by the principal caregiver the youngster has alternative caregivers to turn to and possibly to choose between, increasing both its own and the group's survivabilty. By coming into contact with more members of the same class in a relationship of dependence the possibility of forming attachments to these alternative caregivers is increased (Gurski, 1977; Kaufman and Rosenblum, 1968).

CONCLUSIONS

All mammals that have been studied have the capacity to extend maternal behavior to nonrelated offspring. In addition, the anecdotal literature is rife with examples of mothers that have extended maternal care to the young of unrelated species. This capacity is directly related to the process of adoption, which takes place occasionally under natural conditions and is easy to bring about under experimental conditions except in the herd animals such as sheep and goats. The data reviewed here show that not only is multiple mothering a fairly common phenomenon in mammalian societies, but that in those species in which males care for the young, such as wolves and barbary apes, multiple fathering occurs also.

Effects of Culture

Multiple caretakers are commonplace in all human societies that have been studied. In our own culture it has been traditional for maiden aunts to take care of the offspring of their siblings; hence, the metaphorical term "aunting" that many authors have extended to nonhuman animal societies, irrespective of the genetic relationships of the individuals involved. More than one generation may take care of the children, especially including grandparents. In large families, older siblings are frequently drafted to help care for their younger brothers and sisters, and this occurs even in our modern nuclear families. In addition, the same individuals are frequently used as babysitters for nonrelated children.

Multiple mothering is so common in human societies that there should be no problem concerning its extension in new forms of social organization. Indeed in the modern nuclear family, especially if its includes only one or two children, the problem may be lack of multiple caretakers as well as a lack of sibling relationships. From a theoretical standpoint, a child develops a number of dyadic social relationships which act as subsystems of social organization. The number and quality of these social relationships determines the place in the larger and social community, both insofar as these are stable and continuing and so provide security, and as they can be extended to relationships with previously nonrelated persons. The basis of all these relationships is deep emotional contacts maintained over long periods and, in some cases, developed during critical periods when the child is particularly capable of developing new relationships. On the basis of this theory, we would predict that a single child brought up in a nuclear family with no other caretakers than the two parents would develop quite strong dyadic relationships with the father and mother and relatively weak and superficial relationships with other individuals. These child-parent relationships could be extended to other older persons, but with more difficulty than the child who has experience with many caretakers. It would therefore be desirable to provide such a child with opportunities for both multiple caretakers and with multiple peer relationships.

Comments on Social Experiments with Multiple Caretakers

The kibbutz is in effect a stable extended family very similar to primitive tribal organization (where every individual is related to every other in some way) except that the basis of organization is not completely dependent on family relationships. The effect of this system of care, in which children spend the majority of their waking hours with peers, should be to strengthen peer relationships and should make it easy for such children to extend relationships to other peers. Indeed, some of the earlier findings concerning the social adaptation of children reared in a kibbutz indicates that they make very good soldiers. On the other hand, such an intensely regulated and closely knit community, where almost everyone has a deep dyadic relationship with everyone else, is not an ideal environment for a creative, artistic, or intellectual person. Creative activity implies a certain amount of escape from social control.

Day-care centers are becoming a permanent part of present-day American culture. A general principle of social organization among human beings is that the dominant form of social organization within the culture tends to affect and dominate every aspect of life. In our culture the strongest and most pervasive form of social organization is that of politico-economic institutions. We would therefore predict that this type of organization would attempt to meet the problem of multiple caretakers, and this effort has been carried out through day-care centers. As these centers currently operate, both caretaker and peer relationships are quite unstable and should lead to no deep on-going relationships, although the possibility of this type of relationship is not obviated and in fact sometimes occurs in individual instances. Communes provide a setting where stronger relationships may more easily develop because the participants are involved with each other at a deeper level than are most day-care participants; additionally communal groups share a common philosophy, which would encourage a more active educational involvement between adults and children, setting the stage for the development of stronger personal relationships.

REFERENCES

Altmann, M. Patterns of herd behavior in free-ranging elk of Wyoming, *Cervus canadensis nelsoni. Zoologica 41*(2), 65–71 (1956).

Baldwin, B. A., and Shillito, E. E. The effects of ablation of the olfactory bulbs on parturition and maternal behavior in soay sheep. *Animal Behav. 22*, 220–223 (1974).

Beit-Hallahmi, B. and Rabin, A. I. The kibbutz as a social experiment and as a child-rearing laboratory. *Am. Psychol. 32*(7), 532–541 (1977).

Bekoff, M. Social behavior and ecology of African canidae. In *The Wild Canids*, M. W. Fox, ed. Van Nostrand Reinhold, New York (1975), pp. 120–142.

Bertram, B. C. R. The social system of lions. *Scient. Am. 232*(5), 54–65 (1975).

Bettelheim, B. *Children of the Dream.* Collier-Macmillan Ltd., London (1969).

Bowlby, J. *Attachment*. Basic Books, New York (1969).

Brueggeman, J. A. Parental care in a group of free-ranging Rhesus monkeys (*Macaca Mulatta*). *Folia Primat. 20*, 178–210 (1973).

Burton, F. D. The integration of biology and behavior in the socialization of *Macaca sylvana* of Gibraltar. In *Primate Socialization*, Frank E. Poirer, ed. Random House, New York (1972), pp. 29–62.

Cairns, R. B. Attachment behavior of mammals. *Psychol. Rev. 73*(5), 409–426 (1966).

Caldwell, B. M., Wright, C. M., Honig, A. S., and Tannenbaum, J. Infant day care and attachment. *Am. J. Orthopsychiat. 40*(3), 397–412 (1970).

Caldwell, M. C. and Caldwell, D. K. Epimeletic (care-giving) behavior in Cetacea. In *Whales, Dolphins, and Porpoises*, K. S. Norris, ed. University of California Press, Berkeley (1966), pp. 755–788.

Caldwell, D. K., Caldwell, M. C., and Rice, D. W. Behavior of the sperm whale *Physeter catodon L.* In *Whales, Dolphins, and Porpoises*, K. S. Norris, ed. University of California Press, Berkeley (1966).

Caldwell, D. K. and Caldwell, M. C. The dolphin observed. *National History 77*, 58–65 (1968).

Campbell, B. *Human Evolution*, 2nd Ed. Aldine, Chicago (1974).

Cohen, L. J. and Campos, J. J. Father, mother, and stranger as elicitors of attachment behavior in infancy. *Develop. Psychol. 10*(1), 146–154 (1974).

Crook, J. H. The socio-ecology of primates. In *Social Behavior in Birds and Mammals*, J. A. Crook, ed. Academic Press, New York (1970), pp. 103–166.

Crook, J. H. Sources of cooperation in animals and man. In *Man and Beast: Comparative Social Behavior*, J. F. Eisenberg and W. S. Dillon, eds. Smithsonian Institution Press, Washington, D. C. (1971).

Crowcroft, P. and Rowe, F. P. Social organization and territorial behavior in the wild house-mouse (*Mus musculus*). *Proc. Zool. Soc. Lond. 140*, 517–531 (1963).

Davidar, E. R. C. Ecology and behavior of the Dhole or Indian wild dog *Acron alpinus* (Pallas). In *The Wild Canids*, M. W. Fox, ed. Van Nostrand Reinhold, New York (1975) pp. 109–119.

Deag, J. M. and Crook, J. H. Social behavior and 'agonistic buffering' in the wild barbary macaque *Macacus sylvanus. Folia Primat. 15*, 183–200 (1971).

Denenberg, V. H., Hudgens, G. A., and Zarrow, M. X. Mice reared with rats: Modification of behavior by early experience with another species. *Science 143*, 380–381 (1964).

Denenberg, V. H., Ottinger, D. R. and Stephens, M. W. Effects of maternal factors upon growth and behavior of the rat. *Child Dev. 33*, 65–71 (1962).

Denenberg, V. H., Paschke, R. E., and Zarrow, M. X. Mice reared with rats: Effects of prenatal and postnatal maternal environments upon hybrid offspring of C57BL/10J and Swiss albino mice. *Dev. Psychobiol. 6*(1), 21–31 (1973).

DeVore, I. Mother-infant relations in free-ranging baboons. In *Maternal Behavior in Mammals*, H. L. Rheingold, ed. John Wiley & Sons, New York (1963).

Eiduson, B. N., Cohen, J., and Alexander, J. Alternative in child-rearing in the 70's. *Am. J. Orthopsychiat. 43*(5), 720–731 (1973).

Emerson, J. B. Observation of infant-sharing in captive *Colobus polykomos. Primates 14*(1), 93–100 (1973).

Etzioni, A. Editorial: Science and the future of the family. *Science 196* (4289), 487 (1977).

Evans, W. E. and Bastian, J. Communication: Social and ecological factors. In *The biology of marine mammals*, H. T. Andersen, ed. Academic Press, New York (1969) pp. 425–475.

Fox, M. W. Evolution of social behavior in canids. In *The Wild Canids*, M. W. Fox, ed. Van Nostrand Reinhold, New York (1975), pp. 429–460.

Fullerton, C., Berryman, J. C., and Porter, R. H. On the nature of mother-infant interactions in the guinea-pig (*Cavia porcellus*), *Behavior 48*, 145–156 (1974).

Gandelman, R., Paschke, R. E., Zarrow, M. X., and Denenberg, V. H. Care of young under communal conditions in the mouse (*Mus musculus*). *Dev. Psychobiol. 3*, 245–250 (1970).

Gewirtz, J. L., ed. *Attachment and Dependency*. V. H. Winston & Sons, Washington, D. C. (1972).

Gier, H. T. Ecology and social behavior of the coyote. In Fox, M. W. (Ed.) *The Wild Canids*. Van Nostrand-Reinhold Co., New York p. 247–262 (1975).

Griffin, G. A. The effects of multiple mothering on the infant-mother and infant-infant affectional systems. Unpublished Ph.D. dissertation (1966), University of Wisconsin, University Microfilms Inc., Ann Arbor, Michigan.

Gurski, J. C. Multiple mothering in mice: A laboratory study. Unpublished doctoral disseration (1975), Bowling Green State University, Bowling Green, Ohio.

Harlow, H. F., Harlow, M. K., and Hansen, E. W. The maternal affectional system of Rhesus monkeys. In *Maternal Behavior in Mammals*, H. L. Rheingold, ed. John Wiley & Sons, New York (1963), pp. 254–281.

Hazan, B. Introduction. In *Collective Education in the Kibbutz*, A. I. Rabin and B. Hazan, eds. Springer Publishing Co., New York (1973), pp. 1–8.

Hersher, L., Richmond, J. B., and Moore, A. U. Maternal behavior in sheep and goats. In *Maternal Behavior in Mammals*, H. L. Rheingold, ed. John Wiley & Sons, New York (1963), pp. 203–232.

Hinde, B. A. Analyzing the role of the partners in a behavioral interaction—mother-infant relations in Rhesus macaques. *Ann. New York Acad. Sci. 159* Art. 3, 651–667 (1969).

Hrdy, S. B. Care and exploitation of nonhuman primate infants by conspecifics other than the mother. In *Advances in the Study of Behavior*, Vol. 6, J. A. Rosenblatt, R. A. Hinde, E. Shaw, and C. Beer, eds. Academic Press, New York (1976) pp. 101–158.

Jay, J. and Birney, R. C. Research findings on the kibbutz adolescent: A response to Bettelheim. *Am. J. Orthopsychiat. 43*, 347–354 (1973).

Jay, P. Mother-infant relations in langurs. In *Maternal Behavior in Mammals*, H. L. Rheingold, ed. John Wiley & Sons, New York (1963), pp. 282–304.

Jolly, A. *The Evolution of Primate Behavior*. The Macmillan Co., New York (1972).

Kanter, R. M., Jaffe, D., and Weisberg, D. K. Coupling, parenting, and the presence of others: Intimate relationships in communal households. *Family Coord. 24*(4), 433–452 (1975).

Katz, F. and Lewin, G. Early childhood education. In *Collective Education in the Kibbutz*, A. I. Rabin and B. Hazan, eds. Springer Publishing Company, New York (1973), pp. 11–32.

Kaufman, I. C. and Rosenblum, L. A. Effects of separation from mother on the emotional behavior of infant monkeys. *Ann. New York Acad. Sci. 159*, Art. 3, 681–695 (1969).

Kaufman, I. C. Mother-infant separation in monkeys: An experimental model. In *Separation and Depression*, J. P. Scott and E. Senay, eds. AAAS, Washington, D. C. (1973), pp. 33–52.

King, J. A. Social relations of the domestic guinea pig living under semi-natural conditions. *Ecology 37*(2), 221–228 (1956).

King, J. A. Maternal behavior in *Peromyscus*. In *Maternal Behavior in Mammals*, H. L. Rheingold, ed. John Wiley & Sons, (1963), pp. 58–93.

Kleiman, D. G. Some aspects of social behavior in the *Canidae*. *Am. Zoologist 7*, 365–372 (1967).

Kuehme, W. Communal food distribution and division of labor in African hunting dogs. *Nature 205*, 443–444 (1965).

Kunkel, P. and Kunkel, I. A contribution to the ethological analysis of the guinea pig (*Cavia aperea f. poecellus*). *Zeitschrift für Tierpsychologie 21*(5), 602–641 (1964).

Lancaster, J. B. Play-mothering: The relations between juvenile females and young infants among free-ranging vervet monkeys. *Folia Primat. 15*, 161–182 (1971).

Lancaster, J. Play-mothering: The relations between juvenile females and young infants among free-ranging vervet monkeys. In *Primate Socialization*, F. E. Poirer, ed. Random House, New York, (1972), pp. 83–104.

Levine, S. V., Carr, R. P., and Horenblas, W. The urban commune: Fact or fad, promise or pipedream? *Am. J. Orthopsychiat. 43*(1), 149–163 (1973).

Lindburg, D. G. Grooming behavior as a regulator of social interactions in Rhesus monkeys. In *Behavioral Regulators of Behavior in Primates*, C. R. Carpenter, ed. Bucknell University Press, Lewisburg (1973), pp. 124–148.

Lindsay, D. R., and Fletcher, I. C. Sensory involvement in the recognition of lambs by their dams. *Animal Behav. 16*, 415–417 (1968).

McBride, A. F. and Kritzler, H. Observations in pregnancy, parturition, and postnatal behavior in the bottlenose dolphin. *J. Mammalogy 32*(3), 251–266 (1951).

Mitchell, G. and Brandt, E. M. Paternal behavior in primates. In *Primate Socialization*, F. E. Poirer, ed. Random House, New York (1972), pp. 173–206.

Morris, D. *The Mammals*. Hodder & Stoughton, London (1965).

Moltz, H. Otongeny of maternal behavior in some selected species. In *The Ontogeny of Mammalian Maternal Behavior*, H. Holtz, ed. Academic Press, New York (1971), pp. 265–314.

Murie, A. *The Wolves of Mt. McKinley*. U. S. Government Printing Office, Washington, D. C. (1944).

Ottinger, D. R., Denenberg, V. H., and Stephens, M. W. Maternal emotionality, multiple mothering, and emotionality at maturity. *J. Compar. Physiol. Psychol. 56*, 313–317 (1963).

Pettijohn, T. F. Reaction of parents to recorded infant guinea pig distress vocalization. *Behav. Biol. 21*, 438 (1977).

Poirer, F. E. Introduction. In *Primate Socialization*, F. E. Poirer, ed. Random House, New York (1972), pp. 3–28.

Rabb, G. B., Woolpy, J. H., and Ginsburg, B. E. Social relationships in a group of captive wolves. *Am. Zoologist 7*, 305–311 (1967).

Rabin, A. I. *Growing up in the Kibbutz*. Springer Publishing Company, New York (1965).

Reading, A. J. Effect of maternal environment of behavior of inbred mice. *J. Comp. Physiol. Psychol. 62*(3), 437–440 (1966).

Richards, M. P. M. Maternal behavior in rodents and lagomorphs. In *Advances in Reproductive Physiology*, Vol. 2, A. McLaren, ed. Academic Press, New York (1967).

Rosenberg, K. M., Denenberg, V. H., and Zarrow, M. X. Mice (*Mus musculus*) reared with rat aunts: The role of rat-mouse contact in mediating behavioral and physiological changes in the mouse. *Animal Behav. 18*, 138–143 (1970).

Rosenblum, L. A. Infant attachment in monkeys. In *The Origins of Human Social Relations*, H. R. Schaffer, ed. Academic Press, New York (1971) pp. 85–113.

Rosenblum, L. A. Maternal regulation of infant behavior. In *Behavioral Regulators of Behavior in Primates*, C. R. Carpenter, ed. Bucknell University Press, Lewisburg (1973), pp. 195–217.

Rowell, T. E. On the retrieving of young and other behavior in lactating golden hamsters. *Proc. Zool. Soc. Lond. 135*, 265–282 (1960).

Rowell, T. E. Maternal behavior in non-maternal golden hamsters (*Mesocricetus auratus*). *Animal Behav. 9*, 11–15 (1961).

Rudnai, J. *The Social Life of the Lion.* Washington Square East, Wallingford, Pennsylvania (1973).

Sayer, A. and Salmon, M. Communal nursing in mice: Influence of multiple mothers on growth of the young. *Science 164*, 1309–1310 (1969).

Sayer, A. and Salmon, M. An ethological analysis of communal nursing by the house mouse (*Mus musculus*). *Behavior 40*, 60–85 (1971).

Schaller, G. B. *The Serengeti Lion*. University of Chicago Press, Chicago (1972).

Schwarz, J. C., Krolick, G., and Strickland, R. G. Effects of early day-care experience on adjustment to a new environment. *Am. J. Orthopsychiat. 43*, ???? (1973).

Scott, J. P. *Early Experience and the Organization of Behavior*. Wadsworth, Belmont, California (1968).

Scott, J. P. and Fuller, J. L. *Genetics and the Social Behavior of the Dog*. University of Chicago Press, Chicago (1965).

Sedoun, K., Schmidt, V., and Schultz, E. *Storefront Day Care Centers: The Radical Berlin Experiment*. transl. by C. Lord and R. N. Watkins. Beacon Press, Boston (1973).

Shapira, A. and Madsen, M. C. Between- and within-group cooperation and competition among kibbutz and nonkibbutz children. *Develop. Psychol.* ? ? (1974).

Shillito, E. E. and Hoyland, V. J. Observations on parturition and maternal care in Soay sheep. *Proc. Zool. Soc. Lond. 165*, 509–512 (1971).

Sidel, R. *Women and Child Care in China*. Hill & Wang, New York (1974).

Smith, F. V. Instinct and learning in the attachment of lamb and ewe. *Animal Behav. 13*, 84–86 (1965).

Smith, F. V., Van-Toller, C., and Boyes, T. The 'critical period' in the attachment of lambs and ewes. *Animal Behav. 14*, 120–125 (1966).

Southwick, C. H. Population dynamics and social behavior of domestic rodents. In *Biology of Populations*, B. K. Sladen and F. B. Ban, eds. Elsevier, New York (1969) pp. 284–298.

Spiro, M. E. *Children of the Kibbutz*. Harvard University Press, Cambridge, Massachusetts (1958).

Tavolga, M. C. Behavior of the bottlenose dolphin (T. truncatus): Social interactions in a captive colony. In *Whales, Dolphins, and Porpoises*, K. S. Norris, ed. University of California Press, Berkeley (1966), pp. 718–730.

Tizard, J. and Tizard, B. The social development of two-year-old children in residential nurseries. In *The Origins of Human Social Relations*, H. R. Schaffer, ed. Academic Press, New York (1971), pp. 147–161.

Werboff, J., Steg, M., and Barnes, L. Communal nursing in mice: Strain specific effects of multiple mothers on growth and behavior. *Psychonomic Science 19*(5), 269–271 (1970).

Wilson, E. O. *The Insect Societies*. The Belknap Press of Harvard University, Cambridge, Massachussetts (1971).

INDEX